PROFOUND INTELLECTUAL AND MULTIPLE DISABILITIES

NURSING COMPLEX NEEDS

We dedicate this book to the many individuals living with profound intellectual and multiple disabilities, their families and those who support them.

It has been a great privilege and at times a considerable emotional challenge to create the book. Today (Tuesday, 29 July 2008), in response to *Death by Indifference* (Mencap, 2007) the *Independent Inquiry into Access to Healthcare for People with Learning Disabilities* (Michael, 2008) was published. The inquiry makes several key recommendations including:

- Compulsory learning disability training for healthcare professionals
- The involvement of family carers in care and treatment
- Reasonable adjustments for people with a learning disability by health services, including regular health checks and liaison staff across services
- Identify and assess the needs of people with learning disabilities and their carers
- Better inspection of how the NHS treats people with a learning disability
- A confidential inquiry into the avoidable deaths of people with a learning disability and a permanent public health observatory to promote good practice

It is heartening to read the reports, recommendations and in particular the following statement by Sir Jonathan Michael:

> *An annual health check; support when a visit to hospital is needed; help to communicate; better information, and tighter inspection and regulation will all work to reduce inequalities in access to and outcomes from healthcare services* (Michael, 2008, p. 11).

With these recommendations at the forefront of our minds, we hope that the examples presented in this book act to inspire you all, whether carers, students or qualified health or social care practitioners, to develop and share your knowledge, skills and expertise to deliver an excellent service to people with profound intellectual and multiple disabilities.

Michael, J. (2008) *Independent Inquiry into Access to Healthcare for People with Learning Disabilities* is available from http://www.iahpld.org.uk/.

Mencap (2007) *Death by Indifference* is available from http://www.mencap.org.uk/deathbyindifference.

PROFOUND INTELLECTUAL AND MULTIPLE DISABILITIES

NURSING COMPLEX NEEDS

Edited by

Jillian Pawlyn, BA (Hons), PGCE, RNLD
Specialist Practitioner – Community Learning Disabilities Nursing, ENB 978

Steven Carnaby, BSc. (Hons), MSc., Ph.D., D. Clin. Psy., C. Psychol., ILTM

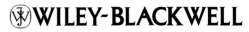
WILEY-BLACKWELL
A John Wiley & Sons, Ltd., Publication

This edition first published 2009
© 2009 by Blackwell Publishing Ltd

Blackwell Publishing was acquired by John Wiley & Sons in February 2007. Blackwell's publishing programme has been merged with Wiley's global Scientific, Technical, and Medical business to form Wiley-Blackwell.

Registered office
John Wiley & Sons Ltd, The Atrium, Southern Gate, Chichester, West Sussex, PO19 8SQ, United Kingdom

Editorial offices
9600 Garsington Road, Oxford, OX4 2DQ, United Kingdom
350 Main Street, Malden, MA 02148-5020, USA

For details of our global editorial offices, for customer services and for information about how to apply for permission to reuse the copyright material in this book please see our website at www.wiley.com/wiley-blackwell.

The right of the author to be identified as the author of this work has been asserted in accordance with the Copyright, Designs and Patents Act 1988.

Library of Congress Cataloging-in-Publication Data

Profound intellectual and multiple disabilities: nursing complex needs / edited by Jillian Pawlyn and Steven Carnaby.
    p. ; cm.
  Includes bibliographical references and index.
  ISBN 978-1-4051-5170-2 (pbk. : alk. paper)   1. People with mental disabilities–Rehabilitation.
2. Learning disabilities–Nursing.   I. Pawlyn, Jillian.   II. Carnaby, Steven.
  [DNLM: 1. Mentally Disabled Persons–rehabilitation.   2. Evidence-Based Medicine.   3. Learning Disorders–nursing.   4. Mentally Disabled Persons–psychology.   5. Quality of Life. WM 308 P964 2009]
  RC570.P697 2009
  616.89′1–dc22

                                                                                              2008022186

A catalogue record for this book is available from the British Library.

Set in 10/12.5pt Sabon by Aptara® Inc., New Delhi, India
Printed in Malaysia by KHL Printing Co. Sdn.Bhd.

1   2009

CONTENTS

CONTRIBUTORS

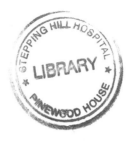

Shirley Budd Continence Lead Nurse, Continence Advisory Service, Sheffield PCT, 722 Prince of Wales Road, Darnall, Sheffield, S9 4EU, Email: shirley.budd@nhs.net

Karen Bunning Senior Lecturer, Queens Building, University of East Anglia, Norwich, Norfolk, NR4 7TJ, Email: k.bunning@uea.ac.uk

Sian Burton Dietician, Bro Morgannwg NHS Trust, 71 Quarella Road, Bridgend CF31 1YE, Email: sian.burton@bromor-tr.wales.nhs.uk

Steven Carnaby Consultant Lead Clinical Psychologist, Westminster Learning Disability Partnership, 215 Lisson Grove, London, NW8 8LW, Email: Steve.Carnaby@westminster.pct.nhs.uk

Mary Codling Primary Care Liaison Nurse, Wokingham Hospital, Wokingham, Berkshire, RG41 2RE, Email: mary.codling@berkshire.nhs.uk

Sue Cox Ridgeway Partnership NHS Trust, Slade House, Horspath Driftway, Headington, Oxford OX3 7JH, Email: sue.cox@ridgeway.nhs.uk

Hannah Crawford Specialist Advisor, Sniperley House, Earls House, Lanchester Road, Durham, DH1 5RD, Email: hannah.crawford@cddps.northy.nhs.uk

Liz Goldsmith Postural Care Skills, The Sharratts, School Lane, Hopwas, Tamworth, Staffs B78 3AD, Email: johnandliz.goldsmith@btopenworld.com

Katie Hickson Ridgeway Partnership NHS Trust, Slade House, Horspath Driftway, Headington, Oxford OX3 7JH

Sarah Hill Postural Care Skills, The Sharratts, School Lane, Hopwas, Tamworth, Staffs, B78 3AD, Email: sarahhill@posturalcareskills.com

James Hogg White Top Research Unit, Springfield House, 15/16 Springfield, University of Dundee, Dundee, DD1 4JE, Email: j.h.hogg@dundee.ac.uk

Sarah King Ridgeway Partnership NHS Trust, Slade House, Horspath Driftway, Headington, Oxford OX3 7JH

Gill Levy Information and Advisory Service, SeeAbility, SeeAbility House, Hook Road, Epsom, Surrey, KT19 8SQ, Email: g.levy@seeability.org

Nicky MacDonald Health Facilitator Learning Disabilities, Berkshire West Primary Care Trust, Northcroft Wing, Avonbank House, West Street, Newbury RG14 1BZ, Email: Nicky.MacDonald@berkshire.nhs.uk

Bea Maes Centre for Disability, Special Needs Education and Child Care, K.U. Leuven, Vesaliusstraat 2, 3000 Leuven, Belgium, Email: bea.maes@ped.kuleuven.ac.be

Melanie Nind School of Education, University of Southampton, University Road, Southampton, SO17 1BJ, Email: man@soton.ac.uk

Jillian Pawlyn Lecturer/Practitioner, Ridgeway Partnership NHS Trust, Slade House, Horspath Driftway, Headington, Oxford OX3 7JH, Email: jill.pawlyn@ridgeway.nhs.uk

Katja Petry Centre for Disability, Special Needs Education and Child Care, K.U. Leuven, Vesaliusstraat 2, 3000 Leuven, Belgium, Email: katja.petry@ped.kuleuven.be

Jan Roast 32 Crecy Walk, Woodstock, Oxon OX20 1US

Sue M. Sandham Freelance Dietitian, The Willows, Barecroft Common, Magor, Caldicot, Monmouthshire, NP26 3EB, Email: susan.sandham@virgin.net

Laura Waite Lecturer in Special Needs, Liverpool Hope University, Education Deanery, Hope Park, Liverpool L16 9JD, Email: waitel@hope.ac.uk

Colin Wallis Consultant Respiratory Paediatrician, Respiratory Unit, Great Ormond Street Hospital for Children NHS Trust, Great Ormond Street, London WC1N 3JH, Email: c.wallis@ich.ucl.ac.uk

Pauline Watt-Smith Honorary Secretary BSDH, Tyndalls, 174 Woodstock Road, Oxford OX5 1PW, Email: pwattsmith@yahoo.co.uk

FOREWORD

The period since the end of World War II has seen a progressive, but as yet far from complete, transformation in the lives of people with profound intellectual and multiple disability and their families. The first studies demonstrating their potential to benefit from systematic interventions were undertaken in the 1940s, 1950s and 1960s (Fuller, 1949; Rice, 1968), as were the first attempts to understand their development rather than emphasise the consequences of developmental delays (Woodward, 1959). In parallel, the changing international emphasis on the rights of people with disabilities and their entitlement to live as full citizens led to significant progress in the engagement of people with profound intellectual and multiple disabilities in their communities. This included their integration, if not inclusion, into educational systems in many (but not all) developed countries and acknowledgement of their right to engage in a fulfilling adult life.

The present volume brings together essential perspectives and information on these positive developments and contributes significantly to their consolidation and further realisation; the volume also highlights, the barriers that people with profound intellectual and multiple disabilities and those who support them face in attaining equal human rights. Central among these barriers are society's fundamental attitudes towards people with profound intellectual and multiple disabilities and the implicit negative assumptions that underpin them. Such attitudes are directly opposed to the positive values which underpin the carefully argued position articulated by Jillian Pawlyn and Steven Carnaby.

It is important when engaging with the constructive ideas presented here to bear in mind a backdrop of intense negativity towards people with profound intellectual and multiple disabilities. At one extreme their very right to life has been denied, most explicitly by certain philosophers. Self-styled bioethicists argue that the assumed lack of self-awareness and cognitive development of people with profound intellectual and multiple disabilities preclude them from being considered as persons. This view asserts that personhood defines what it means to be human, and hence people with profound intellectual and multiple disabilities cannot be considered to be human beings with their attendant human rights. This position has led in recent years to the bioethicist, Peter Singer, arguing that non-persons such as those with profound intellectual and multiple disabilities should be subject to a policy of euthanasia (Singer, 1993). Negative eugenics is indeed alive and indeed well.

Mere disagreement with Singer's clearly formulated views does not take us very far in refuting them, nor do simplistic assertions of the rights of people with profound intellectual and multiple disabilities anymore, than does advocacy of person-centred planning. We need to articulate our views as clearly as have the bioethicists, challenging their definition of personhood as too narrow a view of what constitutes a person. The potential to develop as a person is also an essential part of personhood, while we should acknowledge that personhood is not a simple attribute of the individual but is determined by the interwovenness of the person's relationship with those around them. The very presence of a person with profound intellectual and multiple disabilities affects others interpersonally and is an assertion of personhood in a social context. In emphasising this position, the present volume actively argues for a view that is entirely counter to that expressed by Singer.

The euthanasia of people with profound intellectual and multiple disabilities becomes a reality where the right to life is denied by the assertion that the person's quality of life is too poor to justify their continued existence. Wolfensberger (1994) has cogently characterised the pervasive construct of quality of life as a death-making concept, the use of which to justify euthanasia asserts that no life at all is deemed to be preferable to a poor quality of life. Listen out in the media for how often euthanasia is justified through this quality of life argument: 'If we let her live she'll have an unacceptably poor quality of life!' Quality of life as a constructive concept with potential to benefit people with profound and multiple learning disabilities is considered more fully in this volume, though the dual-edged nature of this construct should always be borne in mind.

If euthanasia is regarded as the extreme counter view to a rights perspective, we should also remind ourselves that the right of people with profound intellectual and multiple disabilities to develop in ways that are typical of other human beings has also in recent years been denied. In the USA, medical interventions have recently been undertaken to restrict the growth of a girl with profound intellectual and multiple disabilities to prevent her development into womanhood, with the agreement of a university medical ethics committee. In what has become known as the 'Ashley case', her uterus, breast buds and appendix were all removed, and high-dose oestrogen hormonal treatment to stunt growth was administered. Gunther & Diekema (2006) refer euphemistically to 'growth therapeutic therapy', though the use of the term 'therapy' is an unacceptable travesty of this term. The justification for this intervention as an aid to caring for the parents as their daughter increased in size and weight must also be rejected. Requests from parents in the UK have recently followed similar lines, and there is little doubt that among parents of daughter and sons with profound intellectual and multiple disabilities there is considerable sympathy for the decisions taken by Ashley's parents. Again, the present volume offers family carers a positive view of what can and should be aimed for.

The above examples of euthanasia and surgical interventions for non-health reasons are stark examples of the possible disadvantaging of people with profound intellectual and multiple disabilities through negative attitudes. Other serious challenges also confront both families and professionals. In a recent longitudinal study of a cohort of individuals (Hogg et al., 2007) over a 10-year period, 21% of the original cohort had died with the principal causes of death – respiratory disease, diseases of the digestive systems and circulatory system disorders. Tube feeding has also been associated with increased mortality (Eyman et al., 1990). Epilepsy, too, invariably affects a majority of people with profound intellectual and multiple disabilities (Hogg, 1992) and has also been implicated in mortality (Chaney & Eyman 2000). The emphasis on meeting complex health care needs in this volume, then, is entirely appropriate and very welcome, with approaches to supporting individuals with each and any of the above health problems, expertly and practically dealt with throughout the book.

Good health is important not only in its own right, but as the basis for personal and social engagement with the world. Fundamental to this engagement is support for communication by and with people with profound intellectual and multiple disabilities. In supporting communication account must be taken of the individual's sensory and motor status. Both the processes involved in effective communication and meeting the sensory needs of individuals are comprehensively reviewed here and practical guidance given. The approaches described provide a constructive basis for maximising the social potential of people with people with profound intellectual and multiple disabilities.

Two important concepts underpinning this book are those of engagement and taking a holistic (but analytical) view of the person with profound intellectual and multiple disabilities. For this reason bringing together a detailed focus on good health, both physical and mental, as a key contributor to the engaged life and ensuring a positive communicative environment for the person with profound intellectual and multiple disability makes this an invaluable resource for all practitioners, among which family carers should occupy a central position.

James Hogg
Universities of Dundee & St. Andrews

References

Chaney, R.H., & Eyman, R.K. (2000). Patterns of mortality over 60 years among persons with mental retardation in a residential facility. *Mental Retardation*, 38(3), 289–293.

Eyman, R.K., Grossman, H.J., Chaney, R.H., & Call, T.L. (1990). The life expectancy of profoundly handicapped people with mental retardation. *New England Journal of Medicine*, 323(9), 584–589.

Fuller, P.R. (1949). Operant conditioning of a vegetative human organism. *American Journal of Psychology*, 62(4), 578–590.

Gunther, D.F., & Diekema, D.S. (2006). Attenuating growth in children with profound developmental disability: a new approach to an old dilemma. *Archives of Pediatrics and Adolescent Medicine*, 160(10), 1013–1017.

Hogg, J. (1992). The administration of psychotropic and anticonvulsant drugs to children and adults with profound and multiple learning disabilities. *Journal of Intellectual Disability Research*, 36, 473–488.

Hogg, J., Juhlberg, K., & Lambe, L. (2007). Policy, service pathways and mortality: a 10-year longitudinal study of people with profound intellectual and multiple disabilities. *Journal of Intellectual Disability Research*, 51, 366–376.

Rice, H.K. (1968). Operant behavior in vegetative patients III: methodological considerations. *Psychological Record*, 18, 297–302.

Singer, P. (1993). *Practical Ethics* (2nd ed.). Cambridge: Cambridge University Press.

Wolfensberger, W. (1994). Let's hang up Quality of Life as a hopeless term. In Goode, D. (ed.), *Quality of Life for Persons with Disabilities: International Perspectives and Issues*. Cambridge, MA: Brooklyn Books; 285–321.

Woodward, W.M. (1959). The behaviour of idiots interpreted by Piaget's theory of sensori-motor development. *British Journal of Educational Psychology*, 29, 60–71.

ACKNOWLEDGEMENTS

We would like to thank our employing organisations for supporting us throughout the development of the book.

To the health care professionals who have given their valuable time to contribute to the book, we thank you.

To our colleagues, families and friends, thank you for granting us the time to complete this 'project'.

Finally, our heartfelt thanks to the individuals with profound intellectual and multiple disabilities, their families and those who support them; thank you for inspiring us to write the book.

Jillian Pawlyn and Steven Carnaby

Section I

ASSESSING COMPLEX NEEDS

Chapter 1

INTRODUCTION

Jillian Pawlyn and Steven Carnaby

> *It is important that everyone understands that people with profound* [intellectual and multiple disabilities] *have the same rights as every other citizen. We must enable each individual to engage with their world and to achieve their potential so that their lives go beyond being 'cared for' to being valued for who they are as people.*
>
> (Mencap, 2007, p. 7)

This statement from the Mencap/PMLD Network paper *Meet the People* is an apt introduction to a book that aims to provide insights for those charged with the responsibility of helping people with profound intellectual and multiple disabilities (PMID) to 'engage with their world' and 'achieve their potential'. This is no easy task. However, by taking a thorough, wide-ranging approach that is advocated by this collection of contributors, we hope to instil confidence and motivate the practitioner striving to implement best practice in this field.

In this introductory chapter we explore definitions and causes of intellectual disability and look at some of the key areas that underpin the remaining chapters: the importance of access to health services, the legal and ethical emphasis on mental capacity and the integration of health and social care philosophies.

About whom are we talking?

The current emphasis on person-centredness in services for people with intellectual disabilities can lead to an arguably inappropriate shying away from diagnosis and categorisation. In this book we will argue that on the contrary, clarity and agreement about the use of accurate terminology – specifically here the term profound intellectual and multiple disabilities – is more likely to lead to the development of person-centred action and the implementation of good person-centred approaches (Mansell & Beadle-Brown, 2005).

Defining intellectual disability

The term intellectual disability has been adopted here in recognition of this book's potentially international readership. In Britain, the term *learning disability* is prevalent in service provision and is one used by professionals. In the USA, *mental retardation* is still in common parlance. *Intellectual disability* is currently used by the academic literature and is likely to move into the provision and professional arena before long.

Intellectual disability is defined by ICD-10 (1996, p. 1) as:

> *...a condition of arrested or incomplete development of the mind, which is especially characterized by impairment of skills manifested during the developmental period, which contribute to the overall level of intelligence, i.e. cognitive, language, motor, and social abilities.*

People with intellectual disabilities have difficulties with learning and have global difficulties on a daily basis with living and coping skills. Like anybody else, people with intellectual disabilities have the potential to develop, but the rate at which this happens is likely to be slower and needs particular supports to be in place for it to happen.

A diagnosis of intellectual disability requires an assessment establishing that the individual meets three main criteria:

1. There is evidence of significant cognitive impairment, measured here as having an IQ of ≤70.
2. There is also evidence that the individual has a significant impairment in adaptive functioning – assessed using standardised tools that measure everyday living and coping skills.
3. Both of these impairments are shown to have been present before the age of 18 years.

All three of these criteria must be met for a diagnosis of intellectual disability to be made.

Intellectual disability encompasses a very wide range of functioning, and this heterogeneity is perhaps one of the main difficulties faced by those responsible for developing service provision (see Chapter 18 for further discussion). ICD-10 also provides further categorisation within the diagnosis of cognitive impairment as shown in Table 1.1.

Causes of intellectual disability

Current thinking and research indicates that intellectual disability can be caused by biological, environmental and social factors. A view was held that mild intellectual

Table 1.1 Levels of cognitive impairment as described by ICD-10.

ICD code	Level of cognitive impairment	Associated IQ
F70	Mild	50–69
F71	Moderate	35–49
F72	Severe	20–34
F73	Profound	<20

disabilities were caused by social and environmental factors and severe and profound disabilities were caused by biological factors. However, evidence now exists to suggest that this distinction cannot be so clearly defined. For example, biological factors can now be shown to account for between one and two in five children with mild intellectual disabilities, as well as for four out of five children with severe intellectual disabilities (Fryers, 1993; Richardson & Koller, 1996).

Social and environmental factors

An early study by Birch et al. (1970) studied a cohort of children in Aberdeen identified as having intellectual disabilities and gathered a range of information via interviews and health and social care records. Their analysis found no relationship between severe intellectual disabilities and either the social class of the parents or family instability, but a strong relationship between parental social class and unstable family background (e.g. abuse, neglect or change of carers) and mild intellectual disabilities. This finding suggests that psychosocial adversity was a major factor contributing to mild intellectual disabilities but not to severe intellectual disabilities (Emerson et al., 2001).

Biological factors

Most of the biological causes of intellectual disabilities operate prenatally and in the majority of cases resulting in severe intellectual disabilities. Two-thirds to three-quarters of cases of severe intellectual disabilities are caused in this way, with the two most common genetic causes being Down's syndrome and Fragile-X syndrome. The most common non-genetic biological cause is cerebral palsy, although it is important to note that not all people with cerebral palsy have intellectual disabilities. Some biological factors can be effectively treated: for example, phenylketonuria is now screened in newborn babies using the heel-prick blood test, enabling treatment with thyroxine followed by a low-phenylalanine diet where indicated (Murphy et al., 1990). Others can be prevented via public health programmes, such as rubella immunisation to protect against pregnancies with rubella embryopathy.

Perinatal factors include birth trauma and cerebral hypoxia; post-natal factors include accidents and infections, such as meningitis.

Prevalence[1]

According to Emerson & Hatton (2004), it is estimated that there are about 985 000 people in England with an intellectual disability (i.e. about 2% of the population), of which 796 000 are aged 20 or over.

[1] These figures are from the Foundation for People with Learning Disabilities, at www.learningdisabilities.org.uk.

There are an estimated 210 000 people with severe and profound intellectual disabilities in England: around 65 000 children and young people, 120 000 adults of working age and 25 000 older people (Department of Health, 2001).

The number of adults with intellectual disabilities is predicted to increase by 11% between 2001 and 2021, raising the number of people in England aged 15 and above with intellectual disabilities to over one million in 2021 (Emerson & Hatton, 2004). The Department of Health (2001) suggests that this increase may be explained by:

- increased life expectancy, especially among people with Down's syndrome;
- growing numbers of children and young people with complex and multiple disabilities who now survive into adulthood;
- a sharp rise in the reported numbers of school age children with autistic spectrum disorders, some of whom will have intellectual disabilities;
- greater prevalence among some minority ethnic populations of South Asian origin.

About 60% of adults with intellectual disabilities live with their families (Department of Health, 2001) while about a third of all people with intellectual disabilities known to services live in care homes and hospitals. About 11 000 of these people live 'out of area', that is away from their home area (Department of Health, 2005).

Defining profound intellectual and multiple disabilities

While a clear, international consensus concerning the precise definition of PIMD is emerging[2], a range of definitions and descriptors have been published in recent times, the details of which can vary from each other. For example, while the World Health Organization (1993) equates profound intellectual disability with an IQ of below 30, the *Diagnostic and Statistical Manual* uses the range of 20–25 (*DSM-IV*; APA, 2000). Hogg & Sebba (1986) suggest that people with profound intellectual disabilities are functioning at five standard deviations below the norm, while Ware (1996) states that people forming this group of individuals have a degree of cognitive impairment so severe that they are functioning at a developmental level of 2 years or less. The World Health Organization (1996), in contrast, sets the criterion of functioning in adults at a level of below 3 years developmentally (see also Royal College of Psychiatrists 2001).

Clinical descriptions of PIMD

These slight variations in definition are academic in the main, although arguably such differences do serve to confuse and distract from the task in hand, that is to carry out thorough and holistic assessment (see Chapter 7). It is perhaps, therefore, easier to employ clinical descriptions of PIMD, which point one in the general

---

[2] See, for example, the work of the IASSID (International Association for the Scientific Study of Intellectual Disability) Special Interest Group at www.iassid.org.

direction as to how individuals functioning at this level might be affected by their various disabilities. For example, the World Health Organization (1996, p. 4) states that people in this range are likely to be:

> ...severely limited in their ability to understand or comply with requests or instructions. Most such individuals are immobile or severely restricted in mobility, incontinent, and capable at most of only the rudimentary forms of non-verbal communication.

It goes on to say:

> They possess little or no ability to care for their own basic needs and require constant help and supervision.

DSM-IV-TR (APA, 2000, p. 44), in a similar vein, states that:

> During the childhood years, they display considerable impairments in sensori-motor functioning... Optimal development may occur in a highly structured environment with constant aid and supervision and an individualised relationship with a caregiver. Motor development and self-care and communication may improve if appropriate training is provided. Some can perform simple tasks in closely supervised and sheltered settings.

Studies in the Netherlands have reported that at least 85% of people with PIMD have some form of visual impairment, in most cases caused by damage to the visual cortex in the occipital lobe (e.g. Van Splunder et al., 2003), and between 25 and 35% experience hearing loss (e.g. Evenhuis et al., 2001). Dysfunctions of taste and smell can be common (Bromley, 2000), along with impaired sense of touch, pressure, temperature and pain (e.g. Oberlander et al., 1999). Seizure disorders are reported to be 50% higher than that mentioned in the literature (e.g. Arts, 1999), and people with PIMD have a higher risk of developing medical complications (e.g. Zijlstra & Vlaskamp, 2005).

Without exception, these clinical descriptions take a deficit approach; in focusing on what individuals with PIMD are unable to do and the areas of life with which they have most difficulty, the reader is faced with a daunting list of problems and challenges. Indeed, the person is often noticeably absent. The medical model continues to be criticised for its diagnostic approach, and more recent thinking about the social construction of disability is often vehement in its condemnation of approaches that appear to consider people in terms of their perceived 'deviance' from social norms. Rapley (2004) reminds us that the word 'diagnosis' in talking about intellectual disability leads directly to a medicalisation of the individual. Rapley (2004, p. 43) refers to the work of Boyle (e.g. Boyle 1999) in summarising that:

> ...it has been by the appropriation of the language of medicine (with all of the supposed scientificity that goes with it ...) to talk of unwanted conduct that the psy professions [i.e. psychiatry and psychology] have assumed authority over the management and control of those who, in one way or another, trouble the social order.

The debate concerning labelling, categorisation and the inevitable wielding of power that results from this process provides a tension between the call for clarity that enables discourse about need and a respectful acknowledgement of subjective perspective and dignity that we hope will be at least in part reflected by some of the contributors in this book. Our stance is to use language as the first step in establishing clarity, but as importantly to symbolically raise the profile of a population at risk of being at best ignored and at worst made to suffer through neglect. Throughout the chapters presented here, contributors use the term 'profound intellectual and multiple disabilities'. In 2008, this has emerged as the most accurate way of describing a heterogeneous group of individuals who share the common experience of experiencing the world using skills that can be conceptualised as functioning at the very early stages of development in conjunction with both (usually a range of) additional physical and sensory disabilities and vulnerability to complex physical and mental health problems. Nakken & Vlaskamp (2007) have also championed this term, arguing for a clear definition of the 'target group' in order to prevent misunderstandings and improve dissemination of good practice. They observe that at an international congress in 2004, no fewer than 11 different terms were used to describe (apparently) similar groups of people in order to discuss treatment and support.

There is a view that the term 'profound intellectual disabilities and multiple impairment' is stigmatising a group of people that are already stigmatised enough. Perhaps as a way of avoiding this, *Valuing People* (Department of Health, 2001) made no specific reference to people with PIMD, instead using terms such as 'complex needs' and 'high support needs'. This is arguably problematic as other groups within society – who do not have profound intellectual disabilities coupled with additional physical disabilities – could also be described using these terms. Examples include people experiencing significant and chronic mental health problems, such as treatment-resistant schizophrenia and other forms of psychotic illness, or people with a 'dual diagnosis' of mental illness and long-term substance misuse. Person-centred planning and person-centred action (see Chapter 6) place the individual at the centre of our thinking in order to identify what is going well in their life and then identify needs in order for these needs to be met. Lack of clarity – arguably aimed at making ourselves feel more comfortable with the language we are using – does not enable this process to unfold effectively.

Prevalence rates for people with PIMD

Figures for the population of people with PIMD understandably vary with the definition adopted. *DSM-IV-TR* (APA, 2000, p. 44) states:

> ...*the group with profound mental retardation constitutes approximately 1–2% of people with mental retardation.*

However, Cooper et al. (2007) worked with an adult intellectual disability population from which they identified 18% as having profound intellectual disabilities. This study used the ICD-10 criterion of functioning at ≤3 years in contrast to the *DSM-IV-TR* criterion (ICD-10, 1996).

Key areas in working with people with PIMD

This book takes a detailed approach to a range of issues pertinent to the lives of people with PIMD. These issues are underpinned or determined by a number of key areas as described briefly below.

Health

According to the Disability Rights Commission (2006), people with intellectual disabilities are 2.5 times more likely to have health problems than do other people, with 4 times as many people with intellectual disabilities dying of preventable causes as do people in the general population. This is clearly of concern when considering the evidence that people with PIMD are very likely to experience a wide range of complex health issues, often associated with particular conditions (e.g. issues with the digestive system linked with Cornelia de Lange syndrome and diseases of the nervous system seen in Angelman syndrome) and sometimes requiring significant intervention (Berg et al., 2007).

The development of better supports combined with advances in medical care means that the number of individuals with profound intellectual disabilities combined with fragile health is increasing in the developed world (Nakken & Vlaskamp, 2007). This increase brings with it the concept of 'older' people with PIMD; while there is increasing acknowledgement of the ageing nature of the wider intellectual disability population, there also needs to be recognition that people with PIMD are also reaching adulthood and beyond, with individuals now needing ever-increasing levels of complex technology to ensure that they not only survive, but do so enjoying an acceptable quality of life.

Capacity

The Mental Capacity Act (2005) and its consequent implementation in 2007 has enshrined the concept of capacity in law. It provides a statutory framework for substitute decision making for those who lack capacity, putting into statute common law principles and best practice. In excess of 2 million people in England and Wales lack capacity to make some decisions for themselves (Department for Constitutional Affairs, 2007). According to the Department for Constitutional Affairs (2007), there are 6 million carers and professionals who provide care and treatment, and prior to the Mental Capacity Act there had been no legal requirement for next of kin to be consulted with regard to treatment if their relative is not able to consent. Incapacity could be assumed on the basis of diagnosis alone and there was no clear legal authority for people acting on behalf of an individual without mental capacity. There had also been no statutory way for wishes regarding future care to be stated in advance and being certain that they are listened to.

The Mental Capacity Act has five main principles:

1. *Presumption of capacity.* A person must be assumed to have capacity unless it is established that he lacks capacity.

2. *The right for individuals to be supported to make their own decisions.* A person is not to be treated as unable to make a decision unless all practicable steps to help him to do so have been taken without success.
3. *The right to make 'unwise' decisions.* A person is not to be treated as unable to make a decision merely because he makes an unwise decision.
4. *Best interests.* An act done, or decision made, under this Act for or on behalf of a person who lacks capacity must be done, or made, in his best interests.
5. *Least restrictive option.* Before the act is done, or the decision is made, regard must be paid to whether the purpose for which it is needed can be as effectively achieved in a way that is less restrictive of the person's rights and freedom of action.

Section 2(1) of the Act states that:

For the purposes of this Act, a person lacks capacity in relation to a matter if at the material time he is unable to make a decision for himself in relation to the matter because of an impairment of, or a disturbance in the functioning of, the mind or brain.

Capacity is assessed using a two-part test. Part 1 establishes whether there is an impairment of or disturbance in the functioning of the person's mind or brain. If that threshold is not reached (i.e. no impairment or disturbance is identified) the person cannot be seen to lack capacity within the Act. Part 2 of the test is a functional assessment which explores whether the impairment is sufficient that the person lacks the capacity to make that particular decision. Section 3 of the Act states that the person is then deemed unable to make that specific decision at that particular time if she or he is unable to:

- understand the information relevant to the decision;
- retain that information;
- use or weigh that information as part of the process of making the decision; or
- communicate the decision (talking, signing, other means).

The Act covers a range of decisions related to a person who lacks capacity in the areas of welfare (including health, medical and social care) and property and financial affairs. These can include everyday decisions or major choices (e.g. surgery and moving house). Many people with PIMD are likely to lack capacity, and the development of good practice in this area is essential.

Where an individual lacks capacity, a 'decision maker' needs to be identified whose task is to act in that individual's 'best interests' using the following checklist of considerations or principles:

- Take into account all relevant circumstances
- Encourage the person to participate as fully as possible
- Be aware of past and present wishes, feelings, beliefs and values

- Ensure inclusivity in relation to the views of carers, family members, the person named, local power of attorney or their deputy (if practicable and appropriate)
- Obtain written statements when the individual has capacity
- No discrimination
- Advocating for life-sustaining treatment, that is must *not* be motivated to bring about that person's death
- With regard to day-to-day decisions the person must have 'reasonable grounds for believing' that what they are doing is in the individual's best interest

The implementation of the Mental Capacity Act has a number of implications for clinicians. Clearly, they have a duty to comply with the Act and its Code, and rolling training programmes have been in place in many localities. There is likely to be an increase in demand for clinical psychologists and psychiatrists to carry out capacity assessments, with professionals from other health and social care disciplines requesting consultancy and training in this important area.

Integration of health and social care services

The stance adopted in the following chapters together strive towards a 'both/and' position rather than 'either/or'. For the contributors in this volume, medical interventions and good, effective healthcare in general matter just as much as the acknowledgement of personhood and autonomy. Emotional well-being and positive emphasis on achievement and attainment are just as important as thorough assessment of dysphagia, respiration and postural management. At risk of stating what is clearly apparent, all of these issues are interdependent. Artificial positioning of the social model as being diametrically opposed to the medical model is thankfully outdated when applied to the lives of people with mild or moderate intellectual disabilities; however, it can be the case that when support for people with PIMD is being considered the integration of health and social care becomes more difficult. Local implementation can lead to intervention being primarily about providing clinical input to address identified health concerns to the detriment of considerations about rights and quality of life, *or* such medical issues are hidden beneath the drive towards ensuring that the individual concerned is living an 'ordinary' lifestyle, compromising risk management and appropriate healthcare provision.

The chapters in this book attempt to thoroughly investigate the issues and appropriate related interventions across all areas of functioning for people with PIMD and are organized into two main sections which explore the assessment and meeting of complex needs respectively. The first section begins by mapping the main areas that enable the development of a positive perspective on the lives of people with PIMD. Katja Petry and Bea Maes begin by discussing the concept of quality of life and its application to people with PIMD, an essential starting point for considering what people need and why support is offered in the ways recommended in later chapters. Jan Roast and colleagues extend this by sharing their own stories, grounding these ideas in real life and practical experiences.

The next three chapters together form the core foundation of thinking that underpins the best practice set out in Section 2. Karen Bunning emphasises the essential role of communication partnerships, providing clear and helpful guidance on developing an understanding of the ways in which communication skills can be supported and enhanced. Melanie Nind builds on these ideas in discussing the importance of emotional well-being, arguably an area that has been largely ignored until relatively recently and here taking its rightful place at the very centre of best practice. The third core element, supporting the attainment and maintenance of good health, is discussed in the context of meaningful, person-centred and personally relevant planning of effective healthcare driven by acknowledgement and implementation of appropriate policy and guidance. The final chapter in this section attempts to draw the ideas discussed thus far in highlighting the need for thorough transdisciplinary, rather than merely multidisciplinary, assessment.

With the wider context and value base now established, Section 2 takes a 'head to toe' approach to meeting complex needs, with contributors focusing on key areas and suggesting best practice. Mental health issues for people with PIMD have been largely underresearched, and the first chapter in this section reviews what is reported to be understood about this difficult area at the present time. Mary Codling and Nicky MacDonald then go on to discuss epilepsy, providing a full account likely to be essential reading for practitioners. Sensory loss is discussed firstly by Gill Levy in her chapter on vision and visual impairment and then by Laura Waite's chapter on hearing loss.

Respiratory health is reviewed by Colin Wallis, who provides invaluable information that is both illuminating and reassuring in its practical, measured approach. Similarly, Pauline Watt-Smith's discussion of dental care and oral health emphasises the need for proactive approaches that recognise the essential adoption of specific practices for people with such significant disabilities, as do the chapters by Hannah Crawford on dysphagia and by Sian Burton and colleagues on nutrition, hydration and weight, respectively. Sarah Hill and Liz Goldsmith conclude Section 2 with a detailed and accessible account of good postural management.

Meeting Complex Needs concludes with a review of the themes and arguments raised throughout the book, revisiting some of the discussion set out in this introduction and proposing an agenda for further development of service provision. In doing so, it attempts to join all of its contributors in raising the hidden profile of a group of individuals who in twenty-first-century society are still shamefully at risk of being ignored.

References

APA (2000). *Diagnostic and Statistical Manual of Mental Disorders, 4th edition: Text revision*. Washington, DC: American Psychiatric Association.

Arts, W.F.M. (1999). Epilepsie. In Evenhuis, H., & Nagtzaam, L. (eds) *Wetenschap en geneeskunde voor mensen met een verstandelijke handicap: Een nieuw ontgonnen gebied in de nederlandse gezondheidszorg*. Den Haag, The Netherlands: NOW.

Berg, K., Arron, K., Burbridge, C., Moss, J., & Oliver, C. (2007). Carer-reported contemporary health problems in people with severe and profound intellectual disability and genetic syndromes. *Journal of Policy and Practice in Intellectual Disabilities*, 4(2), 120–128.

Birch, H., Richardson, S.A., Baird, D., Horobin, G., & Illsley, R. (1970). *Mental Subnormality in the Community: A Clinical and Epidemiological Study*. Baltimore, MD: Williams & Wilkins.

Boyle, M. (1999). Diagnosis. In Newnes, C., Holmes, G., & Dunn, C. (eds) *This Is Madness*. Ross-on-Wye, England: PCCS Books.

Bromley, S.M. (2000). Smell and taste disorders: a primary care approach. *American Family Physician*, 61, 337–427.

Cooper, S.-A., Smiley, E., Finlayson, J., Jackson, A., Allan, L., Williamson, A., Mantry, D., & Morrison, J. (2007). The prevalence, incidence and factors predictive of mental ill-health in adults with profound intellectual disabilities. *Journal of Applied Research in Intellectual Disabilities*, 20(6), 493–501.

Department for Constitutional Affairs (2007). *Mental Capacity Act: Code of Practice*. UK: HMSO.

Department of Health (2001). *Valuing People*. London: HMSO.

Department of Health (2005). *Valuing People: What Do the Numbers Tell Us?* London: HMSO.

Disability Rights Commission (2006). *Equal Treatment: Closing the Gap*. UK: Disability Rights Commission.

Emerson, E., & Hatton, C. (2004). *Estimating Future Need/Demand for Supports for Adults with Learning Disabilities in England*. Lancaster, UK: Institute for Health Research, Lancaster University.

Emerson, E., Hatton, C., Felce, D., & Murphy, G. (2001). *Learning Disabilities: The Fundamental Facts*. London: The Foundation for People with Learning Disabilities.

Evenhuis, H., Theunissen, M., Denkers, I., Verschuure, H., & Kemme, H. (2001). Prevalence of visual and hearing impairment in a Dutch institutionalized population with intellectual disability. *Journal of Intellectual Disability Research*, 45, 457–464.

Fryers, T. (1993). Epidemiological thinking in mental retardation: issues in taxonomy and population frequency. *International Review of Research in Mental Retardation*, 19, 97–133.

Hogg, J., & Sebba, J. (1986). *Profound Mental Retardation and Multiple Impairment*. London: Croom Helm.

Mansell, J., & Beadle-Brown, J. (2005). Historical overview and a critical appraisal of person-centred planning. In Cambridge, P. and Carnaby, S. (eds) *Person Centred Planning and Care Management for People with Learning Disabilities*. London: Jessica Kingsley Publishers.

Mencap (2007). *Definition* (PMLD factsheet). Available at: http://www.mencap.org.uk/html/campaigns/PMLD/Meet_the_People_definition.pdf (accessed 23 November 2007).

Murphy, G., Hulse, J.A., Smith, I., & Grant, D.B. (1990). Congenital hypothyroidism: physiological and psychological factors in development. *Journal of Child Psychology and Psychiatry*, 31, 711–725.

Nakken, H., & Vlaskamp, C. (2007). A need for a taxonomy for profound intellectual and multiple disabilities. *Journal of Policy and Practice in Intellectual Disabilities*, 4(2), 83–87.

Oberlander, T.F., O'Donnell, M.E., & Montgomery, C.J. (1999). Pain in children with significant neurological impairments. *Journal of Neurodevelopmental and Behaviour Paediatrics*, 20, 35–243.

Rapley, M. (2004). *The Social Construction of Intellectual Disability*. Cambridge, UK: Cambridge University Press.

Richardson, S.A., & Koller, H. (1996). *Twenty-Two Years: Causes and Consequences of Mental Retardation*. Cambridge, MA: Harvard University Press.

Royal College of Psychiatrists (2001). *DC-LD*. London: Royal College of Psychiatrists.

Van Splunder, J., Stilma, J.S., Bernsen, R.M.D., Arentz, T.G.M.H.J., & Evenhuis, H.M. (2003). Refractive errors and visual impairment in 900 adults with intellectual disabilities in the Netherlands. *Acta Ophthalmologica Scandinavica*, 81, 123–129.

Ware, J. (1996) *Creating Responsive Environments for People with Profound Learning and Multiple Disabilities*. London: David Fulton.

World Health Organization (1993). *International Classification of Diseases, 10th edition: Diagnostic Criteria for Research*. Geneva: World Health Organization.

World Health Organization (1996). *International Classification of Diseases, 10th edition: Guide for Mental Retardation*. Geneva: World Health Organization.

Zijlstra, R., & Vlaskamp, C. (2005). The impact of medical health conditions of children with profound intellectual and multiple disabilities. *Journal of Applied Research in Intellectual Disabilities*, 18, 151–161.

Chapter 2

QUALITY OF LIFE: PEOPLE WITH PROFOUND INTELLECTUAL AND MULTIPLE DISABILITIES

Katja Petry and Bea Maes

Introduction

People with profound intellectual and multiple disabilities (PIMD) assume a specific position with regard to the quality of life (QOL) concept and its measurement. Two decades ago, the idea that people with PIMD experience a QOL and that this is a 'valid' experience would have been scientifically 'suspect' (Goode, 1997). To date, the issue is no longer whether people with PIMD have subjective experiences, but how we can learn about these experiences (Taylor & Bogdan, 1996). The measurement of QOL of people with PIMD remains amongst the most difficult challenges for theorists and practitioners in the field (Campo et al., 1997; Lyons, 2005). QOL researchers have often avoided this challenge and have focused mostly on the experiences of individuals with mild and moderate intellectual disabilities (Campo et al., 1997). As such, limited research is available on the measurement of QOL of people with PIMD.

In this chapter, we attempt to explore the current understanding of the measurement of the QOL of people with PIMD, using five major question forms of QOL measurement (i.e. what, how, who, where and why) as a framework to summarise the current status. In accordance with the consensus document on QOL (Schalock et al., 2002), the term measurement of QOL is used in this chapter to refer to the function in its broad sense (i.e. includes objective and subjective measures, quantitative and qualitative methods, categorical data, description and observation). The term assessment is used to describe how QOL concepts and measures are used as both process and content for helping people to improve their lives.

Learning objectives

In this chapter, readers will learn:

- the importance of the QOL concept;
- widely used definitions of QOL and how it is measured in relation to people with intellectual disabilities; and

- the specific challenges faced when attempting to apply these definitions to people with profound intellectual and multiple disabilities.

What to measure?

This question relates to the conceptualisation of the QOL construct. The term 'quality of life' is constituted of two semantic distinguishable components, namely, 'quality' and 'of life'. The term 'quality' makes us think about the excellence associated with human values, such as happiness, success, wealth, health and satisfaction, whereas 'of life' indicates that the concept concerns the very essence or essential aspects of human existence (Lindstrom, 1992; Schalock et al., 2002). Understanding this semantic meaning is necessary to fully appreciate the importance of the QOL concept (Schalock & Verdugo, 2002). Nevertheless, this does not function as a definition of QOL. Defining and conceptualising QOL is a complex and difficult process. Therefore, QOL researchers have suggested not to define the term but rather to agree about a number of principles that define how QOL should be conceptualised (Schalock & Verdugo, 2002). Four principles were proposed with regard to the conceptualisation of QOL. These principles will be described here and applied to people with PIMD.

The first principle states that the QOL construct is multidimensional and influenced by personal and environmental factors and their interactions (Cummins, 2005). The QOL construct is composed of multiple factors which are generally referred to as domains or dimensions. These domains should be thought of as the range over which the QOL construct extends (Verdugo et al., 2005). Although the specific domains vary somewhat across researchers, most QOL researchers suggest that the actual number of domains is less important than the recognition (1) that any proposed QOL model must recognise the need to employ a multi-element framework, (2) that individuals and families know what is important to them and (3) that any set of domains must represent in aggregate the complete QOL construct (Schalock, 2005). Each domain of QOL is composed of QOL indicators, which are domain-specific perceptions, behaviours or conditions that give an indication of the person's well-being. The measurement of QOL should be based on these QOL domains and indicators (Verdugo et al., 2005).

Recent analyses (Schalock & Verdugo, 2002; Schalock, 2004) of the international QOL literature found considerable agreement regarding the core QOL domains. On the basis of the published work of Hughes et al. (1995), the World Health Organization (1995), Felce & Perry (1996), Schalock (1996), Cummins (1997), Felce (1997), Gardner & Nudler (1997), Gettings & Bradley (1997), Renwick et al. (2000) and Ferdinand & Smith (2003), the most frequently referenced QOL domains (in descending frequency of being reported in the literature review) are interpersonal relations, social inclusion, personal development, physical well-being, self-determination, material well-being, emotional well-being, rights, environment (home/residence/living situation), family, recreation and leisure and safety/security. Schalock et al. (2002) mentioned eight core domains of QOL in their consensus document on QOL: emotional well-being, interpersonal relations, material well-being, personal development, physical well-being, self-determination, social inclusion and rights.

In the extensive literature on QOL, only a small number of studies have specifically engaged in applying a multidimensional framework on QOL to the group of people with PIMD. The core domains that were applied in these studies are similar to those described by Schalock et al. (2002). Campo et al. (1997) used the domains of social inclusion, interpersonal relations and self-determination, while Seifert et al. (2001) and Petry et al. (2005) successfully applied Felce & Perry's (1997) model of QOL to people with PIMD. This model includes the domains of physical well-being, material well-being, social well-being, emotional well-being and productive well-being. These studies cover the core domains of QOL as mentioned in the consensus document on QOL (Schalock et al., 2002), except for the domain of rights. While this might suggest that the core domains are valid for people with PIMD, drawing a conclusion on the basis of three studies is premature.

The second principle states that *the* QOL construct has the same components for all people. This principle represents the idea that there exists an identifiable set of core, essential and fundamental building blocks of life quality that are common to us all (Cummins, 2005). QOL is important for all people and should be thought of in the same way for all people, including individuals with intellectual disabilities. Nevertheless, it is acknowledged that there will be substantial variation in the extent to which the QOL domains are individually valued. The QOL construct is subject to inter- and intrapersonal variability, which means that 'a good quality of life' may mean different things to different people. The domains of well-being will apply to or be experienced variously by different individuals and cultural groups over time (Schalock et al., 2002).

The measurement of QOL needs to be based on a framework which takes into account the common aspects of QOL as well as its inter- and intrapersonal variability. As Borthwick-Duffy (1990) and Hughes et al. (1995) pointed out although the same general dimensions of QOL are important for all individuals, regardless of the severity of disability, differences may exist in the criteria or the indicators used to measure these dimensions. With regard to people with PIMD, the need for a specific operationalisation of QOL is acknowledged in literature (Ouellette-Kuntz & McCreary, 1996; Vlaskamp, 2000). The low level of functioning, the complex and specific needs and the high level of dependency observed in people with PIMD make their daily life, in large part, different from that of people with milder intellectual disabilities or without disabilities. Several authors, therefore, argue that the basic domains of QOL that are relevant for and geared to people with and without disability should be 'translated' into specific indicators that take into account the special needs of people with PIMD in order to make a valid assessment of their QOL (Ouellette-Kuntz & McCreary, 1996; Vlaskamp, 2000).

There is little evidence of such specific operationalisation in the literature. Seifert et al.'s (2001) and Petry et al.'s (2005) models are the only multidimensional models of QOL that use indicators geared to the needs of people with PIMD. Additionally, generic multidimensional models of QOL are sometimes used in research on the

QOL of people with PIMD (Campo et al., 1997). However, these models often contain indicators such as income, status, productivity and autonomy. Viewed from the perspective of people with PIMD these outcomes may be less relevant. In addition, there may be some important aspects for this target group that are not mentioned in generic models of QOL.

The third principle states that QOL has both objective and subjective components (Schalock et al., 2002). QOL exists in two quite different forms: (1) objective features that can be observed and measured within the public domain through such properties as physical quantities and frequencies and (2) a subjective domain that exists only within the private consciousness of each individual and is verified only through repeated responses provided by the person concerned (Cummins, 2005). With regard to the subjective domain, several authors distinguish two components: (1) the individual's general satisfaction with several aspects of his or her life ('satisfaction') and (2) the individual's expressions of positive or negative affects or moods ('happiness') (Marcoen et al., 2002; Schalock & Felce, 2004).

Satisfaction is a commonly used dependent measure because it has a number of advantages (Cummins, 1996, 1998): (1) there is an extensive body of research on the level of satisfaction across populations and service delivery recipients and (2) it allows one to assess the relative importance of individual QOL domains and therefore assign value to the respective domains. The major disadvantages of using only satisfaction as a dependent QOL measure include the following: (1) the reported low correlation between subjective and objective measures of QOL, (2) its trait-like (i.e. stability over time) nature, (3) its tendency to provide only a global measure of perceived well-being and (4) the lack of demonstration to date that it is a sensitive measure of good environmental design and service programmes (Schalock & Felce, 2004; Emerson et al., 2005). Therefore, QOL should not be defined 'primarily' in terms of either its objective or its subjective components. Both are valid indicators of life quality (Cummins, 2005), of which the relative weighting will depend on their anticipated use (Verdugo et al., 2005).

The need for a holistic approach to the measurement of QOL of people with PIMD (i.e. including subjective and objective components of QOL) is strongly promoted in literature (e.g. Edgerton, 1990; Dennis et al., 1993; Goode & Hogg, 1994; Cummins, 1996; Goode, 1997; Schalock, 1994). Nevertheless, very few guidelines are offered on measuring both components of QOL of people with PIMD. With regard to the subjective component of QOL, it is acknowledged that measuring this component for people with PIMD remains amongst the most difficult challenges for QOL researchers (Goode & Hogg, 1994; Goode, 1997; Lyons, 2005). It is problematic to achieve a subjective understanding of the QOL of people with PIMD while also involving them in the process of conceptualisation and measurement because their cognitive impairments limit their levels of understanding, life experiences, communicative capacities and perceptions of QOL (Selai & Rosser, 1993; Oliver et al., 1996; McVilly & Rawlinson, 1998). People with PIMD do not have the required skills to express their subjective experiences verbally (Selai & Rosser, 1993).

Within the limited literature on the subjective component of QOL of people with PIMD, a growing attention has focused on the 'happiness' aspect rather than on the 'satisfaction' aspect. In several studies, researchers have selected behavioural expressions connected to a personal situation of pleasure and contentment as possible indices (measures) of happiness (Favell et al., 1996; Green & Reid, 1996; Ross & Oliver, 2003; Lancioni et al., 2005; Lyons, 2005; Petry & Maes, 2006). Using expressions of positive or negative affects or moods as indices of the subjective component of QOL has some advantages. Expressions of positive or negative affects or moods are potentially more changeable, whereas feelings of satisfaction seem to be rather stable and related to personality.

For a comprehensive estimate of life quality of people with PIMD, measurement of the objective component of QOL is also required. Goode (1997, p. 84) illustrates this need with regard to medical intervention by stating that amongst people with PIMD, development is inherently slow and the presence of additional medical conditions prevalent. Nevertheless, people with PIMD may be entirely unaware of either slow development or additional medical conditions. Indeed, they may even lack any comprehension whatsoever of what a disease is. From the perspective of service providers and that of wider society, a failure to intervene would and should be regarded as culpable. Medical intervention is called for to enhance physical and social interactions in order to extend options for choice, but also to maintain and/or improve functioning and reduce physical distress, which are all important aspects of a person's QOL. The same arguments relating to the subjective and the objective components of QOL in the domain of health also apply to other domains of QOL that are important to people with PIMD.

The fourth principle states that QOL is enhanced by self-determination, resources, purpose in life and a sense of belonging (Cummins, 2005). The QOL construct is based on the assumption that individuals need to have choices and personal control over their interests in activities, interventions and environments. The aims of any QOL programme therefore must be to enhance the individual's self-image and provide empowering environments that increase the individual's opportunities to control aspects of his or her life (Schalock et al., 2002). QOL is thus emancipatory, with self-determination as its central concept.

Self-determination is also an essential aspect in the lives of people with PIMD. It is of great importance for people with PIMD to feel that they control aspects of their life and environment and that they can make choices. Research has demonstrated that people with PIMD are able to make choices (Lancioni et al., 1996; Saunders et al., 2005), although choice and experience may be inextricably bound up in ways that are difficult to assess. The ability to make choices is dependent on experience of choice and is an inherent part of the person's history (Bannerman et al., 1990; Goode, 1997). For instance, the claim that a person with PIMD should be allowed to continue in self-injurious behaviour, 'because it is his choice' is, according to Goode (1997), too simplistic. While this may be a choice existentially speaking, it may be so constrained by lack of experience and/or pathological experience that it is more of a compulsion than a real selection amongst options (Goode, 1997). Support staff are, therefore, expected to adequately build in options in the daily context and to contingently take advantage of preferences (Browder et al., 1998; Green et al., 2000; Cannella et al., 2005). As a result of the opportunity to make choices the person with PIMD takes more initiatives and is more actively involved in activities (Lancioni et al., 1996; Cole & Levinson, 2002; Cannella et al., 2005) and problem behaviour is reduced (Lohrmann-O'Rourke & Yurman, 2001; Cannella et al., 2005).

How to measure?

QOL researchers all over the world agree that QOL is a complex phenomenon to measure because it is elusive, multifaceted and fraught with measurement problems (Schalock & Verdugo, 2002). Nevertheless, efforts to measure QOL have rapidly increased over the past decade because of the great importance given to the concept of QOL in policy.

Historically, six approaches have been used in the area of QOL measurement, according to Schalock & Verdugo (2002). A first approach is multidimensional scaling which measures a person's subjective reactions to life experiences using psychological well-being (e.g. Flanagan, 1982) and personal satisfaction or happiness (e.g. Schalock & Keith, 1993; Cummins, 1997). Ethnographic approaches are a second approach which departs from the idea that the best way to assess one's QOL is through longitudinal research that uses naturalistic, unobtrusive observation to understand people's lives within their natural contexts and through their own eyes (Edgerton, 1990, 1996). Discrepancy analysis focuses on the goodness of fit between individual needs and personal satisfaction of those needs as well as the nature of fit between person and environment (Heal et al., 1995). In a fourth approach, direct behavioural measures such as changes in challenging behaviours (McGill et al., 1994), engagement in activity (Felce, 2000), social interactions, personal freedom and autonomy (Rapley & Hopgood, 1997) are used as an indicator of QOL. In a fifth approach, social indicators are applied in QOL measurement. These social indicators (e.g. health, social welfare, standard of living) may be defined as a statistic of direct normative interest that facilitates concise, comprehensive and balanced judgements about the conditions of major aspects of society (Schalock & Verdugo, 2002; Schyns, 2002). Lastly, there is self-assessment of QOL by people with intellectual disabilities. Participatory Action Research, in which consumers are playing an essential role in measurement of QOL, is rapidly becoming the method of choice amongst QOL researchers (Schalock et al., 2000; Schalock & Verdugo, 2002).

Within the field of intellectual disabilities, the use of quantitative QOL measurement techniques is predominant (Schalock & Verdugo, 2002). Scales, questionnaires and interviews have most often been applied (Hughes et al., 1995) and inventories, indexes and observations of objective indicators are also frequently used (Schalock & Verdugo, 2002). Qualitative QOL measurement techniques are less frequently applied. Nevertheless, several authors share the opinion that QOL can only be measured using qualitative techniques such as document analysis, focus groups, life history, in-depth interviewing or participatory observation (Edgerton, 1990, 1996; Taylor & Bogdan, 1996). These techniques allow one to grasp and understand the person's subjective experiences, perspectives and value systems in a deeper sense. The choice for a quantitative or qualitative measurement technique is inextricably bound up with the focus of measurement. Qualitative techniques are almost exclusively used to measure the subjective component of QOL, whereas quantitative techniques are applied to measure the subjective as well as the objective components of QOL (Maes & Petry, 2000).

In published literature, limited measurement techniques are described that are developed for or have been applied in the measurement of QOL of people with PIMD. With regard to the measurement of the subjective QOL of people with PIMD, we were able to find examples of three approaches. The first approach, used in several studies (Goode, 1994, 1997; De Waele & Van Hove, 2005), is an ethnographic approach. The starting point of these studies is that we need better descriptions of the lives of people with PIMD in order to better understand their QOL. To this end, Goode (1994) utilised participant observation and ethnomethodological techniques that gather data about the everyday social lives of two children and how they experience them. De Waele & Van Hove (2005) in their study of the perspectives of staff and the lived experiences of clients from a QOL frame of reference also used participatory observation in one living unit of people with very severe intellectual disabilities and seriously challenging behaviour in a residential care facility.

The second approach to assessing subjective QOL of people with PIMD is related to the ethnography. While both approaches apply observation as a core measurement technique, the ethnographic approach focuses solely on behavioural expressions of happiness. The majority of studies within this second approach are research studies aimed at measuring and increasing indices of happiness of people with PIMD such as smiling, laughing, yelling while smiling, and excited movements with or without vocalisations (Lancioni et al., 2005). In the context of preference assessment, observations are made of elicited affective responses to different items or situations (Lancioni et al., 1996; Logan & Gast, 2001; Hagopian et al., 2004; Hatton, 2004). Lyons (2003, 2005) also focused on preferences and indices of happiness. He developed the Life Satisfaction Matrix, an instrument and procedure that is designed for measuring the subjective QOL of people with PIMD. The procedure consists of three steps. First, the individual's most familiar communication partner describes to the (unfamiliar) researcher the individual's affective profile. The communication partner then identifies 10 activity periods/experiences that routinely occur in the person's day: 5 are chosen because they are preferred, 3 as non-preferred and 2 of neutral preference. These activities are then ranked from most to least preferred. Second, the next most familiar communication partner does the same. Third, the researcher observes the individual using the affect profile to assess the individual's preferences for the aforementioned and other activities. By triangulating these observations with the preference rankings provided by the communication partner, the affect profile can be validated as a very reasonable indicator of the person's internal state and preferences for these activities. In the procedure that Petry & Maes (2006) developed for drafting individualised profiles of how people with PIMD express pleasure and displeasure, there were also two familiar communication partners and one (unfamiliar) researcher involved. This procedure involves a rating scale for parents and support workers and an observational analysis of videotaped critical incidents by an external researcher. Both data sources are combined in order to draft an individualised profile of expressions of pleasure and displeasure. Such a profile can be used in an assessment of subjective QOL of people with PIMD.

A third approach is found in Ross & Oliver (2003), who developed the Mood, Interest and Pleasure Questionnaire (MIPQ), which is a questionnaire with two subscales (Mood and Interest, and Pleasure) designed to measure affect in adults with severe and profound intellectual disabilities. According to its developers, the MIPQ can offer valuable information on the subjective component of QOL of people with PIMD, given that satisfaction might be reflected in the kinds of behaviours addressed in the MIPQ. This approach differs from the other in that it uses a questionnaire, but there are also similarities. The MIPQ measures levels of mood, interest and pleasure by asking informants to rate operationally defined observable behaviours, which relate to the constructs of mood, interest and pleasure. As such, the MIPQ is based on informants' observation of behavioural expressions of affect.

Questionnaires are often used when attempting to measure the objective component of QOL of people with PIMD. The questionnaire that was developed by Seifert et al. (2001) is a questionnaire where indicators are specifically geared to people with PIMD. However, according to its developers, the purpose of this questionnaire is to act as a checklist in the process of drawing up a support plan for a person with PIMD and not to be used as a 'stand-alone' questionnaire. Consequently, the authors did not check the questionnaire's psychometric properties, unlike the QOL-PIMD, another questionnaire with indicators specifically geared to people with PIMD. The QOL-PIMD was constructed in several phases using interviews with parents and direct support staff (Petry et al., 2005) and a Delphi-procedure with international experts (Petry et al., 2007). The results of an analysis of its psychometric properties were good (Petry et al., submitted).

Other questionnaires that are used in studies to measure the objective QOL of people with PIMD are generic QOL questionnaires, which pretend to be suited for all people with intellectual disabilities. Campo et al. (1997) used the Quality of Life Index (Schalock et al., 1989; Campo et al., 1996) as a QOL measure. This is a questionnaire consisting of 28 items divided in three subscales: environmental control, social relations and community involvement. However, another study by Campo et al. (1996) showed that the Quality of Life Index subscale scores had particularly limited reliability when the tool was administered to a population consisting exclusively of people with severe or profound mental retardation.

Besides questionnaires, direct behavioural measures can also be used as an indicator of the objective QOL of people with PIMD. In the limited body of research on this topic, engagement in activities (Felce et al., 2002; Lancioni et al., 2005) is the most frequently applied direct behavioural measure.

Who should be involved?

In the case of people with intellectual disabilities, QOL has traditionally been evaluated by others or on the basis of social indicators (Verdugo et al., 2005). However, the paradigm shift in the field of intellectual disabilities and the advocacy movement have altered QOL researchers' vision regarding who should be involved in the measurement of one's QOL. The emerging consensus is that people with intellectual disabilities should be involved directly in the measurement of their own QOL. The first priority, therefore, should be to utilise all available and effective methods to enable people with intellectual disabilities to express their own views (Verdugo et al., 2005). Examples of such methods are using alternative or augmentative communication, providing pictorial response alternatives and simplifying the wording of questions and responses. Schalock et al. (2000) showed that with adaptations to survey techniques and the language used in the survey, 81% of participants were able to respond for themselves, despite having significant cognitive, physical and language limitations.

Notwithstanding these serious efforts to enable people to speak for themselves about QOL, there remains a group of individuals with intellectual disabilities who are currently unable to do so, including people with PIMD. A frequently applied method to measure the QOL of this group of people is to involve knowledgeable proxies such as support staff or relatives (Verdugo et al., 2005). These proxies report in an interview or a questionnaire on the objective or subjective component of the QOL of a person with PIMD whom they know very well. The literature however yields conflicting results concerning the value of using a proxy approach. Several researchers have attempted to evaluate consumer-proxy agreement by comparing proxy responses about people who can respond for themselves with self-reports from these same people. In some of these studies, the answers given by people with intellectual disabilities regarding their QOL turned out to strongly disagree with the answers given by proxies (Heal & Sigelman, 1996; Stancliffe, 1995, 2000; Rapley et al., 1998; Cummins, 2002). Others find a greater concordance (Stancliffe, 1999; McVilly et al., 2000). Prominent authors further criticised proxy reporting for distancing the subject person (Brown, 1997) and placing the person in a passive role (Goode, 1997). Because of these problems, the use of proxy measurement is discouraged in the consensus document on QOL for the measurement of the objective as well as of the subjective components of QOL (Schalock et al., 2002). However, the concordance between subjective and proxy ratings seems to be more of a problem in evaluations of emotional experiences and personal preferences than for more objective issues (Borthwick-Duffy, 1996; Perry & Felce, 2002).

For the measurement of the subjective component of QOL of people with PIMD, researchers often rely on observation as a method rather than on proxy reports in interviews or questionnaires. However, this does not entirely solve the validity problem. Goode (1997) argues that all 'subjective' data about people who cannot express themselves in formal languages are 'reputational' data, since the individual cannot be asked in so many words 'How do you feel about ...?' The rater or observer uses his or her opinion in considering how the person with disabilities feels in order to assign 'a subjective state' based on their observations or empathic responses. Reid & Green (2002) found that ratings of preferences of people with PIMD by proxies differed from the preferences that were identified by observation of indices of happiness/unhappiness in reaction to different stimuli. A study by Hogg et al., (2001) also showed a lack of agreement between respondents when interpreting the affective communication of people with PIMD.

A major problem in involving proxies in QOL measurement of people with PIMD is a lack of 'reciprocity of perspectives' between both parties (Keith, 1996; Goode, 1997; Lyons, 2003). QOL measurement depends on the experiences and perceptions of the person(s) designing and performing the measurement as much as it does on those of the person with PIMD. Both parties share a great deal but there are also very real, sometimes insurmountable differences: for example, being a symbolic language user or not. If people do not have shared experiences or culture and one cannot assume reciprocity of perspectives or intersubjectivity (Luckasson et al., 1992; Keith, 1996; Goode, 1997), then communication and understanding may be unreliable and/or invalid (Heal & Sigelman, 1996). While this need for mutual understanding has been widely discussed in the literature, little research has been published in this area (Golden & Reese, 1996; Lyons, 2003).

At this point in time, the question of who should be involved in QOL measurement of people with PIMD remains unresolved. Consequently, QOL researchers face a quandary in relation to individuals who cannot communicate their own views about their QOL: either ignore these individuals because they cannot self-report or obtain data from proxies that may be biased and invalid (Verdugo et al., 2005). If one decides to take a proxy approach, several guidelines to enhance its value are proposed. McVilly & Rawlinson (1998) reviewed the literature on proxy responses with regard to health-related QOL and drew conclusions from this about how proxy responses should be considered in the field of intellectual disabilities. They noted that as questions increased in detail and subjectivity, proxy-subject agreement decreased. Furthermore, the complexity, observability and salience of the issue all affected concurrence (Hensel, 2001). Triangulation of methods and multiple sources of information can also enhance the validity and reliability of measurements (Hughes et al., 1995). This multi-perception aspect is central to an understanding of one's QOL and provides a new challenge to the field of QOL measurement of people with PIMD. Suggestions, choices and perceptions of parents and service and support providers are taken into account. However, it should be recognised that these may differ markedly and centrally from the individual's own perceptions (Schalock et al., 2002).

Where to measure?

An important principle in QOL measurement states that measurement should consider the context of physical, social and cultural environments that are important to people, as people are best understood within the context of these environments (Schalock et al., 2002; Verdugo et al., 2005). In other words, QOL measurement takes on a systems perspective, viewing the individual in interaction with his or her living environment. This systems perspective integrates micro (individual or family), meso (organisation and service delivery network) and macro systems (society and culture) in which individuals and families live.

From a systems perspective, environments are regarded as changeable to accommodate the person's interests, needs and values. An essential idea is that people, places and surroundings can promote and enhance a good life. In turn, an individual's interests and values can emerge in part from the environment in which they live (Schalock et al., 2002). A major advantage of adopting a systems perspective is that it allows us to better understand the predictors of QOL that extend beyond the person to the family, organisation, service delivery system and society (Schalock, 2005). A whole strand of research is focused on investigating these predictors of QOL (Thompson et al., 1996; Felce, 1998, 2000; Stancliffe & Lakin, 1998). These studies clearly indicate that personal characteristics (e.g. health status and adaptive behaviour level), care/supports provider characteristics (e.g. worker stress scores, job satisfaction ratings, staff training, motivation) and environmental variables (e.g. type of residential setting, group size, staffing level, number of household activities participated in and integrated activities) are significant predictors of QOL.

Adopting a systems perspective is also important with regard to people with PIMD. Because of the severity and the complexity of their disabilities, people with PIMD need support in almost every activity of daily life. This support involves many people: family, volunteers and professional support staff from different disciplines and often from different support settings. The environment in which people with PIMD are supported is as such very predictive for their QOL (Renwick et al., 1996). In measuring their QOL, it is important to expand the scope of the measurement from the individual to the systems in which the person is supported. Several studies have investigated which support characteristics are associated with high QOL outcomes for people with PIMD. Initially, the attention was on the impact of service features such as large size, atypical architectural design, barren material circumstances, low staffing levels and outmoded staff remits, training and operational philosophies (Thompson et al., 1996; Felce, 1998). In general, these studies found that a decent, homely, well-located, reasonably staffed environment is a necessary but not sufficient condition for good QOL outcomes. Real life opportunities appear to be dependent on the coming together of three factors at the settings's micro-organisation level: available activity, available personal support and effective assistance (Felce, 1998). What carers do in relation to people with extremely limited independence is of central importance (Jones et al., 1999). In measuring the QOL of people with PIMD, these characteristics of the setting should be taken into account.

Why measure QOL?

In QOL literature, a consensus exists that the main purpose of measuring QOL must be to maintain and enhance the things that already, or could, add worth to people's lives and to take action to improve the things that currently detract from the quality of people's lives. All people, with and without disabilities, share the human experience together and every human being is entitled to live a good life within his or her environment (Schalock et al., 2002). By adopting this value as a central tenet in QOL measurement, the application of QOL in ethical decisions on life and death or in refusing to treat certain people is discarded as an abuse (Wolfensberger, 1994; Borthwick-Duffy, 1996; Hatton, 1998).

Historically, the QOL concept was primarily used as a sensitising notion that gave us a sense of reference and guidance as to what is valued and desired from the individual's perspective. During the last decade, its role has expanded to include (1) a conceptual framework for assessing quality outcomes, (2) a social construct that guides quality enhancement strategies and (3) a criterion for assessing the effectiveness of those strategies (Verdugo et al., 2005). As such, it has become an agent for social change that makes us think differently about people with intellectual disabilities and how we might bring about change at both the individual and the societal level to enhance quality outcomes and reduce their exclusion from the mainstream of society (Schalock et al., 2002; Schalock, 2005).

The application of the QOL concept can be approached at three levels, namely, the individual level, the organisational level (e.g. education, health care and social service programmes) and the societal level (Schalock & Verdugo, 2002). The application of QOL is most apparent at the individual level, but is increasingly found at the organisational and societal levels (Schalock, 2005).

At the individual level, the QOL concept acts as a useful paradigm that can contribute to the identification, development and evaluation of supports, services and policies for individuals. It has the potential to allow a new perspective on people and to be a positive influence on those who work in the fields of education, health and social services, because it steers us in the right direction: towards self-determination, person-centred planning, supporting people's needs and desires and asking people what they think and how they feel (Schalock, 1996; Schalock & Verdugo, 2002). Several principles play an important role in implementing the QOL framework in planning and setting up support for an individual with learning disabilities. These principles are described by many authors (e.g. Bach & Rioux, 1996; Brown, 1996; Renwick et al., 1996; Schalock, 1996; Bradley et al., 1997; Butterworth et al., 1997; Wehmeyer & Schwartz, 1998) and can be summarised by the following concepts:

- *Person-centredness*: In a QOL frame of reference, each person with a disability is regarded and acknowledged as an individual with unique possibilities and needs. As a consequence, support needs to be as individualised and 'person-centred' as possible.
- *Participation*: The QOL of people with intellectual disabilities increases by being able to fully participate in community life. This means that they get the opportunity to live, work, learn and recreate along with people without disabilities in ordinary settings and that they receive the support that is necessary to accommodate their specific needs.
- *Appreciation and respect*: QOL is associated with a fundamental respect for and appreciation of the diversity in individual perspectives and lifestyles.

- *Choice and control*: Making your own choices and decisions is one of the core elements of QOL, as mentioned in the description of the first interrogatory.
- *Relationships*: Of crucial importance for a person's QOL is having interpersonal relations that are characterised by a strong affective involvement, interdependency and mutual respect and appreciation.
- *Competence*: In a QOL frame of reference, the emphasis is on a person's preferences, possibilities and desires rather than on needs and limitations. Support is directed both at making people with intellectual disabilities and the people in their environment conscious of their own possibilities and at stimulating individuals in their growth towards independence.

Adopting these principles and a QOL frame of reference in general is regarded in literature as meaningful in setting up support for people with PIMD. In the past, people with PIMD were called and approached as 'bedridden' (Zijlstra, 2003). Their limitations were stressed instead of their possibilities. Currently, people with PIMD are viewed as individuals that, similar to any other person, have the need to lead a life of their own, in which they feel good and can develop optimally. It is acknowledged that they are able to build up meaningful relations, to express their needs, wishes and preferences and to exert influence on their environment. This change in perspective on people with PIMD is in accordance with the principles in the QOL frame of reference. Applying this frame of reference to a further extent in regard to this target group will allow the new perspective on people with PIMD to grow and to be a positive influence on those who work in the fields of education, health and social services.

Once QOL is assessed at an individual level, it is possible for service providers to evaluate their programmes and to implement a number of quality enhancement techniques at *the* organisational level (Schalock et al., 2002). In others words, QOL application should be the basis for intervention and supports (Brown & Brown, 2005). A key point is person-centred planning (Butterworth et al., 1997). The nature and the intensity of support is no longer determined by the existing system ('system-centred'), but are directed by the needs, wishes and possibilities of the person with a disability ('person-centred').

Person-centred planning is acknowledged as being important in supporting people with PIMD. Procedures for individualised planning and scheduling of activities seem to be crucial for establishing a high quality of support (Hatton et al., 1996; Emerson et al., 2000). Such procedures were associated with higher levels of staff assistance and higher levels of positive contact between clients and staff. They also resulted in an improved participation of clients in daily, leisure and community activities. The positive effects of person-centred planning incite service providers in the field of people with PIMD to use this method (Sanderson, 2002). Interventions need to be set up according to the QOL principles and implemented using person-centred planning methods.

At the societal level, there is a consensus in literature that discussions of QOL for people with disabilities should not be separated from discussions about QOL for people without disabilities (Schalock et al., 1990; Goode, 1994, 1997; Cummins,

2005). Therefore, objective indicators for a defined group of interest may be compared to total population norms and ranges to establish the social equity of that group's circumstances. In several studies a comparison is made of objective life circumstances between people with and without disabilities with regard to work and leisure, level of control and choices, social networks, participation in activities and services in the community, physical health and income (e.g. Newton et al., 1994; Sands & Kozleski, 1994; Wehmeyer & Metzler, 1995). Such a comparison mostly reveals a rather negative picture for people with disabilities. Therefore, a social policy of equal opportunities should be installed that responds to the assessed differences in QOL between people with and without disabilities (Felce & Perry, 1996). For instance, the low representation of people with intellectual disabilities in the workforce and their relative state of poverty may occasion social policy initiatives to develop techniques and processes that broaden the opportunity of paid work at levels of remuneration at or above the minimum wage (Schalock et al., 2002). Principles on QOL can guide policymakers in designing a social policy which enhances disability prevention, rehabilitation and equalisation of opportunities of individuals with disabilities to further their full and effective participation at all levels of society (Schalock et al., 2002). As such QOL becomes, according to Schalock (1996, p. 123), '...a principle that is applicable to the betterment of society as a whole ...'.

In several comparative studies it has become apparent that people with PIMD are a vulnerable group. Personal ability was found to be the single most powerful predictor of variation in QOL outcomes (Hatton et al., 1996; Stancliffe & Lakin, 1998; Emerson et al., 1999; Felce et al., 2000; Perry et al., 2000). Higher ability is related to a greater variety of community settings used, more social activities, better personal integration into the community, more contact with family members, greater choice, greater participation in activities and a more active lifestyle. The consistency of these findings across different groups of research participants suggests that the severity of developmental disability constrains the achievement of a variety of common life experiences (Felce et al., 2002). Therefore, social policy should focus their attention specifically on people with PIMD and take steps towards the elimination of the differences between people with PIMD and people without disabilities or with a milder disability.

Conclusion

In this chapter we attempted to summarise the current understanding in literature on the measurement of QOL of people with PIMD. In general, we can say that measuring the QOL of this target group is a difficult challenge. When thinking about 'what' to measure, the need for a specific operationalisation of QOL becomes clear. However, the question on what this operationalisation should look like remains unanswered. There is also a suggestion of taking a holistic measurement of the QOL of people with PIMD, including its objective as well as subjective components. Several attempts have been undertaken to develop methods to measure both components of QOL including ethnographic approaches, observation, question-naires and direct behavioural measures. Nevertheless, all these methods are faced with validity problems. The question 'who should be involved in the measurement' remains one of the most difficult aspects in measuring the QOL of people with PIMD, as people with PIMD themselves cannot express their subjective experiences verbally. These issues are further complicated by the idea that the characteristics of the support setting should also be taken into account in the measurement, because quality of support has a crucial impact on QOL. Despite these problems, the use-fulness of applying a QOL frame of reference to the support of people with PIMD is shown in literature on an individual, an organisational and a societal level. Re-searchers need to continue in their search for valid and reliable methods to measure the QOL of people with PIMD.

References

Bach, M., & Rioux, M.H.,(1996). Social well-being: a framework for quality of life research. In Renwick, R., Brown, I., & Nagler, M. (eds), *Quality of Life in Health Promotion and Rehabilitation: Conceptual Approaches, Issues and Applications*. London: Sage Publications.

Bannerman, D., Sheldon, J.B., Sherman, J.A., & Harchik, A.E. (1990). Balancing the right to habilitation with the right to personal liberties: the rights of people with developmental disabilities to eat too many doughnuts and take a nap. *Journal of Applied Behavior Analysis*, 23, 79–89.

Borthwick-Duffy, S. (1990). Quality of life of persons with severe or profound mental retardation. In Schalock, R.L. (ed.), *Quality of Life: Perspectives and Issues*. Washington, DC: American Association on Mental Retardation.

Borthwick-Duffy, S.A. (1996). Evaluation and measurement of quality of life: special considerations for persons with mental retardation. In Schalock, R.L. (ed.), *Quality of Life, Vol. I: Conceptualization and Measurement*. Washington, DC: American Association on Mental Retardation.

Bradley, V.J., Taylor, M., Mulkern, V., & Leff, J. (1997). Quality issues and personnel: in search of competent community support workers. In Schalock, R. (ed.), *Quality of Life, Vol. II: Applications to Persons with Disabilities*. Washington, DC: American Association on Mental Retardation.

Browder, D.M., Cooper, K.J., & Lim, L. (1998). Teaching adults with severe disabilities to express their choice of settings for leisure activities. *Education and Training in Mental Retardation and Developmental Disabilities*, 33, 228–238.

Brown, I., & Brown, R.I. (2003). *Quality of Life and Disability: An Approach for Community Practitioners*. London: Jessica Kingsley.

Brown, R.I. (1996). People with developmental disabilities: applying quality of life to assessment and intervention. In Renwick, R., Brown, I., & Nagler, M. (eds), *Quality of Life in Health Promotion and Rehabilitation: Conceptual Approaches, Issues and Applications*. London: Sage Publications.

Brown, R.I. (1997). *Quality of Life for People with Disabilities: Models, Research and Practice*. Cheltenham, UK: Stanley Thornes.

Brown, R.I., & Brown, I. (2005). The application of quality of life. *Journal of Intellectual Disability Research*, 49(10), 718–727.

Butterworth, J., Steere, D.E., & Whitney-Thomas, J. (1997). Using person-centered planning to address personal quality of life. In Schalock, R. (ed.), *Quality of Life, Vol. II: Applications to Persons with Disabilities.* Washington, DC: American Association on Mental Retardation; 5–24

Campo, S.F., Sharpton, W.R., Thompson, B., & Sexton, D. (1996). Measurement characteristics of the Quality of Life Index when used with adults who have severe mental retardation. *American Journal on Mental Retardation,* 100(5), 546–550.

Campo, S.F., Sharpton, W.R., Thompson, B., & Sexton, D. (1997). Correlates of the quality of life of adults with severe or profound mental retardation. *Mental Retardation,* 35, 329–337.

Cannella, H.I., O'Reilly, M.F., & Lancioni, G.E. (2005). Choice and preference assessment research with people with severe to profound developmental disabilities: a review of the literature. *Research in Developmental Disabilities,* 26(1), 1–15.

Cole, C.L., & Levinson, T.R. (2002). Effects of within-activity choices on the challenging behavior of children with severe developmental disabilities. *Journal of Positive Behavior Interventions,* 4, 29–31.

Cummins, R.A. (1996). The domains of life satisfaction: an attempt to order chaos. *Social Indicators Research,* 38, 303–328.

Cummins, R.A. (1997). Assessing quality of life. In Brown, R.I. (ed.), *Assessing Quality of Life in People with Disabilities: Models, Research, and Practices.* London: Stanley Thornes.

Cummins, R.A. (1998). The second approximation to an international standard for life satisfaction. *Social Indicators Research,* 43, 307–334.

Cummins, R.A. (2002). Proxy responding for subjective well-being: a review. *International Review of Research in Mental Retardation,* 25, 183–207.

Cummins, R.A. (2005). Moving from the quality of life concept to a theory. *Journal of Intellectual Disability Research,* 49(10), 699–706.

Dennis, R.E., Williams, W., Giangreco, M.F., & Cloninger, C.J. (1993). Quality of life as context for planning and evaluation of services for people with disabilities. *Exceptional Children,* 59, 499–512.

De Waele, I., & Van Hove, G. (2005). Modern times: an ethnographic study on the quality of life of people with a high support need in a Flemish residential facility. *Disability and Society,* 20, 625–639.

Edgerton, R.B. (1990). Quality of life from a longitudinal research perspective. In Schalock, R. (ed.), *Quality of Life: Perspectives and Issues.* Washington, DC: American Association on Mental Retardation.

Edgerton, R.B. (1996). A longitudinal-etnographic research perspective on quality of life. In Schalock, R.L. (ed.), *Quality of Life, Vol. I: Conceptualization and Measurement.* Washington, DC: American Association on Mental Retardation.

Emerson, E., Robertson, J., Gregory, N., Hatton, C., Kessissoglou, S., Hallam, A., Knapp, M., Järbrink, K., Netten, A., Walsh, P., Lineham, C., Hillery, J., & Durkan, J. (1999). *Quality and Costs of Residential Support for People with Learning Disabilities: A Comparative Analysis of Quality and Costs in Village Communities, Residential Campuses and Dispersed Housing Schemes.* Manchester, UK: University of Manchester, Hester Adrian Research Centre.

Emerson, E., Robertson, J., Gregory, N., Kessissoglou, S., Hatton, C., Hallam, A., Knapp, M., Järbrink, K., Netten, A., & Linehan, C. (2000). The quality and costs of community-based residential supports and residential campuses for people with severe and complex disabilities. *Journal of Intellectual and Developmental Disability,* 25, 263–279.

Emerson, E., Robertson, J., Hatton, C., Knapp, M., Walsh, P.N., & Hallam, A. (2005). Costs and outcomes of community residential supports in England. In Stancliffe, R.J., & Lakin, K.C. (eds), *Costs and Outcomes of Community Services for People with Intellectual Disabilities*. Baltimore, MD: P.H. Brookes Publishers.

Favell, J.E., Realon, R.E., & Sutton, K.A. (1996). Measuring and increasing the happiness of people with profound mental retardation and physical handicaps. *Behavioral Interventions*, 11, 47–58.

Felce, D. (1997). Defining and applying the concept of quality of life. *Journal of Intellectual Disability Research*, 41(2), 126–135.

Felce, D. (1998). The determinants of staff and resident activity in residential services for people with severe intellectual disability: moving beyond size, building design, location and number of staff. *Journal of Intellectual & Developmental Disability*, 23, 103–119.

Felce, D. (2000). Engagement in activity as an indicator of quality of life in British research. In Keith, K.D., & Schalock, R.L. (eds), *Cross-Cultural Perspectives on Quality of Life*. Washington, DC: American Association on Mental Retardation.

Felce, D., Jones, E., & Lowe, K. (2002). Active support: planning daily activities and support for people with severe mental retardation. In Holburn, S., & Vietze, P.M. (eds), *Person-Centered Planning: Research, Practice and Future Direction*. Baltimore, MD: P.H. Brookes Publishers.

Felce, D., Lowe, K., Beecham, J., & Hallam, A. (2000). Exploring the relationships between costs and quality of services for adults with severe intellectual disabilities and the most severe challenging behaviours in Wales: a multivariate regression analysis. *Journal of Intellectual and Developmental Disability*, 25, 307–326.

Felce, D., & Perry, J. (1996). Exploring current conceptions of Quality of Life: a model for people with and without disabilities. In Renwick, R., Brown, I., & Nagler, M. (eds), *Quality of Life in Health Promotion and Rehabilitation: Conceptual Approaches, Issues and Applications*. London: Sage Publications.

Felce, D., & Perry, J. (1997). Quality of life: the scope of the term and its breadth of measurement. In Brown, R.I. (ed.), *Quality of Life for People with Disabilities: Models, Research, and Practice* (2nd edition). Cheltenham, UK: Stanley Thornes.

Ferdinand, R., & Smith, M.A. (2003). *2003 Nebraska Development Disabilities Provider Profiles*. Lincoln, NE: The ARC of Nebraska.

Flanagan, J.C. (1982). Flanagan, 1982 measurement of quality of life: current state of the art. *Archives of Physical Medicine and Rehabilitation*, 63, 56–59.

Gardner, J.F., & Nudler, S. (1997). Beyond compliance to responsiveness: accreditation reconsidered. In Schalock, R. (ed.), *Quality of Life, Vol. II: Applications to Persons with Disabilities*. Washington, DC: American Association on Mental Retardation.

Gettings, R.M., & Bradley, V.J. (1997). *Core Indicators Project*. Alexandria, VA: National Association of State Directors of Developmental Disabilities Services, Inc.

Golden, J., & Reese, M. (1996). Focus on communication: improving interaction between staff and residents who have severe or profound mental retardation. *Research in Developmental Disabilities*, 17(5), 363–382.

Goode, D. (1994). *A World Without Words: The Social Construction of Children Born Deaf-Blind*. Philadelphia, PA: Temple University Press.

Goode, D. (1997). Quality of life as international disability policy: implications for international research. In Schalock, R.L. (ed.), *Quality of Life, Vol. II: Application to Persons with Disabilities*. Washington, DC: American Association on Mental Retardation.

Goode, D.A., & Hogg, J. (1994). Towards an understanding of holistic quality of life in persons with profound intellectual and multiple disabilities. In Goode, D. (ed.), *Quality of Life for Persons with Disabilities: International Perspectives and Issues*. Cambridge, MA: Brookline Books.

Green, C.W., Middleton, S.G., & Reid, D.H. (2000). Embedded evaluation of preferences sampled from person-centered plans for people with profound multiple disabilities. *Journal of Applied Behavior Analysis*, 33, 639–642.

Green, C.W., & Reid, D.H. (1996). Defining, validating, and increasing indices of happiness among people with profound multiple disabilities. *Journal of Applied Behavior Analysis*, 29(1), 67–78.

Hagopian, L.P., Long, E.S., & Rush, K.S. (2004). Preference assessment procedures for individuals with developmental disabilities. *Behavior Modification*, 28(5), 668–677.

Hatton, C. (1998). Whose quality of life is it anyway? Some problems with the emerging quality of life consensus. *Mental Retardation*, 36, 104–117.

Hatton, C. (2004). Choice. In Emerson, E., Hatton, C., Thompson, T., & Parmenter, T.R. (eds), *The International Handbook of Applied Research in Intellectual Disabilities*. Chichester, UK: John Wiley & Sons.

Hatton, C., Emerson, E., Robertson, J., Henderson, D., & Cooper, J. (1996). Factors associated with staff support and user lifestyle in services for people with multiple disabilities: a path analytic approach. *Journal of Intellectual Disability Research*, 40, 466–477.

Heal, L.W., Rubin, S.S., & Park, W. (1995). *Lifestyle Satisfaction Scale*. Champaign-Urbana, IL: University of Illinois, Transition Research Institute.

Heal, L.W., & Sigelman, C.K. (1996). Methodological issues in quality of life measurement. In Schalock, R.L. (ed.), *Quality of Life, Vol. I: Conceptualization and Measurement*. Washington, DC: American Association on Mental Retardation.

Hensel, E. (2001). Is satisfaction a valid concept in the assessment of quality of life of people with intellectual disabilities? A review of literature. *Journal of Applied Research in Intellectual Disabilities*, 14, 311–326.

Hogg, J., Cavet, J., Lambe, L., & Smeddle, M. (2001). The use of 'Snoezelen' as multisensory stimulation with people with intellectual disabilities: a review of the research. *Research in Developmental Disabilities*, 22, 353–372.

Hughes, C., Hwang, B., Kim, J., Eisenman, L.T., & Killian, D.J. (1995). Quality of life in applied research: a review and analysis of empirical measures. *American Journal on Mental Retardation*, 99, 623–641.

Jones, E., Perry, J., Lowe, K., Felce, D., Toogood, S., Dunstan, F., Allen, D., & Pagler, J. (1999). Opportunity and the promotion of activity among adults with severe mental retardation living in community residences: the impact of training staff in Active Support. *Journal of Intellectual Disability Research*, 43, 164–178.

Keith, K.D. (1996). Measuring quality of life across cultures: issues and challenges. In Schalock, R.L. (ed.), *Quality of Life, Vol. I: Conceptualization and Measurement*. Washington, DC: American Association on Mental Retardation.

Lancioni, G.E., O'Reilly, M.F., & Emerson, E. (1996). A review of choice research with people with severe and profound developmental disabilities. *Research in Developmental Disabilities*, 17, 391–411.

Lancioni, G.E., Singh, N.N., O'Reilly, M.F., Oliva, D., & Basili, G. (2005). An overview of research on increasing indices of happiness of people with severe/profound intellectual and multiple disabilities. *Disability and Rehabilitation*, 27(3), 83–93.

Lindstrom, B. (1992). Quality of life: a model for evaluating health for all. *Soz Praventivmed*, 37, 301–306.

Logan, K.R., & Gast, D.L. (2001). Conducting preference assessments and reinforcer testing for individuals with profound multiple disabilities: issues and procedures. *Exceptionality*, 9(3), 123–134.

Lohrmann-O'Rourke, S., & Yurman, B. (2001). Naturalistic assessment of and intervention for mouthing behaviors influenced by establishing operations. *Journal of Positive Behavior Interventions*, 3, 19–27.

Luckasson, R., Coulter, D.L., Polloway, E.A., Reiss, S., Schalock, R.L., Snell, M.E., Spitalnik, D.M., & Stark, J.A. (1992). *Mental Retardation: Definition, Classification and Systems of Supports*. Washington, DC: American Association on Mental retardation.

Lyons, G. (2003). *Life Satisfaction for Children with Profound Multiple Disabilities*. Unpublished Ph.D. Thesis, The University of Newcastle, New Castle.

Lyons, G. (2005). The Life Satisfaction Matrix: an instrument and procedure for assessing the subjective quality of life of individuals with profound multiple disabilities. *Journal of Intellectual Disability Research*, 49(10), 766–769.

Maes, B., & Petry, K. (2000). Naar een groeiende consensus over de betekenis van het concept 'kwaliteit van leven'. In Ghesquière, P., & Janssens, J.M.A.M. (reds), *Van zorg naar ondersteuning: ontwikkelingen in de begeleiding van personen met een verstandelijke handicap*. Houten, The Netherlands: Bohn Stafleu Van Loghum.

Marcoen, A., Van Cotthem, K., Billiet, K., & Beyers, W. (2002). Dimensies van subjectief welbevinden bij ouderen. *Tijdschrift voor gerontologie en geriatrie*, 33(4), 156–164.

McGill, P., Emerson, E., & Mansell, J. (1994). Individually designed residential provision for people with seriously challenging behaviours. In Emerson, E., McGill, P., & Mansell, J. (eds), *Severe Learning Disabilities and Challenging Behaviours*. London: Chapman & Hall.

McVilly, K.R., Burton-Smith, R.M., & Davidson, J.A. (2000). Concurrence between subject and proxy ratings of quality of life for people with and without intellectual disabilities. *Journal of Intellectual and Developmental Disabilities*, 25, 19–40.

McVilly, K.R., & Rawlinson, R.B. (1998). Quality of life issues in the development and evaluation of services for people with intellectual disability. *Journal of Intellectual and Developmental Disability*, 23(3), 199–218.

Newton, J.S., Horner, R.H., Ard, W.R., LeBaron, N., & Sappington, G. (1994). A conceptual model for improving the social life of individuals with mental retardation. *Mental Retardation*, 32, 392–402.

Oliver J., Huxley, P., Bridges, K., & Mohamad, H. (1996). *Quality of Life and Mental Health Services*. London: Routledge.

Ouellette-Kuntz, H., & McCreary, B. (1996). Quality of life assessment for persons with severe developmental disabilities. In Renwick, R., Brown, I., & Nagler, M. (eds), *Quality of Life in Health Promotion and Rehabilitation: Conceptual Approaches, Issues and Applications*. London: Sage Publications.

Perry, J., & Felce, D. (2002). Subjective and objective quality of life assessment: responsiveness, response bias, and resident. Proxy concordance. *Mental Retardation*, 40, 445–456.

Perry, J., Felce, D., & Lowe, K. (2000). *Subjective and Objective Quality of Life Assessment: Their Interrelationship and Determinants*. Cardiff, UK: University of Wales College of Medicine, Welsh Centre for Learning Disabilities.

Petry, K., & Maes, B. (2006). Identifying expressions of (dis)pleasure by persons with profound multiple disabilities. *Journal of Intellectual and Developmental Disability*, 31(1), 28–38.

Petry, K., Maes, B., & Vlaskamp, C. (2005). Domains of quality of life of people with profound multiple disabilities: the perspective of parents and direct support staff. *Journal of Applied Research in Intellectual Disabilities*, 18, 35–46.

Petry, K., Maes, B., & Vlaskamp, C. (2007). Operationalizing quality of life for people with profound intellectual and multiple disabilities: a Delphi study. *Journal on Intellectual Disability Research*, 51(5), 334–349.

Petry, K., Maes, B., & Vlaskamp, C. Psychometric evaluation of a questionnaire to measure the quality of life of people with profound multiple disabilities (QOL-PMD). *Intellectual and Developmental Disabilities*, submitted.

Rapley, M., & Hopgood, L. (1997). Quality of life in a community-based service in rural Australia. *Journal of Intellectual & Developmental Disabilities*, 22(2), 125–141.

Rapley, M., Ridgeway, J., & Beyer, S. (1998). Staff:staff and staff:client reliability of the Schalock & Keith (1993) Quality of Life Questionnaire. *Journal of Intellectual Disability Research*, 42(1), 37–42.

Reid, D.H., & Green, C.W. (2002). Person-centered planning with people who have severe multiple disabilities: validated practices and misapplications. In Holburn, S., & Vietze, P.M. (eds), *Person-Centered Planning: Research, Practice and Future Directions*. Baltimore, MD: P.H. Brookes Publishers.

Renwick, R., Brown, I., & Raphael, D. (2000). Person-centered quality of life: contributions from Canada to an international understanding. In Keith, K.D., & Schalock, R.L. *Cross-Cultural Perspectives on Quality of Life*. Washington, DC: American Association on Mental Retardation.

Renwick, R., Brown, I., Rootman, I., & Nagler, M. (1996). Conceptualization, research, and application: future directions. In Renwick, R., Brown, I., & Nagler, M. (eds), *Quality of Life in Health Promotion and Rehabilitation: Conceptual Approaches, Issues and Applications*. London: Sage Publications.

Ross, E., & Oliver, C. (2003). The assessment of mood in adults who have severe or profound mental retardation. *Clinical Psychology Review*, 23, 225–245.

Sanderson, H. (2002). A plan is not enough: exploring the development of person-centered teams. In Holburn, S., & Vietze, P.M. (eds), *Person-Centered Planning: Research, Practice and Future Directions*. Baltimore, MD: P.H. Brookes Publishers.

Sands, D.G., & Kozleski, E.B. (1994). Quality of life differences between adults with and without disabilities. *Education and Training in Mental Retardation and Developmental Disabilities*, 29, 90–101.

Saunders, M.D., Saunders, R.R., Mulugeta, A., Henderson, K., Kedziorski, T., Hekker, B., & Wilson, S. (2005). A novel method for testing learning and preferences in people with minimal motor movement. *Research in Developmental Disabilities*, 26(3), 255–266.

Schalock, R.L. (1994). Quality of life, quality enhancement, and quality assurance: implications for program planning and evaluation in the field of mental retardation and developmental disabilities. *Evaluation and Program Planning*, 17(2), 121–131.

Schalock, R.L. (ed.) (1996). *Quality of Life, Vol. I: Conceptualization and Measurement*. Washington, DC: American Association on Mental Retardation.

Schalock, R.L. (2004). Quality of life: what we know and do not know. *Journal of Intellectual Disability Research*, 48, 203–216.

Schalock, R.L. (2005). Guest editorial: introduction and overview. *Journal of Intellectual Disability Research*, 49(10), 695–698.

Schalock, R.L., Bartnik, E., Wu, F., Konig, A., Lee, C.S., & Reiter, S. (1990). *An International Perspective in Quality of Life: Measurement and Use*. Paper presented at the Annual Meeting of the American Association on Mental Retardation, Atlanta, GA. Available at: http://eric.ed.gov/ERICDocs/data/ericdocs2sql/content_storage_01/0000019b/80/22/79/21.pdf (accessed 1 October 2007)

Schalock, R.L., Bonham, G.S., & Marchand, C.B. (2000). Consumer based quality of life assessment: a path model of perceived satisfaction. *Evaluation and Program Planning*, 23, 77–88.

Schalock, R.L., Brown, I., Brown, R., Cummins, R.A., Felce, D., Matikka, L., Keith, K.D., & Parmenter, T. (2002). Conceptualization, measurement, and application of quality of life for people with intellectual disabilities: report of an international panel of experts. *Mental Retardation*, 40(6), 457–470.

Schalock, R.L., & Felce, D. (2004). Quality of life and subjective well-being: conceptual and measurement issues. In Emerson, E., Hatton, C., Thompson, T., & Parmenter, T. (eds), *Handbook of Applied Research in Intellectual Disabilities*. West Sussex, UK: John Wiley & Sons.

Schalock, R.L., & Keith, K.D. (1993). *Quality of Life Questionnaire*. Worthington, OH: IDS Publishing.

Schalock, R.L., Keith, K.D., Hoffman, K., & Karan, O.C. (1989). Quality of life: its measurement and use. *Mental Retardation*, 27(1), 25–31.

Schalock, R.L., & Verdugo, M.A. (2002). *Handbook on Quality of Life for Human Service Practitioners*. Washington, DC: American Association on Mental Retardation.

Schyns, P. (2002). Wealth of nations, individual income and life satisfaction in 42 countries: a multilevel approach. *Social Indicators Research*, 60, 5–40.

Seifert, M., Fornefeld, B., & Koenig, P. (2001). *Zeilperspektive Lebensqualität. Eine Studie zur Lebenssituation von Menschen mit schwerer Behinderung im Heim*. Bielefeld, Germany: Bethel-Verlag.

Selai, C.E., & Rosser, R.M. (1993). Good Quality Quality? Some methodological issues. *Journal of the Royal Society of Medicine*, 86, 440–443.

Stancliffe, R.J. (1995). Assessing opportunities for choice making: a comparison of self- and staff reports. *American Journal on Mental Retardation*, 99, 418–429.

Stancliffe, R.J. (1999). Proxy respondents and the quality of life questionnaire empowerment factor. *Journal of Intellectual Disability Research*, 43, 185–193.

Stancliffe, R.J. (2000). Proxy respondents and quality of life. *Evaluation and Program Planning*, 23, 89–93.

Stancliffe, R.J., & Lakin, K.C. (1998). Analysis of expenditures and outcomes of residential alternatives for persons with developmental disabilities. *American Journal on Mental Retardation*, 102, 552–568.

Taylor, S.J., & Bogdan, R. (1996). Quality of life and the individual's perspective. In Schalock, R.L. (ed), *Quality of Life, Vol. I: Conceptualization and Measurement*. Washington, DC: American Association on Mental Retardation.

Thompson, T., Robinson, J., Dietrich, M., Farris, M., & Sinclair, V. (1996). Interdependence of architectural features and program variables in community residences for people with mental retardation. *American Journal on Mental Retardation*, 101, 315–327.

Verdugo, M.A., Schalock, R.L., Keith, K.D., & Stancliffe, R.J. (2005). Quality of life and its measurement: important principles and guidelines. *Journal of Intellectual Disability Research*, 49(10), 707–717.

Vlaskamp, C. (2000). De betekenis van het 'nieuwe paradigma' in de zorg voor mensen met ernstig meervoudige beperkingen. In Ghesquière, P., & Janssens, J.M.A.M. (eds), *Van zorg naar ondersteuning: ontwikkelingen in de begeleiding van personen met een verstandelijke handicap*. Houten, The Netherlands: Bohn Stafleu Van Loghum.

Wehmeyer, M.L., & Metzler, C.A. (1995). How self-determinated are people with mental retardation? The national consumer survey. *Mental Retardation*, 33, 111–119.

Wehmeyer, M.L., & Schwartz, M. (1998). The relationship between self-determination and quality of life for adults with mental retardation. *Education and Training in Mental Retardation and Developmental Disabilities*, 33, 3–12.

Wolfensberger, W. (1994). Let's hang up 'Quality of Life' as a hopeless term. In Goode, D., *Quality of Life for Persons with Disabilities: International Perspectives and Issues*. Cambridge, MA: Brookline Books.

World Health Organization Quality of Life Group (1995). The World Health Organization Quality of Life Assessment (WHOQOL): position paper from the World Health Organization. *Social Science Medicine*, 42, 1403–1409.

Zijlstra, R. (2003). Dansen met olifanten: Een onderzoek naar de implementatie van het opvoedingsprogramma in de zorg voor mensen met ernstige meervoudige beperkingen. Groningen, The Netherlands: Stichting Kinderstudies.

Chapter 3

SUPPORTING A PERSON WITH PROFOUND INTELLECTUAL AND MULTIPLE DISABILITIES TO MAINTAIN THEIR HEALTH: A PARENT CARER AND SUPPORT TEAM EXPERIENCE

Jan Roast, Katie Hickson and Sarah King

This chapter presents the experiences of a parent and a team of support workers supporting a young lady through a number of complex health situations. It commences with a presentation from the parent's perspective, where the parent presents the challenges she has faced supporting her daughter's complex health needs. The second part of the chapter presents the experience of a support team supporting the young lady in hospital and the challenges they faced meeting her health needs in an unfamiliar environment. The chapter concludes with a wish list for services and those supporting people with profound intellectual and multiple disabilities.

Parent's perspective

Introduction

My name is Jan and I am mother to 27-year-old Amanda[1] who has been labelled as having profound intellectual and multiple disabilities. She is a wonderful and much loved daughter who has brought great joy and some sadness to my life. Whilst she now lives in her own home independently with a good support network and is having a great life, she continues to direct and influence my life in many ways. She has caused me to be connected with wonderful people in both the health and caring fields and given me a whole new career as a consultant for people with intellectual disabilities. Thank you, Amanda, for being such a great teacher.

---

[1] To maintain confidentiality the name has been changed.

Learning objective

My aim in contributing to this book is to give the reader an insight into what it has been like for a parent of someone like Amanda – the highs and the lows, the successes and frustrations, and above all what can be learned from our experience – what we would keep and what we hope might be different in the future.

My story

The story begins in the late 1970s when Amanda was born apparently normal in every way. However, it was not many weeks before I became very anxious about her development. There was odd behaviour which only lasted seconds but which prompted me to ask our local doctor for help. The first general practitioner (GP) was sure I was being an 'overanxious' mother, but I persisted and a second GP listened more carefully and immediately sent her to a hospital for a scan and other tests.

This was my first taste of the hospital 'process'. Here was a child who looked so 'normal' but so obviously had a problem; what followed was a true nightmare.

The hospital wanted to perform a CT scan on Amanda and told us to come back in the morning. (In those days it was not common practice to stay with your child.) The next morning we arrived in hospital and nobody, and I mean nobody, would make eye contact or speak to us other than to say that we had to wait for the consultant to arrive. We waited for most of the day and during that dreadful time I thought I had mentally prepared myself for what was to come. My daughter must have epilepsy, but I would cope – that was the worst diagnosis I could imagine – how wrong I was. When the consultant eventually arrived, he sat us down and gently told us that Amanda had tuberous sclerosis but that 20% of 'these' children would grow up normally. Could they genetically test our other two children and would we like to see a medical social worker! All I could think was that 80% wouldn't enjoy a normal life, and not only did we have one child with a serious genetic condition but we could have three! The next few days and weeks passed in a complete blur, but I remember nobody was optimistic about her future; she wouldn't walk, wouldn't talk and would probably not live to make double figures, and I really shouldn't spend time looking for a cure. In fact one consultant said, probably because he thought it was what we wanted to hear, that we could be assured that they didn't try too hard with these children. However, amongst all this doom and gloom, I clearly remember one particularly enlightened and empathetic doctor saying that 'nobody could know for sure how she would develop and not to give up'. This was exactly what I needed to hear: the chance to hope without being unrealistic, and I have tried to put this advice to good use ever since. I feel sure that things have moved on enormously in terms of how medical staff explains such news to families, but to me the learning here is never to take away all hope without absolute certainty.

The next few years were spent exploring the unfamiliar world of disability and learning how to get the best life for our daughter. Mostly there were good medical services which linked well with an extremely supportive special school. Everything was coordinated and documented through school or a specialist paediatric assessment centre, including physiotherapy, occupational therapy, medical assessments and interventions, equipment and offers of respite. There were a few difficult times, in particular a visit to dermatology as the consultant wanted everybody to see her 'atypical rash'. I remember feeling very upset and protective of Amanda, she was not a specimen to be viewed – she was a person. But although life wasn't easy, as I look back these were the easiest years.

One of the many hiccups which I remember when Amanda hit teenage and is probably worth recounting as an example of what was to come relates to a referral to the local mobility centre. This was a renowned facility and the waiting list was long. I was clear that what I needed was a lighter, easily foldable wheelchair. As sole carer (my husband having sadly died), I needed to be able to lift my daughter into a car and then stow her wheelchair in the back several times a day without damaging my back. What was actually demonstrated to me was a very heavy, very ugly wheelchair which was said to be light if I took the time to disassemble both wheels, arm rests, foot plates, cushion and various other parts. I was not impressed and said so. Later my GP received a letter from the hospital suggesting that I was an 'angry parent', who would benefit from counselling, not a lighter wheelchair! It seemed clear that there was a budget for counselling but not for a lighter wheelchair. I complained, had the report erased from her notes and eventually got a lighter wheelchair.

I am grateful that Amanda has been reasonably healthy during her life so we have not needed to use inpatient services until recently. However, last year Amanda became very ill, and whilst her GP was reluctant to admit her knowing it wasn't the best place for someone like Amanda, he felt she needed hospital help. Firstly, I must say that the extremely skilled doctors did manage to find out what was wrong and eventually to help her on the road to recovery, but it was an awful experience for everybody. . . .

We had now arrived in the National Health System, a system that does not easily accommodate people who require 24-hour support and who cannot communicate their needs in a conventional way. Amanda's care, it was clear, could not be relinquished to nursing staff, yet the best overnight arrangement that could be found for her now 'essential' care staff was a mattress on the floor in Amanda's room. Furthermore, it seemed to me that Amanda was stripped of every ounce of choice and control the minute she entered hospital. On one occasion, when I asked if the intravenous fluid drip could be administered during the day so that she and her staff could try to sleep at night, I was told that hospital was a 24-hour service and therefore it would be done when it was convenient to the nursing staff. Of course it was no good telling Amanda to go back to sleep once woken – she would not have understood – so often, she and the staff were awake through the night. Nor would it have been worth saying that Amanda's staff weren't paid waking night rates and therefore the whole support budget would have been in jeopardy.

It felt to us all very much like entering a huge slow moving machine and going through the various stages and processes until we reached the end of the production line, and if that end product involved getting her well then so much the better. It seemed to be the 'process and the policies' that mattered most, not Amanda's needs or individual choices.

Such basics as food were not easily available outside mealtimes and since she was eating so little and losing considerable weight, we needed to be able to offer her something more regularly. At one point Amanda was booked for an MRI scan very early one morning at another hospital a few minutes away. Her own wheelchair-adapted vehicle was on hand, and we asked if we could take her for the appointed time. However, 'policy' demanded that she go in an ambulance, leave an hour earlier and detour to other sites to pick up more patients so they could all be transported together. This seemed to me to be rules for the sake of rules, inflexible and not in my daughter's best interests – needless to say, she went in the ambulance and then had to wait several hours for the return trip.

Nevertheless, we found the nursing staff to be very willing and helpful but under such pressure that they didn't have time to learn anything about how to support Amanda even though her person-centred plan (Circles Network, 2005) was by her bed for them to read. In fact they were too busy to perform tasks other than changing drips and cannulas and taking 'observations'. Maybe they relied on Amanda's ever present carer, but I would be very concerned about how she would have fared had she gone into hospital without this support.

Summary

In summary, Amanda's individual needs and wishes were overridden by the hospital system. Person-centred planning, the basis of Amanda's life, was ignored. Having said all this, we are extremely grateful to the hospital that she is now well and continuing her valued life within the community.

Support workers' perspective

Introduction

Our names are Katie and Sarah, and we are support workers employed as part of a nine-piece support team. We support Amanda to live in her own home; Amanda has profound intellectual and multiple disabilities, complex epilepsy and requires full support 24/7.

Our aim is to give the reader some knowledge of our experiences and the challenges we faced as support staff when supporting someone with profound intellectual and multiple disabilities to meet their health needs at home when they were seriously ill and hospital admittance was needed.

Learning objectives

From reading this chapter, the reader will:

- Develop a greater understanding of the challenges faced by support workers supporting a person with profound intellectual and multiple disabilities;
- Develop a greater appreciation of the complexities of meeting the health needs of a person with profound intellectual and multiple disabilities while in hospital.

In early 2005 Amanda seemed unwell, not wanting to eat or drink very much. Our first thoughts as a team were that she had a bug of some kind or just an everyday common cold and felt under the weather, just like any one of us feels if we have a cold. However, after a couple of days Amanda showed no signs of improvement. We made an appointment with her GP; after a few simple checks he decided to prescribe her a course of antibiotics. The antibiotics appeared to be working, and Amanda seemed to show signs of improvement.

One month on Amanda was struggling to eat and drink again, so it was back to the doctors where she had lots of blood tests taken. Throughout this time Amanda's weight became our main concern as she was just under seven stone and dropping rapidly. Unintentional weight loss is usually an indicator of health decline, so it is important that assessments are made quickly so that the right intervention can be made (Johnson et al., 2006). We had been advised by the dietitian that her optimum weight should be around eight stone.

Towards the end of February and the beginning of March, Amanda didn't seem to be getting better; instead, she seemed to be getting worse. She wasn't taking her medication well; she was gagging on food and starting to be violently sick. After going backwards and forwards to the doctors a hospital appointment was made for further tests to be done. The outcome of the first appointment was inconclusive and in our eyes was rather confusing. It was now decided that Amanda needed a kidney scan, the results of that showed nothing to say what was wrong with her. Once again Amanda returned home, and we felt helpless to do anything to help her get better.

Once again Amanda was on antibiotics, and after a doctor's visit to the house Amanda was still not eating or drinking sufficiently. By the end of March we still had no idea of what was wrong with Amanda.

We had another call from the doctors – everyone was at their wits' end. Amanda's mother decided to admit Amanda to hospital, but due to it being a bank holiday and nothing would be done to help her, after one night's admission, she was returned home.

It wasn't until the beginning of April that Amanda was finally admitted to hospital; this would prove to be a frustrating and challenging 2 weeks for us.

Amanda was admitted to a highly infectious diseases ward at a local general hospital, and she was allocated her own room. Because she was so dehydrated she was placed on a drip; now the hard task of getting better had begun. From our point of view it seemed to be a huge relief that Amanda was in a place to make her better.

We, as support staff, had to stay with Amanda during her hospital stay. We appreciate that the priority of the staff was to attend to Amanda's health needs, but we needed to stay to support Amanda because we feared that the hospital staff wouldn't be able to communicate effectively with Amanda and wouldn't support her in the way we would at home. Amanda requires 24/7 support at home and the pressures upon the ward staff meant they couldn't be with her on that basis. Facilities for carers were abysmal. They were unable to adequately cater for carers accompanying a person in hospital 24/7. Sleeping and bathing facilities were inadequate while access to food and drink was exceptionally poor. We had provision for food or drinks on the ward so we either had to bring our own into the hospital or rely on Amanda's mum to bring in food and drink when she visited. We realised that the ward staff were busy with the many patients on the ward and as a result never offered us a break from caring for Amanda. So we would sit with Amanda until the next member of staff came on duty hours later.

At times the approach of the hospital staff left us feeling frustrated; despite Amanda having a comprehensive person-centred plan (Circles Network, 2005), we were frequently required to repeat information, and this often appeared to be disregarded. This let us feeling devalued and unimportant, and we feel it is essential that the hospital staff listen to the information provided by a family member or carers because they know the person best.

Frequently, throughout her stay in hospital, the nurses and healthcare assistants would come in to change the drip and cannula, often during the early hours. This intervention would wake Amanda, and frequently she would remain awake long after the intervention. The ward staff appeared not to take into regard either Amanda's or our need for uninterrupted sleep, and due to the staffing requirements back at the house, we were doing long shifts often more than 24 hours continually to support Amanda and then returning to her home to support her housemate. For Amanda and other people with profound intellectual and multiple disabilities, establishing a sleep wake routine is important to ensure quality sleep is achieved (Espie et al., 1998). Regrettably, hospital interventions can disrupt the sleep wake cycle to detrimental effect, and it can take a considerable length of time before the person's sleep wake cycle returns to normal.

The whole support team were extremely tired and getting stressed. It started to put extreme pressure on us all as a team, and this pressure was heightened as some team members did not participate in providing hospital care. For those who were there, there were the additional demands of travelling to and from the hospital.

Amanda has lots of seizures and not once when they happened did any of the ward staff come to her room to check she was alright, we were left administering her medication and meeting her needs. Exactly who has the duty of care when a person is in hospital? Surely when a person is admitted to hospital, it is the hospital's responsibility to meet their needs and not the responsibility of those visitors who may be carers. Only when the other health professionals began to appreciate our knowledge of Amanda's needs and behaviours did we begin to make progress.

Amanda was away from her own environment in an unfamiliar place, supported by medical and nursing staff who did not know her well and who found it very difficult to communicate with her. She needed us to advocate for her needs, and interpret and communicate to those providing medical and nursing interventions; comfort, consistency and continuity are important to Amanda to help her feel safe and calm. As support workers we tried our best to maintain this by making a home from home in a small hospital room.

The positive outcome of this stay so far was that we felt we were getting through to the doctors and other members of the healthcare team in how to support Amanda's complex needs; the hospital staff were beginning to understand her needs which helped Amanda on her road to recovery.

Eventually after what felt like a lifetime, Amanda slowly but surely began to get stronger, started to eat and drink the food we offered her and began to return to the Amanda we knew. It is a challenge for the ward staff to recognise when Amanda was improving as they did not know how she was when she was well. They relied on us to point out the signs of her improvement. After 2 weeks it was agreed between the care team and doctors that Amanda would continue to improve without hospital intervention and so she was discharged home. We were all very relieved to hear this decision.

Once home in her familiar surroundings, her mood improved rapidly, she was less tense and appeared calmer, and for the first time she welcomed close contact, cuddles, from her carers. This is not something Amanda had previously permitted. We understood this to mean that she wanted comforting and was relieved to be home. Interpreting a person's behaviour and applying meaning to it is essential to meeting the needs of a person who has a profound intellectual and multiple disabilities.

Two years later, reflecting back over the experience, we as a team are able to recognise the direct and indirect impact this health experience has had on the way we support to Amanda; we now monitor Amanda's health and behaviour more rigorously, using charts and recorded observations. Amanda's person-centred plan (Circles Network, 2005) now contains written guidelines in place for; when we observe certain signs or presenting symptoms, we are attempting to identify triggers or patterns of reoccurring health change in an attempt to prevent a relapse occurring.

We make sure new staff have a comprehensive induction into Amanda's support needs so they can support her in the best way possible.

Summary

In summary, we all feel that this has been a major learning curve and we have all gained immense knowledge from the experience and we have gained a greater understanding of how Amanda communicates with us, and in return we feel we are better able to support her to her full needs.

We have full confidence that if this were to happen again, we as a team would know the right channels to go through to ensure Amanda gets the best possible treatment and outcome while ensuring minimal stress and disruption to Amanda's life.

Along with Amanda's devoted mother, we were her lifeline, we were her voice, we are proud to have supported her during her health crisis and we are proud to continue to support her to improve her health.

Having supported Amanda through this experience, we make the following recommendations:

A parent's wish list for the future

- Try not to take away all hope from families even when the future does not look bright.
- Endeavour not to make assumptions about the needs of carers.
- Listen to parents – they are the real experts on their children.

- Try to create more flexibility in the system for the good of the patient. 'Patients' are people with real lives, including those with learning disabilities.
- Ensure that nursing staff have the time to get to know special people like Amanda and utilise their person-centred plan or health action plan when provided.

A support worker's wish list for the future

- While the person is well, help the GPs to get to know them so they can more easily recognise when the person is unwell.
- Prepare a hospital grab sheet containing the essential information about the person which can go into hospital with them in an emergency.
- Prepare a patient passport/hospital book which provides additional information specifically focused on hospital care.
- Contribute to the discharge planning meetings.
- Seek support from your local intellectual disability community team; you don't have to go it alone.
- Petition your local hospital and service commissioner to recognise your needs when supporting a person with profound intellectual and multiple disabilities in hospital.

Resources are available to support people with an intellectual disability on admission to hospital from the 'A2A' (Access to Acute) interest group homepage via http://www.nnldn.org.uk/a2a/index.asp

Editors' comments

Now that you have read about Amanda's experience of health decline and subsequent hospital admission, we are confident you will identify the positive and the negative aspects of her experience. We must emphasise that this is an account of one person's health experience, and the concerns expressed by the authors of the chapter were raised with the individuals and services concerned at the time and were addressed.

In the light of the recent report *Death by Indifference* (Mencap, 2007), the plight of people with an intellectual disability when being admitted to hospital remains an area of grave concern.

Mencap (2008) advises that hospitals and healthcare professionals:

- listen to parents and carers;
- find out the best way to communicate;
- with the individual look for symptoms of serious illness;
- avoid making assumptions about a person's quality of life;
- ensure they have a clear understanding on the law about capacity to consent and the implications of the Disability Discrimination Act; and
- ask community intellectual disability teams to help.

Meeting complex health needs requires strong and genuinely reciprocal partnership working. While medics and allied health professionals have the valuable clinical skills for carrying out health interventions, family members, carers and support workers know the individual with profound intellectual and multiple disabilities best. Good communication and the fostering of mutual respect between all parties is more likely to result in a positive outcome for the person being supported.

We feel it is imperative to emphasise the importance of recognising signs of health decline and implementing both a systematic and person-centred approach to meeting the health needs of people with profound intellectual and multiple disabilities.

References

Circles Network (2005). *What Is Person Centred Planning?* Available at: http://www. circlesnetwork.org.uk/what_is_person_centred_planning.htm (accessed 27 June 2007).

Espie, C.A., Paul, A., McFie, J., Amos, P., Hamilton, D., McColl, J.H., Tarassenko, L., & Pardey, J. (1998). Sleep studies of adults with severe or profound mental retardation and epilepsy. *American Journal on Mental Retardation*, 103(1), 47–59.

Johnson, C., Farley, A., & Hendry, C. (2006). Nurses' role in nutritional assessment and screening. *Nursing Times*, 102(49), 28–29.

Mencap (2007). *Death by Indifference*. London: Mencap.

Mencap (2008). *Hospitals and Healthcare Professionals Checklist*. Available at: http://www.mencap.org.uk/displaypagedoc.asp?id=1472 (accessed 30 June 2008).

Chapter 4

MAKING SENSE OF COMMUNICATION

Karen Bunning

Introduction

Communication is the conduit between the individual and the world. It is the very cornerstone of identity formation, social engagement and human relationships (Bunning, 2004). In this respect, people with profound intellectual and multiple disabilities (PIMDs) are no different to the typically developing population. The real differences lie in the scope and level of sophistication of available skills and the role performed by significant others (the people who engage with them on a daily basis). People with PIMDs are likely to function within the earliest stages of communication development (Ware, 1996; Coupe O'Kane & Godbart, 1998). Self-expression is through the use of subtle communication behaviours such as eye gaze, body language, facial expression and vocalisation, which may not be immediately recognisable by others (Grove et al., 1999, 2001). Significant others draw on personal experience with the individual and cues from the immediate environment in an effort to work out the most likely meaning of such behaviours; however, this is far from straightforward. Research into the identification and measurement of affective responses as potential indicators of satisfaction or preference in the context of service evaluation suggests that individuals vary and show considerable idiosyncrasy in their displays of feeling (Green & Reid, 1996). It appears to be easier to obtain high observer agreement on positive affect, perhaps because it is more likely to be conveyed in conventional ways (e.g. through smiling and laughing) than other emotions. Many individuals emit idiosyncratic behaviour patterns that lack the salience necessary to convey communicative intentionality (Iacono et al., 1998; Carter & Iacono, 2002; Snell, 2002).

Intentionality

Communicative intentionality is defined as a 'purposeful action on the environment' (Coupe O'Kane & Godbart, 1998). The degree to which the individual with PIMDs is consciously aware of his/her own intention to effect change in the environment is a moot point. Awareness may vary from situation to situation and over time. So even when a behaviour is ascribed one meaning by a carer, it may not be clear whether in fact that individual intended the behaviour to be a signal bearer of meaning

(Grove et al., 2000). The behaviour may have been a reflexive response to an internal sensation or external event, such as thirst or someone shouting in the immediate vicinity. Based on the criteria described by Bates et al. (1975), Stamp & Knapp (1990), and others, Grove et al. (2000, p. 5) define the indicators of communicative intent as follows:

- *Alternating eye gaze:* Where a person looks at you, then at something or something else, then back at you again
- *Clear waiting for a response:* Where a person appears to have suspended any ongoing activity in anticipation of a reaction from someone
- *Active seeking of proximity:* Where a person moves to follow or to sit close to someone
- *Systematic variation in behaviour:* Where no response is forthcoming, the person will repeat, elaborate or change the behaviour
- *Persistence and intensity of behaviour:* If a person emits the same behaviour with a number of individuals in different situations and with apparent forcefulness

Whilst certain features in the environment, that is familiar usage of vocabulary and utterances, routine actions and activities may cue in the meanings of communication, exactly how confident can we really be in our interpretation of such ambiguous communication when the individual is not able to contradict an interpretation and say, 'No, that's not what I meant'? (Grove et al., 1999). An added concern is just how much of what we say is understood by the person. Carer's overestimation of an individual's communication skills is a frequently encountered problem with the learning disabled population, let alone those with PIMDs (Bartlett & Bunning, 1997; McConkey et al., 1999; Purcell et al., 2000). The net effect is that people with PIMDs occupy a vulnerable position regarding engagement with the outside world for the purposes of self-expression, self-determination and social recognition (Porter et al., 2001). As such, communication occupies a place of immense importance when considering the question of how best to support the needs of people with PIMDs in all aspects of daily life.

Learning objectives

The learning objectives for this chapter are to:

1. explore the dimensions of communication with people with PIMDs;
2. discuss the challenges of social interaction and communicative inclusion;
3. overview approaches for assessing the communication of people with PIMDs; and
4. critically review some key approaches to positive communication practice.

Dimensions of communication

In order to be a skilful communicator, particularly with people with PIMDs, one needs to appreciate the various dimensions of communication. It is not just about the exchange of words through the conventions of linguistic code, for example, speech, writing or sign, but also includes paralinguistic phenomena, which refers to the prosodic features of communication, such as changes in pitch, stress patterns and intonation – all of which add to the meaning being communicated. Non-verbal behaviours are also integral to communication (Coupe O'Kane & Godbart, 1998). The actions and movements employed by a person can be signal bearers of meaning. For example, the person who stamps a foot in expression of anger; the person who grabs hold of a person's sleeve to attract their attention – all these have the potential to convey meaning.

Process of communication

Communication does not happen in a categorical way such that one person sends a message to the other person for decoding according to a set of shared linguistic rules, and vice versa. A categorical view of communication is characterised by strict demarcation of turns and passivity on the part of the 'receiver'. Its shortcomings lie in its neglect of the active role of the listener and the mutual coordination of interaction between any two interactants. Fogel (1993) rejects this linear conceptualisation of communication in favour of a continuous processing model, which captures the mutuality and co-regulation of interaction in the construction of meaning. It is about two or more people working together and coordinating their actions in ongoing response to each other and the context (Grove et al., 1999; Olsson, 2004). Both the interactants are active contributors in the coding and inference of ideas (Sperber & Wilson, 1995).

What makes the process accessible for both is the use of shared code to facilitate common reference, that is the language in use conveyed through speech sounds, words, grammatical rules, etc. Where a common code is not fully available to one individual because of the nature of the PIMDs, the construction of meaning becomes challenging and even elusive at times (Grove et al., 1999, 2001). The case example of Leda illustrates some of the particular challenges to the communication partners.

Case vignette: Leda

Leda is 25-year old and has profound and multiple intellectual disabilities. She uses a wheelchair but is dependent on her support staff for mobility. Leda was registered blind at birth although staff have observed that she will move items, particularly flashing lights, close to her right eye for inspection. A recent audiometric assessment revealed a profound bilateral hearing impairment. Leda has been observed to engage frequently in moving her head from side to side in a rhythmic motion. During these times she emits a low moaning sound. Sometimes she pushes her body back into her chair with force. The staff think this means that she is unhappy about something but are not sure of the specific reasons underlying the behaviour. One member of staff reports that when she sits down next to her, Leda seems to move slightly as if she knows her, but she's not sure. The support staff are asking all kinds of questions:

- *We know very little about Leda – her likes and dislikes – how do we establish what they are?*
- *How can we let Leda know that someone is present, let alone start interacting with her?*
- *How do we include Leda in activities, given her dual sensory impairment and lack of voluntary motor control?*
- *How can we know if Leda is trying to tell us something through her body language?*
- *How can we let Leda know that she can affect the people and objects in the immediate environment by her own actions?*

Communication characteristics

The case vignette of Leda demonstrates the challenges of communication with a person with PIMD (Remington, 1997; Grove et al., 1999; Olsson & Granlund, 2003). The presence of physical disability can make it difficult to discriminate between a voluntary and an involuntary action, what is an intentional communication act and what is not (Iacono et al., 1998). The increased likelihood of sensory impairments (that may or may not be diagnosed due to the difficulties in acquiring accurate assessment data amongst this population) is another factor (see Chapters 10 and 11). When present, reduced sensory input will undoubtedly affect communication (Yeates, 1992, 1995; Kiernan & Kiernan, 1994; Lavis et al., 1997). Multiple forms of problem behaviour are more likely amongst those people with the more severe cognitive deficits and who are non-verbal or experience particular difficulty with reception and expression of language (Remington, 1997). The presence of stereotypic (repetitive behaviours with an apparent lack of purpose and predictable feedback), for example rocking and hand flapping, or self-injurious behaviour, for example hand biting and head banging, may further interfere with or disrupt the communicative flow (Kiernan & Kiernan, 1994). The frequency and intensity of such behaviours may act as a barrier to social engagement with the individual (Jones et al., 1995). An inverse relationship between the amount of social interaction and the occurrence of stereotypes has been suggested (Lee & Odom, 1996; Bunning, 1998): the more stereotypic behaviour emitted by individuals, the less likely it is that they will engage in spontaneous social interaction. Simply attracting the attention of, or opening an interaction with the individual who is engaged in rhythmic body rocking may prove challenging, when one is competing with the person's absorption in their own repetitive sequences of movements.

Cognition and communication

The relationship between the use of communicative functions and cognitive skills, hearing, vision and motor ability has been reported in earlier research. Dunst (1998) reviewed a series of studies investigating sensorimotor development in children and adults with different aetiology of intellectual disability (e.g. Down's syndrome, cerebral palsy, autistic spectrum disorder, spina bifida, and unknown cause) and also included studies on normal development. It was concluded that, on the whole, children with intellectual disabilities acquire sensorimotor competencies in a stage-like manner that parallels that of normal infants. However, congruence between achievements in different domains of development is greater in typically developing infants than it is for children and adults with intellectual disabilities. Object permanence (OP), means end (ME), spatial relations (SR) tend to show greater congruence than OP, ME and either vocal or gestural imitation (VI or GI). Levels of skill development may vary from one domain to another – a person could be at one level in OP and another in VI, for example. This explains the often reported finding of 'splinter skills' in people with intellectual disabilities – they may develop one skill well in advance of others. Conversely, there may be one area of development that is particularly difficult for them. When we look at the extent to which different skills cluster together in the acquisition of sensorimotor intelligence by individuals with intellectual disabilities, there is a tendency for those relating to objects to cluster together (OP, ME and SR) and for those relating to people (VI, GI and OP) to cluster separately – a dissociation not generally seen in typically developing infants. This suggests that these two underlying orientations may not develop in an integrated way in people with learning difficulties. It is important to recognise that some individuals may show a preference for object-related schemes over person-related schemes, which may have implications for the starting point of intervention.

Case example: Martin

Martin is 12-year old with PIMD. He was born with hydrocephalus and spina bifida. He uses a body mould, matrix wheelchair. He was registered blind as an infant although his parents think he may have some vision for dark–light contrasts. Martin spends a great deal of his day grabbing at his favourite things, such as plastic shakers, and rubs them against his face. When significant others open an interaction with Martin, he appears distracted and continues in his search for his objects.

Parent–child interaction

In studies of parent–infant interaction, parental interaction style has been linked with language development (Murray et al., 1990; Papousek, 1995; Beckwith & Rodning, 1996). Where a disability exists, passivity in the infant appears to go hand in hand with reduced input from the primary carer (Ware, 1996). Furthermore, interactions when they do occur are likely to be short compared to those experienced by the typically developing child (Bradley, 1998). This may be related to the observation that behavioural state is highly variable in people with PIMD, with levels of alertness and activity changing within short periods (Guess et al., 1993). Interactions have been reported to be less synchronous (Berger & Cunningham,

1981), suggesting that parents of children with intellectual disabilities seem to have more difficulties adjusting to their behaviour. Certainly, it has been reported that in infants with Down's syndrome, where vocal development is similar, albeit delayed, to that of typically developing children, there are more 'vocal clashes' with adults (i.e. adults and children vocalising together rather than taking turns) (Jones, 1977). Another feature is the directiveness of interactions, with parents using more imperatives than they would with typically developing children of a similar developmental age. However, Maurer and Sherrod (1987) found that parental use of imperatives was governed by the child's behaviour. Others suggest that parental directiveness reflects a desire to explicitly teach their children particular language and communication skills (Mahoney et al., 1990). So-called 'directiveness' is also seen in the developing behaviour repertoires of the child with PIMD. Ogletree et al. (1992) found that children (aged 6–12 years) with PIMD used more behaviour regulation and less joint attention than their typically developing peers. The significance of this is that behaviour regulation is usually characterised by brief encounters with the communication partner in pursuit of a goal. Joint attention, on the other hand, involves a two-way interaction, sometimes of multiple turns, where there is the sharing of experiences.

Ecological view of communication

An ecological view of communication locates the individual in context by capturing human functioning as a series of dependencies where a person's communication is only as effective as the responses of others (Bunning, 2004). Bronfenbrenner's (2005, 1979) ecological systems theory provides a useful model that emphasises the transactional nature of the individual's development and functioning in context. To illustrate this point, Bronfenbrenner (1979) identifies the individual at the centre of a series of circles that gradually move away from the immediate and familiar contexts and people in the person's life, termed microsystems, to community settings and finally society. Considering communication with people with PIMD, our primary interest lies in the immediate environment or microsystems. Examples of microsystems include the family unit, friendship circles and neighbourhood group. Each microsystem, although not exclusive to the others, has its own 'pattern of activities, roles, and interpersonal relations' (Bronfenbrenner, 2005, p. 148). Thus, an individual is likely to respond variously and have different experiences across the different microsystems in his or her life. Surrounding the microsytems is the mesosystem, which is a layer that represents the degree of interconnectedness across the microsystems. It has the potential to promote the sharing of information across communication partners.

Communication partnership

A communication partnership defines the relationship between two people who contribute to the mutual exchange of ideas and meanings bringing their own knowledge, experience, attitude and cultural identity to the interaction (Bartlett & Bunning, 1997; Bunning, 2004). Any one person may experience a variety of communication partnerships during the course of a day and as their life course progresses. Bradshaw (2001) points out that the nature of PIMD means that as the individuals grow up, they are likely to have a limited number of communication partners and a restricted set of experiences.

Kagan (1998, p. 817) talks about the communication 'equation' which is balanced by the skills, experiences and resources of the interactants. The case of Leda, illustrated earlier, highlights the challenges for this communication equation when extreme differences exist between the skills and experiences that each person can draw on (see Bartlett & Bunning, 1997; Bradshaw, 1998; Grove et al., 1999; Bunning & Grove, 2002). Although Simmons-Mackie & Kagan (1999) were writing about people with aphasia when they observed that the discourse style of the communication partner may promote the skills or alternatively cast doubt on the abilities of the individual, there are obvious resonances for people with learning disabilities. The restricted ability to use formal linguistic code means that people with PIMD are highly reliant on significant others for the interpretation of meaning (Grove et al., 1999). Research has shown the importance of bidirectional influence in the communication partnership. Failure to accommodate people with PIMD in an interaction – by adapting input or the provision of interaction opportunities that are amenable to the person with PIMD – creates barriers to communication (Kaiser & Goetz, 1993; Bunning, 1997). This leads us to view communication and approaches to intervention within an ecological framework where interactions occur between the changing person and the dynamic context.

A deliberate approach

When interacting with a person who has restricted communication skills, the communication partners need to make deliberate changes to their usual way of communicating and embrace other forms of expression (Goldbart, 1994). It demands attunement to subtle changes in the individual's behaviour and the context in which they occur (Olsson, 2004). During interactions with significant others, the potential for all behaviours by people with PIMD to be intentional is considered, whether or not they meet the set criteria for intentionality (Carter & Iacono, 2002; Snell, 2002). The onus is frequently placed on the skills and abilities of the significant other, which includes the ability to observe the person's behaviour in context, to interpret the most likely meaning of the behaviour based on a comprehensive knowledge and experience of the individual, and to 'try out' a response based on that interpretation whilst also checking its validity across different situations and communication partners (Grove et al., 2000). Such critical observation and detection of the frequently idiosyncratic behaviours emitted by individuals with PIMD is a complex proposition. McConkey et al. (1999) found that whilst support staff were able to recognise teaching strategies such as correcting, reinforcing, instructing, pointing and touch, they experienced particular difficulty in identifying non-verbal behaviours that were associated with a more client-sensitive responding style.

Assessing communication

Given the complexities of communication, the question of how best to establish the communicative repertoire and potential of the individual with PIMD points to the need for continuous assessment and avoidance of the one-off test situation. The aim is to reveal the competence of the person and therefore communication should be explored across contexts, interaction partners and time. The contributions made by the carer are critical to the assessment of communication (Arthur et al., 1998). Accordingly, the trend in recent practice has moved away from looking at communication in terms of the individual to a focus on context and the contribution of communication partners (see Hogg, 1998). Singular assessment of the person with PIMD represents only half of the equation and neglects the potential mediating role of significant others and reciprocity of interaction. In short, it is about how utterances are formed and presented, how meanings are accessed and inferred, how active listening and sequential responding occur (Bunning, 2004).

Many assessment approaches recommend the use of observation for determining the skills and abilities of the individual. The advantage of this is there is no baseline requirement for level of functioning. Individual potential can be viewed in the most natural settings to the person and with significant others who are familiar and regular communication partners.

Case vignette: Daniel

Daniel is 9-year old with a profound intellectual disability and a moderate to severe hearing impairment that affects both ears. He is not using any amplification currently. Daniel lives in the family home with his parents and his two older siblings. He attends a school for children with special educational needs. The teacher reports that he seems largely unaware of what is going on in the classroom and engages in frequent and prolonged periods of rocking behaviour, whether seated or standing, during which he will often strike the sides of his head with his hands. Daniel has no spoken words as such and has to be physically guided to perform particular actions, such as sit at the table for dinner. Daniel's mother reports that he responds positively to touch and gives the example of patting him with talcum powder after his bath, to which he will laugh and squeal with delight. He often blows raspberries and will sometimes vocalise using low-vowel sounds.

The case vignette of Daniel illustrates just how difficult it is to make accurate and reliable judgements about the abilities and potential of the individual. It requires sensitivity to a wide range of behaviours that may or may not have a communicative function and consideration of the range of communication partners and contexts.

Affective communication assessment (Coupe et al., 1985)

The Affective communication assessment (ACA) is an assessment based on three identified stages of pre-intentional communication development:

- *Level 1 (pre-intentional)*: Reflexive level, where the individual displays 'a small range of very early behaviours, sounds and reflexes which is produced in response to a limited range of internal and external stimuli' to which the significant other assigns social significance. The response tends to be instinctive with the focus on the relationship rather than caregiving activities, for example reciprocal face gazing.
- *Level 2 (pre-intentional)*: Reactive level, where the individual uses 'repertoires of changes of behaviour, reactive behaviours, produced in response to a wide range of stimuli'. Aspects of the caregiving activity attain importance in the interaction with a focus on encouraging reciprocity of vocalisation and body movement, responding to affect expressed by, for example tone of voice and facial expression.
- *Level 3 (pre-intentional)*: Proactive level, where the individual's 'repertoires of behaviour becomes signals to the communicative partner who then assigns communicative intent and meaning'. The communicative partner uses increasingly selective responses as they are able to discriminate between the person's range of behaviours. There is a shift from caregiving activities to focusing on objects and toys (Source: Coupe O'Kane & Godbart, 1998, pp. 11–12).

The ACA is conducted in three stages starting with observation of a structured situation where the individual is presented with a range of individualised sensory stimuli which have been identified in discussion with significant others. The responses of the individual are noted on an 'observation recording sheet' together with an interpretation of what they mean. Video recording or joint observation in situ by two people as a check on reliability of recorded observations is recommended. Next, the recorded repertoires of behaviour are reviewed and the strongest, most consistent responses are identified in terms of like, dislike, want and reject. Finally, the conditions for intervention are created by 'extending existing repertoires and capitalising on new behaviours' through two-way interaction (ibid, p. 14) that focus on:

- vocalisation;
- facial expression;
- body proximity;
- eye contact/orientation;
- physical contact;
- imitation; and
- turn taking.

Early communication assessment (Coupe O'Kane & Godbart, 1998)

The early communication assessment (ECA) is an assessment that utilises 'communicative landmarks' (p. 59) rather than an exhaustive list of communicative behaviours in checklist format in order to key significant others into the communicative level(s) indicated by the person's observed behaviours. It captures information about the individual against an early communication framework and provides a starting place for intervention. Its strength lies in its facility to plot the individual within a developmental sequence that enables the documentation of even the smallest change.

Manchester pragmatics profile (Coupe O'Kane & Godbart, 1998)

The Manchester pragmatics profile (MPP) represents the outcome of a joint working party of health service personnel and educationalists. The aim was to devise a user-friendly assessment that investigates the pragmatic or functional abilities of people with intellectual disabilities. It provides a structured format for recording the repertoire of behaviours used by an individual to convey communicative intentions within different contexts, to socially organise the interaction (the ways in which social interaction is managed through turn taking, seeking attention, repairing misunderstandings, etc.) and to see the listener's point of view (adjusting own communication to the perceived view point of the other person). The assessment focuses on naturally occurring communications and recommends the use of video for initial data collection, although this is not essential. The recorded observations are analysed for *'evidence of skills in communicative intentions, social organisation and presupposition'* (ibid, p. 93). Once an assessment has been completed, the idea is to develop an intervention that focuses on the individual, communication partners and context using a range of recommended methods including environmental manipulation, prompting and use of feedback to the individual among others.

See What I Mean (Grove et al., 2000)

See What I Mean (SWIM) is a set of guidelines that has been developed for use by significant others of people with PIMD (Grove et al., 1999). It aims to help significant others *'to question and check out or validate the accuracy of the meanings they ascribe'* to individual's communication behaviours (ibid, p. 2). Its starting point is that uncertainty and ambiguity are a part of everyday communication, and therefore the intuitive skills that are used by communication partners should form one thread of the assessment. It comprises a series of steps whereby evidence from the individual's behaviour is gathered to support the different interpretations so that the most likely meaning may be identified. The guidelines have been recommended as an aid to key decision-making situations that involve people with PIMD, for example, annual reviews, transition, response to life events such as bereavement. However, the underlying principles of SWIM have broader application in simply exploring everyday interaction by encouraging carers to observe, question and compare their interpretations of individual behaviour with each other so that difficulties are made explicit and successes shared.

Socially responsive environment

Trad (1994) argues that without the experience of interactions with partners who are sensitive and adaptive in their behaviour, infants may fail to develop the ability to make predictions about events and people, and may respond by withdrawal. Empirical research has shown that contingency awareness (learning the causal link between action and consequence) can be established in infants as young as 3-month old when the distance between action and consequence is less than 3 seconds (Coupe O-Kane & Godbart, 1998). This has formed the underlying principle for interventions focusing on very early communication skills (e.g. see Schweigert & Rowland, 1992; Bunning, 1997, 1998). There is evidence to suggest that giving linguistic input during joint attentional focus promotes the acquisition of nouns (Yoder et al., 1998). So it seems the social responsiveness of the communication partner is of paramount importance to the development of communication. Ware (1996) recommends creating an environment that is sensitive and responsive to the behaviours of the person. There should be opportunities for the person with PIMD to respond to events in the environment and effect change in the people and objects around them.

Multi-sensory environments

Multi-sensory environments (MSEs) are frequently used with people with PIMD and provide a range of sensory stimuli of varying intensity (Cavet & Mount, 1995; Pagliano, 1998). Originally developed as a leisure facility for people with intellectual disabilities (see Hulsegge & Verheul, 1987), 'Snoezelen' is one such place. The question of its therapeutic or educational value has led to a number of research initiatives. Mixed results have been reported with a small increase in communication although not attributed solely to Snoezelen (Lindsay et al., 2001). Vasklamp et al. (2003) concluded that an MSE was only as effective as a responsive learning environment. Porter and Miller (2000) question whether users of MSEs would not be equally served as well by a natural environment with sensory opportunities. Nicola Grove's creative solutions to the English curriculum provide an example of such an approach. Grove (1998) uses multi-sensory approaches in drama and storytelling in supporting access to quite complex texts for people with intellectual disabilities (Grove & Peacey, 1999).

Rich and multiple media

Information and communication technology and rich and multiple media provide some new opportunities for addressing communication (Detheridge, 1997). Communication passports offer one way of facilitating interaction between people with PIMDs and their significant others (Millar & Caldwell, 1997). Originally conceived of by the call centre at Edinburgh University in 1992 (http://www.callcentre.org/), a communication passport is a *'written, videoed or object-based record of how a person communicates and some of the things they might like to communicate about'* (Lord, 2002). The process of making a passport in itself helps to raise awareness of communication issues amongst significant others (Millar & Caldwell, 1997).

Development work in multimedia profiling has been used in similar vein. It uses a combination of digital video, still photography, sound, graphics and text to capture personal life experiences, which are stored on a computer for access in planning and review meetings. They help to convey the personal agenda of the person with PIMDs and can support the development of partnership communication (http://www.acting-up.org.uk/).

Augmentative and alternative communication

Augmentative and alternative communication offers a range of tactics and devices for promoting communication (Hogg, 1998). Jan van Dijk first described the use of objects as a means of communication with people with congenital deaf blindness in the 1960s. Quite simply, it is about using an object to represent a meaning, for example, a set of car keys to convey going out in the car. They are used with children and adults with various degrees of intellectual disability (McLarty, 1995; Park, 1997). However, the literature on its application to people with PIMD is fairly limited. Park (2000) recommends a focus on the developmental process whereby an object becomes an object of reference. To this end he defines the MMF principle for guiding object selection which stands for meaningful, motivating and frequent (Park, 1997). The idea is to scrutinise the ways an individual uses objects in different situations over time and to select ones that hold the greatest relevance for the individual. Objects can be used to support the development of communication in this way. Another use is to facilitate access to storytelling activities. Chris Fuller has produced a series of bag books that provide 'concrete illustrations of objects used in various stories' (Park 1997, p. 7).

Tuning-in

What seems to be important to any intervention is the involvement of significant others and the quality of interaction opportunities (Ware & Healey, 1994). Whatever the chosen approach for intervention with people with PIMDs, supporting the development of social interaction and interest in people, leading to the desire to initiate for joint attention is of high communicative importance (e.g. Nind & Hewett, 1994; Hewett & Nind, 1998; see Chapter 5). This means encouraging observational acuity and response sensitivity amongst communication partners to any behaviour that has the potential to be signal bearers of meaning. It means working with the repertoire that the individual provides by offering interpretations and actively scaffolding interactions in the way of a conversation, albeit without the words. Finally, there must be regular correspondence and negotiation between communication partners for the purposes of checking out interpretations of behavioural repertoires and exploring the most effective ways of communicating with the individual.

References

Arthur, M., Butterfield, N., & McKinnon, D.H. (1998). Communication intervention for students with severe disability: results of a partner training program. *International Journal of Disability, Development and Education*, 45, 97–113.

Bates, E., Camaioni, L., & Volterra, I. (1975). The acquisition of performatives prior to speech. *Merrill Palmer Quarterly*, 21, 205–216.

Bartlett, C., & Bunning, K. (1997). The importance of communicative partners: a study to investigate the communicative exchanges between staff and adults with learning disabilities. *British Journal of Learning Disabilities*, 25, 148–152.

Beckwith, L., & Rodning, C. (1996). Dyadic processes between mothers and preterm infants: development at ages two to five years. *Infant Mental Health Journal*, 17(4), 322–333.

Berger, J., & Cunningham, C. (1981). The development of eye contact between mothers and normal vs. Down's syndrome infants. *Developmental Psychology*, 17, 322–331.

Bradley, H. (1998). Assessing and developing successful communication. In Lacey, P., & Ouvry, C. (eds) *People with Profound and Multiple Learning Disabilities: A Collaborative Approach to Meeting Complex Needs*. London: David Fulton; 50–65.

Bradshaw, J. (2001). Communication partnerships with people with profound and multiple learning disabilities. *Tizard Learning Disability Review*, 6(2), 6–11.

Bronfenbrenner, U. (1979). *The Ecology of Human Development: Experiments by Nature and Design*. Cambridge, MA: Harvard University Press.

Bronfenbrenner, U. (ed.) (2005). *Making Human Beings Human: Bioecological Perspectives on Human Development*. London: Sage Publications.

Bunning, K. (1997). The role of sensory reinforcement in developing interactions. In Fawcus, M. (ed.) *Children with Learning Difficulties: A Collaborative Approach to their Education and Management*. London: Whurr Publishers; 97–129.

Bunning, K. (1998). To engage or not to engage? Affecting the interactions of learning disabled adults. *International Journal of Language and Communication Disorders*, 33, 386–391.

Bunning, K. (2004). *Speech and Language Therapy Intervention: Frameworks and Processes*. London: Whurr Publishers.

Bunning, K., & Grove, N. (2002). Making connections: understanding and promoting communication. In Carnaby, S. (ed.) *Learning Disability Today*. Brighton: Pavilion Publishing; 83–94.

Carter, M., & Iacono, T. (2002). Professional judgements of the intentionality of communication acts. *Augmentative and Alternative Communication*, 18, 177–190.

Cavet, J., & Mount, H. (1995). Multi-sensory environments: an exploration of their potential for young people with profound and multiple learning difficulties. *British Journal of Special Education*, 22(2), 52–55.

Coupe, J., Barton, L., Barber, M., Collins, L., Levy, D., & Murphy, D. (1985). *Affective Communication Assessment*. Manchester: Manchester Education Committee.

Coupe O'Kane, J., & Godbart, J. (1998). *Communication Before Speech: Development and Assessment*. London: David Fulton.

Detheridge, T. (1997). Bridging the communication gap (for pupils with profound and multiple learning difficulties). *British Journal of Special Education*, 24(1), 21–26.

Dunst, C. (1998). Sensorimotor development and developmental disabilities. In Burack, J., Hodapp, R., & Zigler, E. (eds) *Handbook of Mental Retardation and Development*. Cambridge: Cambridge University Press; 135–182.

Fogel, A. (1993). Two principles of communication: co-regulation and framing. In Nadel, J., & Camaioni, L. (eds) *New Perspectives in Communication Development*. London: Routledge; 9–22.

Goldbart, J. (1994). Opening the communication curriculum to students with PMLDs. In Ware, J. (ed.) *Educating Children with Profound and Multiple Learning Difficulties*. London: David Fulton Publishers; 15–62.

Green, C., & Reid, D. (1996). Defining, validating and increasing indices of happiness among people with profound multiple disabilities. *Journal of Applied Behavioral Analysis*, 29, 67–78.

Grove, N. (1998). *Literature For All*. London: David Fulton.

Grove, N., Bunning, K., & Porter, J. (2001). Interpreting the meaning of behavior by people with intellectual disabilities: theoretical and methodological issues. In Columbus, F. (ed.) *Advances in Psychology Research*, Vol. 7. New York: Nova Sciences Publishers; 87–126.

Grove, N., Bunning, K., Porter, J., & Morgan, M. (2000). *See What I Mean: Guidelines to Aid Understanding of Communication by People with Severe and Profound Learning Disabilities*. Kidderminster: BILD & Mencap.

Grove, N., Bunning, K., Porter, J., & Olsson, C. (1999). See what I mean: interpreting the meaning of communication by people with severe and profound intellectual disabilities. *Journal of Applied Research in Intellectual Disabilities*, 12, 190–203.

Grove, N., & Peacey, N. (1999). Teaching subjects to pupils with profound and multiple learning difficulties – considerations for the new framework. *British Journal of Special Education*, 26, 83–86.

Guess, D., Roberts, S., Siegel-Causey, E., Ault, M., Guy, B., Thompson, B., & Rues, J. (1993). Analysis of behavior state conditions and associated environmental variables among students with profound handicaps. *American Journal of Mental Retardation*, 97, 634–653.

Hewett, D., & Nind, M. (1998) *Interaction in action*. London: David Fulton.

Hogg, J. (1998). Competence and quality in the lives of people with profound and multiple learning disabilities: some recent research. *Tizard Learning Disability Review*, 3(6), 6–14.

Hulsegge, J., & Verheul, A. (1987). *Snoezelen Another World: A Practical Book of Sensory Experience Environments for the Mentally Handicapped*. Chesterfield: Rompa.

Iacono, T., Carter, M., & Hook, J. (1998). Identification of intentional communication in students with severe and multiple disabilities. *Augmentative and Alternative Communication*, 14, 102–114.

Jones, O. (1977). Mother-child communication with pre-linguistic down syndrome and normal infants. In Schaffer, H.R. (ed.) *Studies in Mother-Infant Interaction*. London: Academic Press.

Jones, R.S.P., Walsh, P.G., & Sturmey, P. (1995). *Stereotyped Movement Disorders*. Chichester: John Wiley & Sons.

Kagan, A. (1998) Supported conversation for adults with aphasia: methods and resources for training conversation partners. *Aphasiogy*, 12, 817–830.

Kaiser, A.P., & Goetz, L. (1993). Enhancing communication with persons labelled severely disabled. *Journal of the Association for Persons with Severe Handicaps*, 18(3), 137–142.

Kiernan, C., & Kiernan, D. (1994). Challenging behaviour in schools for pupils with severe learning difficulties. *Mental Handicap Research*, 7, 117–201.

Lavis, D., Cullen, P., & Roy, A. (1997) Identification of hearing impairment in people with a learning disability: from questioning to testing. *British Journal of Learning Disability*, 25(3), 100–105.

Lindsay, W.R., Black, E., Broxholme, S., Pitcaithly, D., & Hornsby, N. (2001). Effects of four therapy procedures on communication in people with profound intellectual disabilities. *Journal of Applied Research in Intellectual Disabilities*, 14, 110–119.

Lord, S. (2002). Recipe for conversation. *RCSLT Bulletin*, 602, 10–11.

Mahoney, G., Fors, S., & Woods, S. (1990). Maternal directive behaviour revisited. *American Journal on Mental Retardation*, 94, 398–406.

Maurer, H., & Sherrod, K. (1987). Context of directives given to young children with DS and nonretarded children: development over two years. *American Journal of Mental Deficiency*, 91, 579–590.

McConkey, R., Purcel,l M., & Morris, I. (1999). Staff perceptions of communication with a partner who is intellectually disabled. *Journal of Applied Research in Intellectual Disabilities*, 12, 204–210.

McLarty, M. (1995). Objects of reference. In Etheridge, D. (ed.) *The Education of Dual Sensory Impaired Children: Recognising and Developing Ability*. London: David Fulton; 34–45.

Millar, S., & Caldwell, M. (1997). *Personal communication passports*. Paper first presented at the *SENSE Conference*, Westpark Centre, University of Dundee, 1–3 September 1997.

Murray, A.D., Johnson, J., & Peters, J. (1990). Fine tuning of utterance length to preverbal infants: effects on language development. *Journal of Child Language*, 17, 511–525.

Nind, M., & Hewett, D. (1994). *Access to Communication*. London: David Fulton.

Ogletree, B., Wetherby, A., & Westling, D. (1992). Profile of the prelinguistic intentional communicative behaviors of children with profound mental retardation. *American Journal of Mental Retardation*, 97, 186–196.

Olsson, C. (2004). Dyadic interaction with a child with multiple disabilities: a system theory perspective on communication. *Augmentative and Alternative Communication*, 20(4), 228–242.

Olsson, C., & Granlund, M. (2003). Presymbolic communication intervention. In Sclosser, R.W. (ed.) *The Efficacy of Augmentative and Alternative Communication*. USA: Elsevier Science; 299–322.

Pagliano, P. (1998). *Multisensory Environments*. London: David Fulton.

Papousek, M. (1995). Origins of reciprocity and mutuality in prelinguistic parent-infany 'dialogues'. In Markova, I., Grauman, C.F., & Foppa, K. (eds) *Mutualities in Dialogue*. Cambridge: Cambridge University Press; 58–81.

Park, K. (1997). How do objects becomes objects of reference? A review of the literature on objects of reference and a proposed model for the use of objects in communication. *British Journal of Special Education*, 24(3), 108–114.

Park, K. (2000). Reading objects: literacy and objects of reference. *PMLD Link*, 12(1), 4–9.

Porter, J., & Miller, O. (2000). The use of multisensory environments. *PMLD Link*, 43–44.

Porter, J., Ouvry, C., Morgan, M., & Downs, C. (2001). Interpreting the communication of people with profound and multiple learning difficulties. *British Journal of Learning Disabilities*, 29, 12–16.

Purcell, M., McConkey, R., & Morris, I. (2000). Staff communication with people with intellectual disabilities: the impact of a work-based training programme. *International Journal of Language and Communication Disorders*, 35, 147–158.

Remington, B. (1997). Verbal communication in people with learning difficulties: an overview. *Tizard Learning Disability Review*, 2(4), 6–14.

Schweigert, P., & Rowland, C. (1992). Early communication and microtechnology: instructional sequence and case studies of children with severe disabilities. *Augmentative and Alternative Communication*, 8, 273–286.

Simmons-Mackie, N., & Kagan, A. (1999) Communication strategies used by 'good' versus 'poor' speaking partners of individuals with aphasia. *Aphasiology*, 13, 807–820.

Snell, M.E. (2002). Using dynamic assessment with learners who communicate nonsymbolically. *Augmentative and Alternative Communication*, 18, 163–176.

Sperber, D., & Wilson, D. (1995). *Relevance, Communication and Cognition* (2nd edition). Oxford: Blackwell.

Stamp, G.H., & Knapp, M.L. (1990). The construct of intent in interpersonal communication. *Quarterly Journal of Speech*, 76, 282–299.

Trad, P.V. (1994). Previewing as a remedy for interpersonal failure in the parent-infant dyad. *Infants and Young Children*, 7, 1–13.

Vasklamp, C., de Geeter, K.I., Huijsmans, L.M., & Smit, I.H. (2003). Passive activities: the effectiveness of multisensory environments on the level of activity of individuals with profound multiple disabilities. *Journal of Applied Research in Intellectual Disabilities*, 16, 135–143.

Ware, J. (1996). *Creating a Responsive Environment for People with Profound and Multiple Learning Difficulties*. London: David Fulton.

Ware, J. & Healey, I. (1994). Conceptualising progress in children with profound and multiple learning difficulties. In Ware, J. (ed.), *Educating Children with Profound and Multiple Learning Difficulties*. London: David Fulton.

Yeates, S. (1992). Have they got a hearing loss? A follow up study of hearing in people with mental handicaps. *Mental Handicap*, 20, 126–133.

Yeates, S. (1995). The incidence and importance of hearing loss in people with severe learning disability: the evolution of a service. *British Journal of Learning Disability*, 23, 79–84.

Yoder, P.J., Warren, S.F., McCathren, R., & Leew, S.V. (1998). Does adult responsivity to child behaviour facilitate communication development? In Wetherby, A.M., Warren, S.F., & Reichle J. (eds) *Transitions in Prelinguistic Communication*. Baltimore: Paul H. Brookes; 385–416.

Chapter 5

PROMOTING THE EMOTIONAL WELL-BEING OF PEOPLE WITH PROFOUND AND MULTIPLE INTELLECTUAL DISABILITIES: A HOLISTIC APPROACH THROUGH INTENSIVE INTERACTION

Melanie Nind

Introduction

This chapter addresses the emotional well-being of people with profound intellectual and multiple disabilities and how this can be fostered by using the approach of Intensive Interaction as a holistic intervention. Firstly, emotional well-being is defined and its importance is discussed. Secondly, the problems associated with the emotional well-being and mental health of people with profound intellectual and multiple disabilities are outlined. Thirdly, the case is made for a holistic approach, and finally, Intensive Interaction is presented as one such approach.

Learning objectives

At the end of this chapter the reader will:

- see the importance of emotional well-being for the overall health, development and quality of life for people with profound intellectual and multiple disabilities;
- understand why emotional well-being has been neglected and the dangers of this continuing;
- have an overview of the research evidence on the most effective ways to meet the mental health needs of people with profound intellectual and multiple disabilities (which may be sparse) by seeing the applicability of evidence from the mainstream research on emotionally healthy environments (largely schools);
- understand how the emotional well-being of this population needs to be fostered through holistic intervention; and

- understand the potential of intensive interaction as one such approach to good, research-informed practice in promoting emotional well-being.

What is emotional well-being?

Stewart-Brown (2000, p. 32) defines emotional well-being as:

> A holistic, subjective state which is present when a range of feelings, among them energy, confidence, openness, enjoyment, happiness, calm, and caring are combined and balanced.

Experiencing emotional well-being does not mean being happy all the time, but it does mean feeling okay and not suffering mental distress, depression or anxiety. Emotional well-being is strongly associated with mental health – the ability to grow and develop, to make relationships and to be resilient in the face of difficulties. Unlike mental health, however, emotional well-being as a term has the advantage of being *'positive, salutogenic and non-medicalized' and thus 'clearly the "business" of everyone from parents to professionals and not just doctors'* (Weare, 2004, p. 8).

Emotional well-being is linked with having emotional competence (sometimes referred to as emotional literacy) and engaging in emotional processes (emotional intelligence). Whereas, however, some abilities to understand and use information about the emotional states of oneself and others, and perceiving, appraising, expressing and regulating emotion may be a challenge too far for someone with a profound intellectual disability, having emotional well-being is not. It can be gained from feeling 'uniquely known, recognized, nurtured and valued' (Weare, 2004, p. 25). As Weare (2004) explains, establishing emotional well-being and emotional literacy is about getting feedback, being listened to, experiencing and managing a range of emotions, and experiencing self-efficacy. Helping people with emotional well-being involves increasing their emotional pleasure and satisfaction, their relaxation, fun, joy, their ability to lose themselves in the moment and their experience of engagement or inner peace.

Emotional and social development includes attachment or bonding, which is *'the basis for forming connections with others, the basis on which all social competences are based'* (Weare, 2004, p. 42). Attachment provides trust based on the consistency and reliability of other people. Emotional development includes understanding the causes of emotions or basic contingency – that a particular feeling is linked with an event. It includes expressing emotions in a safe way and not being overwhelmed by them. It is about developing a vocabulary of emotions, managing relationships and communicating effectively, all learned through interactions with others.

Why is emotional well-being important for a person with profound intellectual and multiple disabilities?

Emotional well-being is closely bound up with quality of life issues (Moss et al., 2000). Emerson et al. (1996) included in their definition of a high quality of life: receiving individually tailored support to become full participants in the life of the community, developing skills and independence, being given appropriate choices and control over one's life, and being treated with respect in a safe and secure environment. There is strong overlap here with the things that support emotional well-being, itself an inherent part of establishing meaningful relationships and taking control of one's life.

Emotional well-being is increasingly being linked with the ability to learn, and interest is growing in exploring this as a symbiotic process. We learn better when we feel good and in turn learning makes us feel good. This has long been the instinct of teachers and philosophers and is now being shown by cognitive neuroscience (e.g. LeDoux, 1998; Damasio, 2000). Goleman (1996) has made the case that emotional intelligence is more influential than conventional intelligence for all kinds of personal, career and school success. Emotional well-being makes a difference to the person not just at that time but to their long-term development. This understanding has been influential in increasing the emphasis on emotional literacy in schools and in the education policy agenda.

Emotional well-being is also important for mental health. People with intellectual disabilities are more likely to experience mental health difficulties during their lives than the general population (Hunt & Tarleton-Lord, 1998). Moreover, mental health difficulties are understood to increase in proportion to the severity of multiple disabilities (Sinason, 1994). While studies of the prevalence of mental health problems among people with intellectual disabilities vary greatly depending on definition, methods of identification and population studied, increased levels are to be expected based on their life experiences, circumstances and reduced capacity to cope with everyday challenges (Hatton, 2002). The more severe the intellectual disability, the less is known about the picture of mental health among the population; this, Hatton (2002) argues, is because of the challenges posed to current mental health classification systems, assessment procedures and treatment protocols. There is research evidence though that people with profound intellectual disabilities experience stressful emotions even when overt signs may be absent (Chaney, 1996). A call for interest in the mental health of people with profound intellectual disabilities (Sheehy & Nind, 2005) also produced strong anecdotal evidence from carers that depression and anxiety are suffered.

Historical neglect of emotional well-being

A review of the literature on the emotional well-being and mental health of people with profound intellectual disabilities quickly reveals the short history of work in this area. In 2003, Arthur (p. 25) exclaimed, 'At last, the emotional lives of people with learning disability begin to attract attention'. Moss et al. (2000) date this interest to the last 15 years and identify 'a growing international recognition of the need to respond more adequately to mental health problems in this population' (p. 97). The reasons for the neglect of emotional well-being are important to our understanding of how we might now address this neglect. The context, in the UK at least, is that the emotional lives of people with intellectual disabilities were 'submerged by the behavioural technologies of the 1970s and 1980s' and, with the people themselves, 'incarcerated in large subnormality hospitals' (Arthur, 2003, p. 25). Increased clinical and research attention has come with the process of deinstitutionalisation, but as Arthur (2003) argues, a better physical environment outside the institution is pointless if life is characterised by loneliness, isolation, fear and apathy, if social interactions remain limited, if there is little concern for the subjective quality of the individual's experience and if independent living skills and the treatment of challenging behaviour are prioritised over emotional well-being.

The reasons why the emotional well-being and mental health of people with severe and profound intellectual disabilities have been overlooked are discussed by Sheehy & Nind (2005) and in outline are as follows:

1. The history of seeing this group as subnormal and subhuman – this is at odds with recognising their emotional selves which epitomises their very humanness.
2. People with profound intellectual and multiple disabilities and people with mental health difficulties have largely been seen as separate and distinct groups, provided for by separate services with different cultures (Hatton, 2002). The prominent 'deficit' of the intellectual disability is the lens through which the whole person is viewed, thus masking other needs.
3. The mental health needs of people with profound intellectual and multiple disabilities are not frequently discussed because they are not heard. It is not possible to talk to them about mental health issues and so these issues are shied away from, and the group's powerlessness and low status (which passes on to those who care for them) mean this is not challenged.

Hatton (2002) adds to this list the specific obstacles to the identification of mental health problems:

1. The applicability of standardised classification systems is untested and criteria may need modification if they are applicable at all.
2. The relationship between mental health difficulties and challenging behaviour is unclear – challenging behaviours may be separate to mental health difficulties or an idiosyncratic expression to them, additional to them or a contributory factor in them.
3. The inability to describe mental states needed for some identification.
4. Misattribution of signs of mental health problems such as poor self-care to a person's intellectual disability.
5. Difficulty accessing referral pathways to mental health services.

Staff awareness of emotional states is clearly an issue for both identifying difficulties and preventing them. Moss et al. (2000, p. 98) stress the point that 'the people who are usually first to notice significant signs and symptoms (i.e. immediate carers) are usually the least qualified to undertake this task [recognition of mental disorders]'. Yet, the people they care for have increased risk of developing problems and increased need for basic attention to the quality of their existence. It is for all these reasons that looking after the emotional well-being of people with profound intellectual and multiple disabilities is an important part of looking after their (mental) health and crucial to nursing their complex needs.

Current best practice: a holistic approach to promoting emotional well-being

Stepping away from the world of intellectual disability into the world of health education means a shift from knowing very little about what works in promoting emotional well-being to knowing a great deal. Interest in the link between being emotionally well and learning well has led to a surge of research and attempts to clarify the evidence and implications. The outcome is evidence showing that holistic approaches are more effective (Wells et al., 2003) (but also harder to evaluate as they are more complex). Weare (2004, p. 53) sums up:

> ...there is a growing tendency to look at environments rather than individuals, both as the focus of concern and as the solution to problems, at the relationships between problems rather than at single problems, at clusters of risk factors rather than single causes, and at positive capacities rather than problems and deficits.

This is enormously helpful to work with people with profound intellectual disabilities, pointing towards proactive, preventative work concerned with the whole person and their environment. Moreover, it points to the need for an embedded, coherent, congruent approach across the whole organisation and for social contexts that foster productive, pleasant relationships, teamwork, mutual responsibility and delight in the company of others. Therefore, addressing staff training in mental health issues by itself is insufficient; the emotional well-being of the staff must be addressed. This requires a long-term, developmental approach involving the whole community; the more there are in a community who are socially and emotionally competent, the easier it is to support those with acute problems. Thus, staff need to foster environments where emotions are accepted as normal and unthreatening, discussed freely, expressed in safe ways, written about in policies and considered in decision-making (Weare, 2004).

Returning to the specific concern with profound intellectual disabilities, this holistic approach is entirely compatible with the desired outcome, outlined in the model developed by Moss et al. of 'reduction of symptoms, reduction of staff stress and carer burden, and improvements in quality of life', together with minimisation of difficulties re-occurring through long-term prevention (Moss et al., 2000, p. 104). Multidisciplinary approaches to assessment and multi-modal responses to difficulties are part of an acceptance of clusters of inter-related factors, causes and signs of difficulty. Moreover, a holistic approach can encompass Arthur's (2003) recommendation that we need to facilitate the emotional development of staff, improve relationships and improve the quality of emotional interactions and lives of caregivers, whom people with intellectual disabilities need as allies. Identifying features of enabling and disabling social and physical environments for emotional well-being is also highly compatible with a social model of disability.

Specialist intervention: Intensive Interaction as a holistic approach

Authorities on emotional well-being and emotional literacy, such as Weare, advocate holistic approaches, but they are also keen to disassociate from any connotations of these as unfocused, laissez-faire approaches. Indeed Weare (2004) specifically notes that approaches need to be sustainable, explicit, and developmentally appropriate with clear goals and clear roles. Evaluation of emotional literacy programmes indicates they are most effective when they attempt to teach attitudes and values together and when there are opportunities to learn these in a supportive environment.

Origins of the approach

One such 'programme' or approach for people with profound intellectual and multiple disabilities is Intensive Interaction (Nind & Hewett, 1994, 2001, 2005). Intensive Interaction is most often associated with supporting the social and communication development of people with the most severe and complex intellectual disabilities, but increasingly also with emotional development and well-being as part of this (Nind & Hewett, 2005; Nind, 2006a). Intensive Interaction refers to a way of interacting that facilitates social, communication, emotional and all development based on the style of interaction between caregivers and infants that facilitate such development.

Following Ephraim's (1979) work on 'augmented mothering', Intensive Interaction had its theoretical origins in the psychological research (such as Brazelton et al., 1974; Schaffer, 1977) which showed the rich intuitive teaching and learning (Carlson & Bricker, 1982) found within caregiver's interaction. While work with people with intellectual disabilities was largely dominated by very structured programmes to teach isolated skills and modify behaviour based on behavioural psychology, other psychologists were illustrating how infants learn in a very naturalistic way. The ability to make eye contact is not ordinarily learned as an isolated skill for an extrinsic reward. Babies make eye contact because of the way their parents/caregivers use their faces and voices to attract and hold their attention within the context of them regularly exploring each other's responses while simply enjoying each other. Similarly, learning about facial expressions and their connections with emotions occurs in interaction sequences that illustrate these in safe, meaningful and enjoyable ways. The idea that people with intellectual disabilities do not, however, learn naturally began to be challenged by augmented mothering and Intensive Interaction where naturalistic interaction was used very intensively with people with intellectual disabilities of all ages.

Intensive Interaction itself was developed in the late 1980s at a school within an institutional setting by a group of teachers seeking more effective and humane alternative to the behavioural approaches common at that time. The students were young adults who had not yet learned the fundamentals of early social communication, including individuals with profound and multiple intellectual disabilities. Staff went through a process of learning how to make interactions effective, whatever the extent of the person's intellectual and other impairments, and how to relate to people who had been isolated and difficult to reach for some years. Although originally an educational approach, Intensive Interaction has also evolved as a more generic approach used by parents, carers and practitioners from a range of disciplines (see Hewett & Nind, 1998).

Defining features

Intensive Interaction is characterised by its aim (to facilitate social and communication development) and the processes of interacting, which are nurturing, naturalistic and intensive. It involves regular, frequent interactions between the practitioner and the person with intellectual disabilities, in which there is no focus on the task or outcome, but in which the primary concern is the quality of the interaction itself. These interactions are not about 're-parenting', and tend to differ from naturally occurring caregiver–infant interactions in two important regards. Firstly, they are continuously recorded (in written and/or video form), reflected upon and evaluated as an integral part of the process. Secondly, they are engaged in by a team of practitioners who bring collective strengths and avoid the exclusivity of the caregiver–infant relationship. However, they have much in common with the interactions with infants including the following key features that are known to foster development (see Nind, 1996):

1. The interactions are about mutual pleasure and often involve elements of game playing; they are about being together with the purpose of enjoying each other.
2. They involve the practitioner in adjusting their interpersonal behaviours (gaze, voice, style of talking, body posture, facial expression) to become engaging and meaningful.
3. The interactions are flowing in time with pauses, repetitions, blended rhythms; the practitioner carefully scans the responses and makes constant micro-adjustments, thus achieving optimum levels of attention and arousal.
4. They involve the practitioner in inferring intentionality, that is, crediting the person with intellectual disabilities with thoughts, feelings and intentions and responding to their behaviours as if they are initiations with communicative significance.
5. The practitioner uses contingent responding, following the lead of the person with intellectual disabilities and thus giving them a good share of the control of the activity.

These interactions introduce the person with intellectual disabilities (or infant) to the social world, attending to faces and voices, getting feedback and making things happen. They provide a context for feeling 'uniquely known, recognized, nurtured and valued' (Weare, 2004) and experiencing being listened to as they go through a range of emotions, particularly emotional pleasure and satisfaction.

Mutual pleasure in the interactions helps both parties to feel relaxed and secure and to lose themselves in the interaction. It serves as a motivator to come back for more interactions – sustaining and repeating the cognitive, social and emotional engagement. This enables the person with intellectual disabilities to achieve a state of self-experience such as joy, suspense and excitation (Stern, 1985).

Adjustments in interpersonal behaviour are usually instinctive. Adults do not talk to babies as they do to other adults. Even other children do all kinds of instinctive things like dipping their head, widening their eyes and smiling a lot. Voices are made more sing-song, and little phases are repeated over and over with a playful, questioning tone. Staff interactions with people with intellectual disabilities, however, can cause them great angst in that their instincts might steer them towards amending their interactive style in this way, but internalised rules about how one should behave respectfully might undermine this intuition. This can result in a compromised style of interaction, interacting differently depending on who else is around, or even talking and interacting very little at all. On the whole, staff do not make the adjustments that people with a profound intellectual disability need, but Intensive Interaction gives permission to make appropriate adjustments based on the firm knowledge that they are both effective and necessary.

The careful timing in interaction sequences serves to achieve 'an elaborate interweaving of the participants' behavioural flow' (Schaffer, 1977, p. 5). In this way the timing of the interactions suits both parties, and they can synchronise their rhythms, attention and emotional states. This is achieved through watching, waiting and pausing, so that the initiations of the interactive partner are not missed and their contributions to the interaction are processed. Ultimately, such skilled interaction creates joint attention, turn-taking routines and feelings of being listened to.

Imputing intentionality is fundamental to supporting the transition to intentional communication (Newson, 1979; Harding, 1983). Lock (1978) argued that it is by treating novices as social communicators that they become so. Responding to sounds, facial expressions, body postures as if they are telling us something indicates to the person their communication potential. Two-way dialogue is created by doing something and then treating whatever the interaction partner does as a turn. This creates 'proto-conversations', an important stage of rehearsing the skills needed for real turn taking and dialogue. At first, interpretations of behaviours or sounds will not correspond to any intended meaning, but over time meanings will be co-constructed. Similarly, by treating behaviours as if they have emotional content, the emotional world will become meaningful.

Contingent responding involves responding in time and characteristic to something the other person does. Without contingent responding we would never connect, but instead conduct parallel but separate one-way conversations. Instinctive contingent responding to infants includes mirroring their facial expressions and sounds, blowing bubbles when they do, laughing or showing mock surprise at any sudden movements, and so on. Research has shown that for people with intellectual disabilities the world is often not contingent on them, and their potential initiations of contact are missed so that they develop passivity and self-stimulation (Ware, 1996). Intensive Interaction, in contrast, uses deliberate contingent responding to illustrate social cause and affect, showing that one has an inner locus of control (Field, 1979). This sense of being in control is essential to a desire to explore the environment and for emotional literacy.

Emotional well-being work

Traditionally, across professions, techniques to gain insights into the mental health or emotional states of people with profound intellectual disabilities have been lacking, and an inability to communicate has prevented understanding of changes in how an individual is feeling. Intensive Interaction, however, develops the ability to communicate with people who are functioning at the earliest stages of communication development. Using Intensive Interaction empowers families and practitioners to read and interpret the non-verbal behaviour of people with profound intellectual and multiple disabilities and to attune to idiosyncratic and potential communications. It is these people who live and work with individuals with profound disabilities who have insights into their well-being, but these insights are often underdeveloped, underused and undervalued. Intensive Interaction can provide a whole language and framework for describing how someone typically interacts, how their interactions are developing and therefore, how someone is behaving out of character for them when they may be anxious or depressed.

Intensive Interaction, in common with all good emotional literacy programmes, works on the premise that behaviour has meaning and emotional origins. In this way stereotyped behaviours, such as rocking or hand flapping, are not seen as serving any purpose, detrimental to social acceptance and therefore need to be eliminated. They are seen as part of the limited range of options that the person has for controlling the environment and bringing predictability to their world. Intensive Interaction practitioners might join in with some stereotyped behaviours in contingent responding, sharing that person's rhythms and movements, valuing them and what is important to them. Opting to do this though will depend on it bringing mutual enjoyment or at least a coming together of some kind. Joining in is not about encouraging/reinforcing or discouraging the behaviour, but it is simply using it as a point of connection (see Nind & Kellett, 2002; Nind, 2006b).

A holistic approach

In Intensive Interaction, nurturing, facilitative interactions do not just happen – the practitioner assumes responsibility for making them happen. This will involve learning optimum times when the person with intellectual disabilities is alert and responsive and when they will not be disturbed and how to reach or 'access' that individual (see Nind & Hewett, 2001, 2005). These are the details of Intensive Interaction – the skills and process part of the approach. But more fundamentally, making interactions happen involves creating an ethos where having such interactions is not only welcome but valued as meaningful 'work'. This is the holistic part of the approach. Thus, Intensive Interaction meets the criterion of effective emotional literacy intervention in encompassing attitudes, values and skills, and opportunities to learn these in a supportive environment.

The focus on individuals should not lead to a neglect of the environment, the importance of which is emphasised not just by advocates of holistic approaches to emotional well-being. Siegel-Causey & Bashinski (1997) argue for a triangular framework for communication: the learner/learning disabled person, the communication partner and the environmental context. Similarly, Ware (1996) stresses the importance of a responsive environment *'in which people get responses to their actions, get the opportunity to give responses to the actions of others, and have an opportunity to take the lead in interaction'* (p. 1).

Weare (2004) stresses the importance of emotional literacy programmes being focused with clear aims to avoid the sense of fuzzy and warm 'anything goes'. This is especially true for Intensive Interaction where interactions should not be unfocused but finely tuned to each individual, requiring careful attention to detail and sensitive reflection. Written policies help to focus staff on the purpose and essence of the approach and the coherence between Intensive Interaction and any other imperatives. Policies should refer to safeguards for staff (regarding consent to interact, physical contact, etc.) and processes for keeping records and evaluating progress (see Nind & Hewett, 2001).

Evidence has been accumulating about the effectiveness of Intensive Interaction (Watson & Knight, 1991; Nind, 1996; Watson & Fisher, 1997; Lovell et al., 1998; Samuel, 2003). Kellett's research (Kellett, 2001, Kellett & Nind, 2003) has additionally highlighted some of the critical aspects in implementing Intensive Interaction that substantially affect the outcomes. This work has shown that the micro-politics of the staff environment, how resources are managed, and the approach to staff development, coordination and policymaking all make a significant impact. Thus, the holistic environment cannot be separated from the quality of the interactions – they inevitably affect one another – and the emotional well-being of everyone involved is affected by both.

Intensive Interaction should encompass planning, monitoring and critical reflection, helping to ensure that interactions are not negatively influenced by the fatigue or emotional state of the interactive partner. Research on the interaction patterns of parents and (learning) disabled infants has shown that parents, anxious about the atypical response of their infants, may start 'working' too hard at their interactions – driving them instead of following their child's lead (Field, 1979). But research also shows that the amount of support they receive makes a difference in this respect (Dunste & Trivette, 1986). Intensive Interaction is a team approach which should have in-built support through the shared reflections and problem solving essential for coping positively with the interactive response – or lack of response – of a person with intellectual disabilities. Observing each other's interactions, giving feedback, reviewing video to evaluate the timing and quality of pauses, and so on, are all ways of helping to sustain interactions and (feelings of) efficacy.

This teamwork also allows for continuity in approach and protects the person with intellectual disabilities from the possibility of being isolated from anyone with whom they can successfully interact and relate. Numerous case studies (e.g. Kellett & Nind, 2003) have shown that Intensive Interaction sessions are often the 'high' points when people with intellectual disabilities are at their happiest, most playful and most socially engaged. There is a danger that these feelings of well-being may become equated solely with the interactive partner rather than with a small number of close carers or with their own abilities and actions. It is irresponsible to create a situation in which a person with intellectual disabilities is dependent upon any one professional carer for his or her continued emotional well-being. There is a delicate balance to be achieved between recognising that one cannot support people to develop their communication, social and emotional abilities without 'getting involved' and bonding at some level, and recognising that this is not about replicating *exclusive* parenting-type bonds. A supportive environment is one in which practitioners can feel safe to talk about how they feel about their emotional attachments and feel good rather than precious about sharing with colleagues the elements of their interactions that seem key to their success.

The holistic approach should extend to and encompass family members as part of any team, sharing knowledge about the interaction, likes and dislikes of the individual. Family may want to join in, or least see, the meticulous record keeping that is part of the approach and that helps to demonstrate subtle changes. They should share in the feedback from video, others, the person with intellectual disabilities her or himself, and perhaps use this to alter their interactive style a little, or to simply do more of what they already do well with renewed confidence and enthusiasm. When handled sensitively, active reflection on interactions can supplement intuitive interacting without interfering with natural warmth and spontaneity and without everyday family interactions feeling like 'work' (Taylor & Taylor, 1998).

For Intensive Interaction to work well, staff/families need to have good relationships with each other. The approach is one in which practitioners use themselves (voice, face, physicality, ongoing judgement) as their primary equipment. This can make people feel exposed. Interacting through musical instruments or someone's favourite object, for example, may provide a feeling of security, but ideally the emotional climate should be one in which using objects is a positive, rather than defensive, choice. Creating safe spaces to work, providing time to air disquiet and enabling staff to start with service-users with whom they already have a relationship are all part of attending to emotional needs.

Managers or coordinators have a significant role to play in creating an environment in which it is okay to look or sound 'silly', where everyone understands that this is about creating a good match between the interactions on offer and people's intellectual and emotional readiness. Offering interactions that look acceptable, but fail to connect, should not be seen as an alternative to offering interactions at the level at which people with profound intellectual disabilities can engage. Practitioners who have been in 'intellectual disability' for any length of time will have experienced the swing of the pendulum towards age-appropriate interactions and may feel uncomfortable with its swing back towards developmental appropriateness. Dialogue about this is essential, as is honesty about what the real issues are; concern with age appropriateness can offer a place to hide deeper concerns with self-consciousness, being judged, and so on. (For a full discussion of age appropriateness and developmental appropriateness, see Nind & Hewett, 1996.) This issue is also discussed in the research on emotional literacy, and Weare (2004, p. 88) concludes that effective programmes *take a developmental approach, and attempt to tailor the programme to the stage, rather than just the age, of the learner. They are usually based on an effort to assess where the learner is starting from*.

Another element of Intensive Interaction, making it suitable for promoting well-being, but also requiring sensitive handling, is that it often uses touch. Making physical contact as part of interacting with people with limited understandings is almost inevitable, whether this be patting hands, stroking a cheek, or rough and tumble. This is an enjoyable, natural, irreplaceable aspect of communicating with someone who is pre-verbal. But more than this, touch has a deep emotional and psychological significance as an aspect of non-verbal interacting; it is one of the underpinning experiences to all areas of human development. At whatever age, touch is a primary means for providing comfort and for communicating empathy. In Intensive Interaction, physical contact may be incidental to interactions or the central focus for what is happening. Practitioners have to be comfortable with this amidst a culture of continuing revelations about sexual abuse of children and vulnerable adults and an associated 'moral panic' about touch (Johnson, 2000). Responses to this culture need to be measured and balanced with an understanding of the potential dangers of denying children (and adults) touch (see Piper & Smith, 2003, for an excellent discussion of this).

Issues concerning physical contact can arouse deep emotional responses, but this needs to be balanced with knowledge of the positive effects of physical contact. Touch through massage therapy, for example, has been linked with weight gain in preterm babies (Scafidi et al., 1996); the sociability and interaction behaviour of babies of depressed mothers (Field et al., 1996); the cognitive performance of preschool children (Hart et al., 1998); aggressive adolescents showing reductions in aggressive behaviour (Diego et al., 2002); children with autism displaying improvements in attentiveness (Field et al., 1997); and reductions in stereotyped behaviour and improvements in sociability (Escalona et al., 2001). In massage, there is the risk that touch becomes 'technical' instead of 'natural' (Piper & Smith, 2003), and this is where the less-formalised touch of Intensive Interaction is advantageous. Touch is a fundamental factor in health, well-being and cognitive development (Montagu, 1995). It provides a direct and understandable form of contact with another person and a fundamental experience in the development of communication powers. Approaches that involve touch also require an atmosphere that is open and trusting and therefore a clear ethos.

The holistic Intensive Interaction environment facilitates committed colleagues and supports them in their practice such that a critical mass of emotionally supportive work can develop. Staff who are less emotionally secure with the approach might be encouraged to engage in cooperative teamwork to free other staff for one-to-one interactive time or to video record interactions adopting a safe, 'invisible' position behind a camera as a non-threatening introduction. Sharing success and enabling all staff to feel a sense of ownership in the progress that people make is a key part of successful implementation of the approach (Kellett & Nind, 2003) as well as crucial to the emotional well-being of the whole team.

Sustaining the emotional well-being of Intensive Interaction practitioners has been found to be important to the effectiveness of the approach. In all six of the case studies reported in Kellett & Nind (2003), the detailed patterns of progress or otherwise of the children were found to reflect the patterns of the emotional state, fatigue and burn out of the staff who were their main interactive partners (evident in staleness, missed cues, increased directiveness and failure to make contingent responses and modifications to language or interactive style). It is tempting, when fatigued, to skip reflection time, but this is when it is particularly important. The reflective part of Intensive Interaction, in which the practitioners ask themselves about what happened, the significance of this and how they felt about the interaction, might help to highlight difficult periods to be addressed, usually through a team response. Because Intensive Interaction works at optimum levels when staff enjoy emotional well-being, strategies need to be put in place to help foster this well-being, such as sharing the emotional highs and lows of progress and setbacks. Strategies are also needed to enable Intensive Interaction to happen when the practitioner is feeling good about themselves rather than forcing interactions when they are feeling low, stressed or overtired.

Conclusion

The emotional well-being of people with profound intellectual disabilities has been neglected for far too long. Awareness about emotional states and mental health has been raised, and methods of assessment and intervention need to catch up with awareness and need. Inevitably, there will be huge barriers to assessing mental illness in people with intellectual disabilities and complex issues in relation to identifying difficulties and making effective responses. But these are the problems of what to do in a specific sense when things go wrong. There is much that we can all do to prevent difficulties arising in the first place through being proactive in promoting emotional well-being. This chapter has made the case that Intensive Interaction, known for facilitating social and communication development, also offers an effective way of working for anyone wanting to support the emotional development and well-being of people with profound intellectual disabilities. Repeatedly accounts of Intensive Interaction practitioners dwell not just on the progress made by people with intellectual disabilities but on how the approach makes them feel good. This is in keeping with the essence of all good approaches to emotional well-being, which need to address the well-being of the whole community.

References

Arthur, A.R. (2003). The emotional lives of people with learning disability. *British Journal of Learning Disabilities*, 31, 25–30.

Brazelton, T.B., Koslowski, B., & Main, M. (1974). The origins of reciprocity: the early mother-infant interaction. In Lewis, M., & Rosenblum, L.A. (eds) *The Effect of the Infant on its Caregiver*. New York: John Wiley & Sons; 49–76.

Carlson, L., & Bricker, D.D. (1982). Dyadic and contingent aspects of early communicative intervention. In Bricker, D.D. (ed.) *Interventions with at Risk and Handicapped Infants*. Baltimore: University Park Press; 291–308.

Chaney, R.H. (1996). Psychological stress in people with profound mental retardation. *Journal of Intellectual Disability Research*, 40(4), 305–310.

Damasio, A. (2000). *The Feeling of What Happens*. London: Vintage.

Diego, M., Field, T., Hernandez-Reif, M., Shaw, J., Rothe, E., Castellanos, D., & Mesner, L. (2002). Aggressive adolescents benefit from massage therapy. *Adolescence*, 37, 597–607.

Dunste, C.J., & Trivette, C.M. (1986). Looking beyond the parent-infant dyad for the determinants of maternal styles of interaction. *Infant Mental Health Journal*, 7, 69–80.

Emerson, E., Cullen, C., Hatton, C., & Cross, B. (1996). *Residential Provision for People with Learning Disabilities: Summary Report*. Manchester: Hester Adrian Research Centre.

Ephraim, G.W.E. (1979). *Developmental Process in Mental Handicap: A Generative Structure Approach*. Unpublished Ph.D. thesis, Brunel University, Uxbridge.

Escalona, A., Field, T., Singer-Strunck, R., Cullen, C., & Hartshorn, K. (2001). Brief report: improvements in the behavior of children with autism following massage therapy. *Journal of Autism and Developmental Disorders*, 31, 513–516.

Field, T.M. (1979). Games parents play with normal and high risk infants. *Child Psychology and Human Development*, 10(1), 41–48.

Field, T., Grizzle, N., Scafidi, F., Abrams, S., Richardson, S., Kuhn, C., & Shanberg, S. (1996). Massage therapy for infants of depressed mothers. *Infant Behavior and Development*, 19, 109–114.

Field, T., Lasko, D., Mundy, P., Henteleff, T., Talpins, S., & Dowling, M. (1997). Autistic children's attentiveness and responsivity improve after touch therapy. *Journal of Autism and Developmental Disorders*, 27, 333–338.

Goleman, D. (1996). *Emotional Intelligence*. London: Bloomsbury.

Harding, C. (1983). Setting the stage for language acquisition: communication development in the first year. In Golinkoff, R. (ed.) *The Transition from Pre-Lingusitic to Lingusitic Communication*. New Jersey: Lawrence Erlbaum Associates.

Hart, S., Field, T., Hernandez-Reif, M., & Lundy, B. (1998). Preschoolers' cognitive performance improves following massage. *Early Child Development and Care*, 143, 59–64.

Hatton, C. (2002). Psychosocial interventions for adults with intellectual disabilities and mental health problems: a review. *Journal of Mental Health*, 11(4), 357–373.

Hewett, D., & Nind, M. (eds) (1998). *Interaction in Action: Reflections on the Use of Intensive Interaction*. London: David Fulton.

Hunt, G., & Tarleton-Lord, D. (1998). Snapshots of the mind. *Nursing Times*, 94(16), 55–56.

Johnson, R.T. (2000). *Hands Off! The Disappearance of Touch in the Care of Children*. New York: Peter Lang.

Kellett, M. (2001). *Implementing Intensive Interaction: An Evaluation of the Efficacy of Intensive Interaction in Promoting Sociability and Communication in Young Children who have Severe Learning Difficulties and of Factors Affecting its Implementation in Community Special Schools*. Unpublished Ph.D. thesis, Brookes University, Oxford.

Kellett, M., & Nind, M. (2003). *Implementing Intensive Interaction in Schools: Guidance for Practitioners, Managers and Coordinators*. London: David Fulton.

LeDoux, J. (1998). *The Emotional Brain*. London: Phoenix.

Lock, A. (1978). *Action, Gesture and Symbol*. London: Academic Press.

Lovell, D.M., Jones, S.P., & Ephraim, G. (1998). The effects of intensive interaction on a man with severe intellectual disabilities. *International Journal of Practical Approaches to Disability*, 22(2/3), 3–9.

Montagu, A. (1995). Animadversions on the development of a theory of touch. In Field, T. (ed.) *Touch in Early Development*. New Jersey: Lawrence Erlbaum; 1–10.

Moss, S., Bouras, N., & Holt, G. (2000). Mental health services for people with intellectual disability: a conceptual framework. *Journal of Intellectual Disability Research*, 44(2), 97–107.

Newson, J. (1979). Intentional behaviour in the young infant. In Shaffer, D., & Dunn, J. (eds) *The First Year of Life*. New York: John Wiley & Sons; 91–96.

Nind, M. (1996). Efficacy of intensive interaction: developing sociability and communication in people with severe learning difficulties using an approach based on caregiver-infant interaction. *European Journal of Special Needs Education*, 11(1), 48–66.

Nind, M. (2006a). *Beyond Access to Communication. Keynote address*. Intensive Interaction Conference 2006. Leeds.

Nind, M. (2006b). Stereotyped behaviour: resistance by people with profound learning disabilities. In Mitchell, D., Traustadottir, R., Chapman, R., Townson, L., Ingham, N., & Ledger, S. (eds) *Exploring Experiences of Advocacy by People with Learning Disabilities: Testimonies of Resistance*. London: Jessica Kingsley; 202–211.

Nind, M., & Hewett, D. (1994). *Access to Communication: Developing the Basics of Communication with People with Severe Learning Difficulties through Intensive Interaction*. London: David Fulton.

Nind, M., & Hewett, D. (1996). When age-appropriateness isn't appropriate. In Coupe O'Kane, J., & Goldbart, J. (eds) *Whose Choice? Contentious Issues for those Working with People with Learning Difficulties*. London: David Fulton; 48–57.

Nind, M., & Hewett, D. (2001). *A Practical Guide to Intensive Interaction*. Kidderminster: British Institute of Learning Disabilities.

Nind, M., & Hewett, D. (2005). *Access to Communication: Developing the Basics of Communication with People with Severe Learning Difficulties through Intensive Interaction* (2nd edition). London: David Fulton.

Nind, M., & Kellett, M. (2002). Responding to individuals with severe learning difficulties and stereotyped behaviour: challenges for an inclusive era. *European Journal of Special Needs Education*, 17(3), 265–282.

Piper, H., & Smith, H. (2003). 'Touch' in educational and child care settings: dilemmas and responses. *British Educational Research Journal*, 29(6), 879–894.

Samuel, J. (2003). *An Evaluation of Intensive Interaction in Community Living Settings for Adults With Profound Learning Disability*. Unpublished D.Clin Psychology thesis. Open University.

Scafidi, F.A., Field, T.M., Wheeden, A., Schanberg, S., Kuhn, C., Symanski, R., Zimmerman, E., & Bandstra, E.S. (1996). Cocaine-exposed preterm neonates show behavioral and hormonal differences. *Pediatrics*, 97, 851–855.

Schaffer, H.R. (ed.) (1977). *Studies in Mother-Infant Interaction*. London: Academic Press.

Sheehy, K., & Nind, M. (2005). Emotional well-being for all: mental health and people with profound and multiple learning disabilities. *British Journal of Learning Disabilities*, 33, 34–38.

Siegel-Causey, E., & Bashinski, S.M. (1997). Enhancing initial communication and responsiveness of learners with multiple disabilities: a tri-focus framework for partners. *Focus on Autism and Other Developmental Disabilities*, 12(2), 105–120.

Sinason, V. (1994). *Mental Handicap and the Human Condition*. London: Free Association Books.

Stern, D.N. (1985). *The Interpersonal World of the Infant*. New York: Basic Books.

Stewart-Brown, S. (2000). Parenting, wellbeing, health and disease. In Buchanan, A., & Hudson, B. (eds) *Promoting Children's Emotional Well-being*. Oxford: Oxford University Press; 28–47.

Taylor, B., & Taylor, S. (1998). Gary's story: parents doing Intensive Interaction. In Hewett, D., & Nind, M. (eds) *Interaction in Action: Reflections on the Use of Intensive Interaction*. London: David Fulton.

Ware, J. (1996). *Creating a Responsive Environment for People with Profound and Multiple learning Difficulties*. London: David Fulton.

Watson, J., & Fisher, A. (1997). Evaluating the effectiveness of Intensive Interaction teaching with pupils with profound and complex learning difficulties. *British Journal of Special Education*, 24(2), 80–87.

Watson, J., & Knight, C. (1991). An evaluation of intensive interactive teaching with pupils with severe learning difficulties. *Child language Teaching and Therapy*, 7(3), 10–25.

Weare, K. (2004). *Developing the Emotionally Literate School*. London: Paul Chapman.

Wells, J., Barlow, J., & Stewart-Brown, S. (2003). A systematic review of universal approaches to mental health promotion in schools. *Health Education*, 103, 197–204.

Chapter 6

ACHIEVING AND MAINTAINING HEALTH

Jillian Pawlyn

Introduction

This chapter presents an outline of recent approaches which have informed and influenced the way we support people with profound intellectual and multiple disabilities (PIMDs) to achieve and maintain optimum health.

This chapter begins by introducing the reader to person-centred planning (PCP) and its various approaches, models and tools. The reader will then be presented with an overview of health profiling and health action planning, with an explanation of how this can assist in identifying health needs and supporting the person with PIMD to maintain and achieve health gains. The final part of this chapter focuses on health facilitation, identifying what we mean by the term and how it is achieved for people with PIMD.

Learning objectives

At the end of this chapter the reader will:

- develop knowledge of the key aspects of PCP;
- develop knowledge of the key aspects of health action planning; and
- be able to recognise factors that contribute to the success of health facilitation.

Valuing People identifies the:

> ... *need to develop a new approach to delivering better life chances for people with learning disabilities ... promote effective partnership working at all levels to ensure a really person-centred approach to delivering quality services*
> (Department of Health (DH), 2001c, p. 22).

Initially the white paper *Valuing People* (DH, 2001c) sets us the task of achieving several key objectives. Within these there are four objectives which relate to person-centred approaches and to meeting health needs of people with PIMD (Figure 6.1);

Objective 3: Enabling people to have more control over their own lives
To enable people with learning disabilities to have as much choice and control as possible over their lives through advocacy and a person-centred approach to planning the services they need.

Objective 5: Good health
To enable people with learning disabilities to access a health service designed around their individual needs, with fast and convenient care delivered to a consistently high standard and with additional support where necessary.

Objective 9: Quality
To ensure that all agencies commission and provide high-quality, evidence-based and continuously improving services which promote both good outcomes and best value.

Objective 11: Partnership working
To promote holistic services for people with learning disabilities through effective partnership working between all relevant local agencies in the commissioning and delivery of services.

Figure 6.1 Government objectives for intellectual disability services (abridged) (DH, 2001 C, p. 26).

to achieve these objectives, it is essential for all of us to work in partnership. These objectives provide the focus for local action to implement the proposals set out in joint investment plans. Joint investment plans are developed through partnership working, where health and local authorities, together with partner agencies, assess the service needs of local people and compare this with existing services and identify where there are shortfalls in the service and how these shortfalls will be met by identifying the investment and reinvestment needed to reshape services.

Within *Valuing People* (DH, 2001c) several targets were applied to these and other objectives. Mansell & Beadle-Brown identified that *'these were extremely ambitions targets for public policy'* (Mansell & Beadle-Brown, 2004, p. 2) given that these targets are being applied to shaping the support and service provision for people with intellectual disabilities and complex needs. Progress towards the achievement of these targets is reported upon later in this chapter.

Following the implementation of *Valuing People* to ensure clarity, a definition of person-centred approaches was sought.

Person-centred approaches

Person-centred approaches are ways of commissioning, providing and organising services rooted in listening to what people want and to help them live in their communities as they choose. These approaches work to use resources flexibly, designed around what is important to a person from their own perspective and work to remove any cultural and organisational barriers to this. People are not simply placed in pre-existing services and expected to adjust, rather the service strives to adjust to the person. Person-centred approaches look to mainstream services and community resources for assistance and do not limit themselves to what is available within specialist intellectual disability services. They strive to build a person-centred organisational culture (DH, 2001a, p. 16).

Having now defined what we mean by person-centred approaches, it is necessary to consider what is meant by the term person-centred planning:

> *Person centred planning is a process of life planning for individuals, based around the principles of inclusion and the social model of disability.... Person centred planning replaces more traditional outmoded styles of assessment and planning which are based on a medical model approach to people's needs*
>
> (Circles Network, 2005).

According to Pearpoint et al. (undated) and Webb & Sanderson (2002), PCP is where the person is at the centre of planning their lives. PCP means planning with people – not doing to them. The person is central to their own plans, and facilitators/supporters will do what it takes to give them the maximum possible safe management of their own planning and lives. The person in the centre is the most important person in the plan.

The DH (2001a, pp. 13–14) identified five features of PCP which distinguish it from other forms of assessment or planning:

1. The person is at the centre.
2. Family members and friends are full partners.
3. PCP reflects the person's capacities, what is important to the person (now and for their future) and specifies the support they require to make a valued contribution to their community.
4. PCP builds a shared commitment to action that will uphold the person's rights.
5. PCP leads to continual listening, learning and action, and helps the person to get what they want out of life.

It is essential that the person with PIMD is meaningfully involved in the process of developing their person-centred plan (DH, 2002b).

There are several approaches available to assist with developing person-centred plans, including:

- *essential lifestyle planning* (Smull & Harrison, 1992);
- *group action planning* (Turnbull & Turnbull, 1996; Blue-Banning et al., 2000);
- *individual service design* (Forest & Pearpoint, 1992);
- *McGill action planning system (MAPS)* (Vandercook et al., 1989; Forest & Pearpoint, 1992);
- *personal futures planning* (O'Brien, 1987; Mount & Zwernick, 1988);

- *planning alternative tomorrows with hope (PATH)* (Pearpoint et al., 1993); and
- *whole life planning* (Butterworth et al., 1993).

Several of these approaches feature a graphical component which is designed to help people find direction and build strength, while others feature questions through which individuals can develop to a plan of action to head towards their *dream* and away from their *nightmare*. Others combine both approaches with a flexible set of questions and graphical maps from which the individuals, their advocate and the facilitator can build a sense of the individual's strengths and gifts and how they could be better utilised.

All of the approaches provide a powerful means of gathering information to identify what is and what is not working in the person's life right now. At the heart of all these processes is the belief that every individual has their own life to lead, a life that is right for them. Sometimes it is difficult to work out what is best to do and sometimes we need people to help us work out what is best to do. PCP is the process of helping people work out the best thing for themselves to do which informs how the person needs and wants to be supported.

Although each of these approaches has unique features, they share a number of basic values and strategies; one key aspect is that of a circle or network of support:

- Central to PCP is a circle of friends and supporters, including the person with in- tellectual disabilities, family members, friends, peers and other service providers. The richness of this circle is especially important when planning with a person with PIMD. It is essential that several members of the circle know the person well and have an established rapport and effective system of communication to be able to explore and identify their strengths, gifts, dreams and nightmares.
- This circle meets a number of times to build relationships with the person with intellectual disabilities, to explore their strengths and interests and to develop team unity.
- Then, in a major planning session the circle develops a comprehensive plan for the individual's future.
- Then the plan is reviewed on a regular basis agreed by the circle of support.

Another approach to supporting the person with PIMD is referred to as active support – originally conceptualised to address the issue of ensuring the provision of high-quality support to people with severe learning disabilities and challenging behaviour (see Emerson & Hatton, 1994). This approach is composed of:

- planned and focused support which emphasises its 'active' component;
- engaging the person in being active participant;
- on a daily basis this requires the systematic planning of service users' daily 'activities' and deployment of staff;
- training of staff to equip them with the necessary skills to effectively engage with service users as active participants in activities;

- requires clearly defined goal or opportunity planning; and
- requires monitoring and evaluation, monitoring the level of active engagement by service users.

(Adapted from Sanderson et al., 2002)

Active support is valuable because it provides a systematic approach to planning and delivering daily activities, and unlike other approaches it specifically focuses on the role of the paid carer and the training they require in supporting the person. A systematic approach to planning and documenting interventions by paid carers is advocated by Clark & Gates (2006), who promote the use of a nursing model as this might assist in care being delivered in a more organised and guided way for people with PIMD.

Person-centred planning – strategic context

O'Brien & Towell (2003) identify the need for thinking about PCP in the strategic context. They defined this context as identifying what needs to change in specialist services and what needs to change in mainstream services (such as housing, transportation, education, benefits and services that help people get into jobs) if large numbers of people are going to be able to turn good plans into better lives.

O'Brien & Towell (2003) also indicated the need for a number of key results:

1. the development of local capacity to provide people with an intellectual disability the assistance they require to say how they want to live their lives, and what assistance and opportunities will make a positive difference;
2. the development of local capacity of specialist services so they can deliver assistance in a way that meets the requirements of the individuals, informed through their person-centred plan.
3. for people with an intellectual disability to participate and contribute to their communities.

One term which is common to these three 'key results' is the presence of the term capacity: 'capacity is used in this context to stand for all that it takes to do something well, including peoples knowledge and skills, authorization, time, and investments of money' (O'Brien & Towell, 2003, p. 1); together these three results create the strategic context for PCP. O'Brien & Towell (2003, pp. 4–5) also identify the desire to develop local capacity in mainstream services so that people with intellectual disabilities benefit from the services to which their citizenship entitles them:

> Person Centred Planning is one of the ways to direct these changes. Working in partnership mainstream services will learn how to include people with learning disabilities and specialist services will learn how to assist people to have the lives they want by responding to what they request based on their person-centred plans. More people will have a good chance to have better lives.

Challenges

With each new approach to supporting people with an intellectual disability to meet their needs and dreams, there have been casualties along the way. All too often services have neglected to fully evaluate what has gone before, and risk 'throwing the baby out with the bathwater[1]'. They may implement new approaches because they are directed to do so or may want to be seen doing the 'right thing'. Kendrick (2004) advises caution regarding the apparent overemphasis and overreliance on formal PCP within intellectual disability services. He encourages us to consider the inherent limitations and risks within each of the formal PCP systems before cultivation by a person or within an organisation.

Challenges faced by services supporting people with PIMD include the need for the following:

- Individuality of planning 'versus' standardisation of person-centred plans to ensure integration within other recording systems.
- Resource-driven constraints within services and service planning 'versus' delivering on individual dreams and desires.
- Professional/service control 'versus' individual control (empowered). How much opportunity do people have to develop their own plans? Services need to consider how they embrace the role of the advocate in the development of person-centred plans for people with PIMD.

Does formal PCP lead to a 'better life'?

Kinsella (2000) reported that there was no evidence of the effectiveness of PCP when compared to other care planning processes. Five years on PCP was reported to be having a positive benefit on the life experiences of people with intellectual disabilities (Emerson et al., 2005b). However, Emerson et al. also caution that:

> While PCP was associated with benefits in some domains of 'quality of life', it had no apparent impact on others (e.g., more inclusive social networks, employment, physical, activity, medication) and there were three areas (risks, physical health, emotional and behavioural needs) where there was evidence of change in a 'negative' direction (Emerson et al., 2005b, p. iii).

Given this result it is essential that services consider how to reverse this negative direction through improving the quality of life of a person with PIMD (see Chapter 2).

There is a risk that services have made PCP overly complicated, and subsequently it is a challenge to ensure plans are implemented and dreams are realised. To meet government targets (DH, 2001c), it is important for organisations supporting people with PIMD that they invest in resources to develop person-centred plans. However

---

[1] English proverb loosely meaning those who by trying to rid themselves of a bad thing succeed in destroying whatever good there was as well.

with a reduction in personal income (state benefits (UK)) and reduced investment in services at both strategic and local authority level, it is a perpetual challenge to ensure sufficient funds are available to implement plans and realise dreams. Regrettably, there remains little involvement from independent advocates to ensure the voice of the person with PIMD is heard (McNally, 2007). Some interpretations have led to overemphasis on the social components of an individual's life, leading to acquisition and maintenance of 'good' health being devalued, often an afterthought. Services need to be ever mindful of the goals of PCP and refer to the five key features which underpin any PCP approach (DH, 2001a).

It is essential that the person-centred plan clearly identifies the supports that the person requires, in particular identifying what is important for them to stay healthy and safe (Sanderson & Smull, 2005). This component of a PCP is sometimes referred to as a health action plan.

Health action planning

A health action plan (HAP) is a personal plan about what a person with an intellectual disability needs to do to be in good health.

Health action plans are not new; Fitton (1994) discussed the importance of individual plans and care books for people with an intellectual disability. She stressed that the care book is a valuable tool that could be used to empower people in communicating information about them and as a reminder, reference and guidance document for the person's carers. The DH has shown an increased recognition of and support for the health needs of people with intellectual disabilities (DH, 2001b, c, 2002a).

The DH (2002a) identified five principles of health action planning, stating that it:

1. should support the white paper's values of rights, independence, choice and inclusion;
2. will be about more than individual plans – it should include strategic actions to support and sustain their implementation;
3. should address both individual and societal influences on the health of people with intellectual disabilities;
4. is a shared responsibility, with each person and agency playing a role appropriate to their skills and experience; and
5. will support the mainstream health agenda and the drive to reduce health inequalities.

It is envisaged that with the right support and facilitation at many levels, health action planning will assist people to identify their health needs and detail the actions needed, and the services required to maintain and improve health and identify any further help needed to complete these actions.

A survey undertaken by the PMLD Network (2006) sought to identify how many people have a health action plan. Results indicated that 52% of respondents said that the person/people they support have a health action plan that meets the person's needs. As impressive as this appears, that means that 48% either do not have a health action plan or have a plan that does not meet the person's needs. Given this response it is clear that there is room for improvement in this area. Some people have health action plans but find they are not used to share information about the persons' health needs; their use is of limited success. Other respondents identified concerns over the apparent lack of investment for the development and delivery of HAPs and the substantial support needed to implement these initiatives:

> *A Health Action Plan details the actions needed to maintain and improve the health of an individual and any help needed to accomplish these. It is a mechanism to link the individual and the range of services and supports they need, if they are to have better health .... Health Action Plans need to be supported by wider changes that assist and sustain this individual approach. The Plan is primarily for the person with learning disabilities and is usually co-produced with them* (DH, 2002a, p. 5).

Health action plans are individualised and the format and presentation will vary from person to person. There is no set format but guidelines on application can be followed. A health action plan should detail the actions needed to maintain and improve the health of a person and any help needed to accomplish this (DH, 2002a). It is a tool that can be used to link people and the services and support they require to ensure good health. The functions and benefits of the plan are to identify health concerns and how to address them, while improving the involvement and coordination of services for the person. Howatson (2005) emphasised that the health action plan acts as evidence that the person's service provider is working within the boundaries to meet their individual needs.

The DH goes on to identify useful (secondary) functions of health action plans. These might include:

- *to educate or inform the individual and people working with them about health;*
- *to improve the co-ordination of services for the individual;*
- *to influence services and other structures that affect the person's life (including the collection of data to inform change).*

(DH, 2002a, p. 5)

One of the challenges for those responsible for strategic developments is to ensure that the information held in health action plans is handled sensitively, and that the information is used to inform and influence service developments to better meet the needs of people with PIMD.

Other tools which have been developed to assist with health planning include the personal health profile (PHP). The introduction of hand-held health records is relatively new in the area of intellectual disabilities; however, their use is long standing in the field of maternity and child health:

> The personal child health record (PCHR) is a booklet given to new parents in the United Kingdom, to be used as the main record of their child's growth, development, and uptake of preventive health services (Walton et al., 2006, p. 269).

The PCHR provides extensive and valuable information about the child's health and development, in a format which is easy to access and enhances communication between parents and health service providers. The information contained within a PCHR is valuable in informing services of the support a child needs and can be used to influence service development.

Given the successes the PCHR has on recording and monitoring the health of children, it is perhaps surprising that as yet there is no approved health record format for adults with PIMD (living in the UK) in which to record their health needs and uptake of preventive health services. Several services and organisations have been developing their own documents to profile the health needs of the person with intellectual disabilities (Turner et al., 2003; Oxleas National Health Service Trust, 2004).

Health profiling to meet health needs

Health profiling assists in identifying areas of health need, beginning with undertaking a comprehensive assessment (see Chapter 7). Wilkinson (2001) emphasised the importance of a systematic gathering of relevant and important client data, used to identify health problems, plan nursing care and evaluate client outcomes.

A study undertaken by Turk & Burchell (2003) endorsed the use of PHPs as valuable tools to put right the inequality in healthcare faced by people with an intellectual disability. They state that 'PHPs have raised the overall focus on health and we hope will improve communication between adults with learning disabilities, carers and health staff' (Turk & Burchell, 2003, p. 40). A similar positive response was noted in the study by Turner et al; participants identified the Personal Health Profile to be a useful means of storing their health information and providing an individually held health record which could be taken to health appointments (Turner et al, 2003, p. 16).

The PMLD Network (2006) survey also sought to identify the uptake of PHPs for people with PIMD; 46% of people who responded to the survey said that the person/people they support have a PHP. Although substantial this means that 54% of people do not have a PHP. The implications of this are likely to be that health issues remain unidentified and continue as unmet health needs, this affords the possibility of a substantial and detrimental impact on the health and well-being of the person concerned.

There is a risk that services return to a former expectation, when specialist health services or families lead on the implementation of health initiatives for people with

PIMD; this is despite previous guidance to primary care in *Once a Day* (NHSE, 1999) which identified how they could develop to address this imbalance.

One recommendation was that primary care teams:

> ... *support the development of personal health records ... identify patients who have difficulty in drawing attention to their needs and consider ways in which their access to health promotion might be facilitated and any health problems detected ...* (NHSE, 1999, p. 19).

Developing PHPs and delivering accessible health promotion continue to pose considerable challenges for the service development within Primary Care Trusts (PCTs).

The Department of Health (NHSE, 1999) identifies the following action that primary healthcare teams can take:

- Encourage and support people with intellectual disabilities and their carers to attend screening clinics by enabling them to access pictorial and other information and to have preparatory visits on an individual or group basis.
- Encourage local clinics and screening centres to develop their sensitivity and experience so that there is no discrimination and sufficient flexibility in their approach. Alert them to people's special needs such as disabled access facilities and longer appointment times.
- Where screening clinics are not available, services need to encourage the individual to attend local health facilities so that opportunistic health screening can take place.
- Where an individual is unable to attend the local facilities, only then should a domiciliary visit be considered. This should be carried out in consultation with the client and their community nurse (primary healthcare team or community intellectual disability team).

Our actions are to support people with PIMD to access services available to the wider population and not recreate services which are already present in an attempt to overcome service deficit. Our actions should enable, not disable.

Health screening/health checks

As previously indicated, a significant concern for people with PIMD relates to identifying health needs. In one study of a group of people with PIMD who were given a health check, 92% were found to have a previously undetected but treatable condition (Meehan et al., 1995). Provision of health checks remains an area of contention for families and service providers alike.

Matthews (1998) identified that health screening should include as shown in Table 6.1.

Once a Day (NHSE, 1999) identified that some primary care teams had established regular health checks as a way to support the person to identify and meet their health needs. The Department of Health recently strengthened its commitment for introducing comprehensive health checks for people who have an intellectual

Table 6.1 Health screening checklist.

Body measurements (height, weight, waist, etc.)	Breast health
Cervical	Circulation and breathing
Dental and oral hygiene	Digestion and elimination
Dysphagia	Ears and hearing
Epilepsy	Eyes and vision
Experience of pain	Feet
Lifestyle risks (i.e. smoking)	Medication
Menstruation/menopause	Physique and mobility
Podiatry	Sexuality
Sleep	Skin health
Testicular health	Urinary system and bowels
Weight	

Adapted from Matthews (1998).

disability by promising to review the best way to deliver this commitment (DH, 2006). The Royal College of General Practitioners (2007) stipulate that these health checks are to be comprehensive and to be able to be administered by general practitioners (GPs) and practice nurses, with support from intellectual disability community nurses if available. They advocate annual health checks for people with an intellectual disability and are currently piloting annual health checks nationally.

Respondents reported that for those who receive regular, comprehensive health checks, these checks were provided by the person's GP and/or wider primary healthcare team, including community intellectual disability nurses (PMLD Network, 2006); respondents reported an inequality in access to primary care services, in particular the lack of provision of annual health checks to people with an intellectual disability, and the lack of use of an annual health checklist as part of the reviewing process. Concerns regarding inequalities in accessing services to meet health needs of people with intellectual disabilities are widely acknowledged (Kerr et al., 2005).

Where screening services exist, people with an intellectual disability face a further challenge – when is screening required? There is no single standard applied to the various components of health screening either nationally or internationally. It is widely recognised that people with an intellectual disability attend their GP less frequently than the general population, and in acknowledgement of this *Better Metrics* (OSHA, 2006) applied the following objective:

All GPs have a system for ensuring that patients with learning disabilities are invited to attend for health screening if they have not visited the surgery in the last 3 years (OSHA, 2006, p. 111).

While a 3-year recall will reduce the possibility of people being 'lost in the system' or 'overlooked', it does not provide an adequate frequency of health screening or health assessment for people with PIMD. The PMLD Network (2002) recommends that children and adults with PMLD [PIMD] should have annual health checks and should be given priority in establishing the use of health facilitators. They state:

It would be very beneficial for people with [PIMD] to have access to regular health screening. Establishing the norm for someone with [PIMD], which can be complex in itself, will provide an important baseline in understanding the often subtle changes indicating the need for further investigation. Self injuring behaviour, loss of appetite or a decrease in interaction for example, may all be vital pieces of information indicating a change in physical or emotional well being. The role of the proposed health facilitators could be extremely useful here (PMLD Network 2002, p. 21).

Recognising the importance of identifying the patient population more accurately OSHA (2006) set the following objective: '*All GP Practices have a system for identifying patients who have a learning disability*' (2006, p. 108); subsequently the READ CODE system was introduced.

READ CODES are coded clinical terms which enable clinicians to make effective use of electronic patient record systems. These codes are used to identify symptoms, examinations, investigations, diagnoses and medication. By applying standard codes it enables more accurate reporting, auditing and research, automation of repetitive tasks, electronic communication and decision support. For people with a PIMD, the potential benefit of READ CODES relates to accurately diagnosing the intellectual disability and any presenting health conditions etc. through data analysis; it would be possible to identify the population of people with intellectual disabilities and the specific support they require, thus affording a more focused allocation of funding. With the implementation of READ CODES, there is a greater incentive for GPs to register and more accurately identify the health needs of those people registered with their practices; greater accuracy in identifying the health needs of the patient population frequently leads to increases in targeted health investment.

READ CODES work well for those individuals known to a GP; however, services are faced with a further challenge that of ensuring that all people with an intellectual disability are registered with a GP. The Royal College of General Practitioners (2007) and the Department of Health identified this deficit and set a goal that all people with an intellectual disability are to be registered with a GP by June 2004 (DH, 2001c, p. 61). Emerson et al. (2005a) identified in a survey of people with intellectual disabilities – that 99% of respondents said they were registered with a GP and 78% said they had seen their doctor in the last year. In the survey 2,898 people took part; however, their level of intellectual disability was not presented in the report. Therefore, it is difficult to ascertain to what degree these results reflect the health experience of people with PIMD.

Health facilitation

As previously indicated within this chapter, PHPs and HAPs are within and part of the PCP process. The South East PC and HAP Meeting (2005) identified that PHPs and HAPs should not be a separate set of plans but should be informed by information contained within PCP tools, that is MAPS, PATHS, personal futures plans, essential lifestyle plans, circles of support or your own form of planning.

To ensure appropriate support and facilitation is available for the development of person-centred plans, personal health profiles and health action plans, the Department of Health (DH, 2001c) tasked commissioning services to provide health facilitation.

Valuing People (DH, 2001c) stated that each person with an intellectual disability would be offered a health facilitator by 2003. The role of the health facilitator is to support people with intellectual disabilities in getting the healthcare they need. The Department of Health tasked PCTs to have a system in place to identify 1:1 health facilitators/navigators to primary care for people with intellectual disabilities and their families (OSHA, 2006, p. 110).

According to the DH:

Health Facilitation has evolved from roles developed by family carers, practitioners and others wishing to improve the health of people with [intellectual] disabilities. It has also emerged from the wishes of people with [intellectual] disabilities and their relatives and support workers who wanted someone to help support and navigate them through the NHS to access the best and most appropriate healthcare (DH, 2002a, p. 8).

They recognise that:

Health Facilitation involves both case work to help people access mainstream services and also development work within mainstream services to help all parts of the NHS to develop the necessary skills. The impetus for both is to help ensure good health care is delivered in primary and secondary care as well as by specialist [intellectual] disabilities services (DH, 2002a, p. 8).

The Department of Health identifies that the health facilitation role needs to be developed at two levels:

Level 1 – Service development work and informing planning and commissioning;
Level 2 – Person to person work with people with [intellectual] disabilities.

(DH, 2002a, p. 8)

Many health services have appointed people specifically to develop and implement health facilitation and health action plans in their local area. These roles have the responsibility to work with other health service providers to ensure that health facilitation and health action plans are successful. Despite having specific people in post to support the delivery of this initiative, a number of challenges remain in the implementation of health action plans. Several people have criticised the apparent lack of engagement from primary care services engaging in the development and delivery of HAPs.

Research into the impact of health facilitation on the health of people with an intellectual disability is increasing. Whitehead (undated) indicated that preliminary findings identify that the professional background, age, number of years of experience, and level of education of health facilitators influence the way in which they interpret their role. In her study Whitehead (undated) reports that many health facilitation posts are short term and temporary in nature; therefore, time constraints can influence the facilitators' priorities, and that poor or constantly changing management is a feature in the lives of health facilitators and affects how they see their role. Health facilitators indicate they have experienced some degree of difficulty when expected to function at both a strategic and a person-to-person level.

Whitehead identifies that there remains a degree of confusion at the person-to-person level in relation to the role of the health facilitator and the differences between healthcare and nursing care.

Through her research, Whitehead (undated) identified that health facilitators think that when working at a strategic level, they would be more effective if placed within a generic primary care environment. They are also reported as indicating that the concept of 'person centeredness' is not fully understood in relation to health action plans. Results from the study also indicate that for those living independently or with family carers there is little provision to help the person achieve and maintain healthy lifestyles. Whitehead also indicates that encouraging primary health practices to take on board the 'valuing people' targets has been for the most part ineffective. The study conducted by Whitehead focuses on the more formalised role of health facilitator and does not appear to include the experiences of friends and family members in the role of health facilitator, which remains an unexplored role.

Health facilitation is still in its infancy, there is a currently a lack of serious monitoring of the impact that health facilitation has made to date on: the health and well-being of people with intellectual disabilities; their quality of life (see Chapter 2); the primary and secondary care sector, and the commissioning process. As the provision of health facilitation increases, there is an increasing urgency for further research in this area.

Valuing people with profound intellectual and multiple disabilities

In relation to meeting the health needs of people with PIMD, the progress in implementing valuing people has been slow to address their needs.

In the review into the progress of implementation of *Valuing People*, Greig (2005a) reported that there was evidence of excellent work to address health inequalities at a local level. Areas of particular note include the following: local plans for improving peoples' health, led by PCTs and developed through partnership boards; initiatives where the health needs of people with intellectual disabilities are considered as part of all mainstream health plans; health action planning being linked in with PCP; and increased government spending on the National Health Service (NHS) is being used to benefit people with intellectual disabilities. Further positive developments include the introduction of health checks for those who have not seen a GP for 3 years (DH, 2004, p. 27) and the expectation that GP practices make sure that people with a learning disability are not left out of screening pro-grammes (DH, 2005, p. 34). Greig (2005a) identified that the needs of people with intellectual disabilities are usually not thought about when the NHS's main priorities are being delivered, and that NHS strategy and planning as a whole frequently remains unsupported by senior managers. The report indicated that this lack of support and planning and perceived lack of priority is due to a result of several key deficits:

- The decision not to include the *Valuing People* health targets in the NHS's 'must do' targets makes those targets 'optional' for senior managers.
- Lack of data collection and performance indicators about NHS performance on intellectual disabilities to check up on how people are doing.
- Intellectual disabilities not prioritised in the GP contract, so it is difficult for PCTs to put pressure on GPs to do more.

The progress of local authority and NHS services in England, delivering the targets laid down in *Valuing People*, was further scrutinised in a report entitled *Valuing People – What Do the Numbers Tell Us?*[2] (Greig, 2005b). With regards to progress in addressing health needs, the report paints a gloomy picture stating:

> *We found no information about the health of people with* [intellectual] *disabilities. We know that people have worse health than the general population, but we don't know whether things are getting better* (Greig, 2005b, p. 15).

It is disappointing that there is so little evidence of measurable progress in addressing the health inequalities faced by people with PIMD; however, it is heartening to see that services are continuing to develop roles and systems to support such a vulnerable group of people.

Conclusion

This chapter has identified many challenges in meeting the health needs of people with PIMD. There are many tools which can be utilised in planning and delivering person-centred care – remember the strength is in the plan! Profiles can help us to document the health needs of the person; the strength in these tools is their accuracy. An out-of-date profile poses a risk to the person, whilst an up-to-date profile is a useful and valuable tool to inform others in meeting the person's health needs. Health action plans draw all the health planning aspects together. HAPs are most valuable when they are reviewed and updated regularly, a minimum of once a year. The strength of the HAP is in the action which is implemented to meet the identified health need. Finally, the chapter identified the role of health facilitator

---

[2] The report analysed statistical data about people with intellectual disabilities collected by the government from councils and the NHS across England, and statistical data sent by local councils to the Commission for Social Care Inspection. The report only considered data for England.

as health facilitators. We are in a privileged position, where we will be expected to advocate for the person with PIMD. As health facilitators we are ideally placed to work collaboratively with other agencies to ensure the voice of the person with PIMD is heard. We have the opportunity to inform and influence at many levels, including service commissioning, development and delivery, to improve the quality of life for people with PIMD.

Further reading

Hogg, J., Sebba, J., & Lambe, L. (1990). *Profound Retardation and Multiple Impairment: Medical and Physical Care and Management*, Vol. 3. London: Chapman & Hall.

Lacey, P., & Ouvry, C. (eds) (1998). *People with Profound and Multiple Learning Disabilities: A Collaborative Approach to Meeting Complex Needs*. London: Fulton.

Michael, J. (2008). *Healthcare for All: Independent Inquiry into Access to Healthcare for People with Learning Disabilities*. Available at: http://www.iahpld.org.uk/ (accessed 22 July 2008).

Samuel, J. (1997). *The Ignored Minority: Meeting the Specialist Health Needs of People with Profound Learning Disability*. Oxford: Oxfordshire Learning Disability NHS Trust.

Sanderson, H., Kennery, J., Ritchie, P., & Godwin, G. (1997). *People, Plans and Possibilities*. Edinburgh: Scottish Human Services Trust.

Person-centred planning

DH (2002). *Planning with People: Accessible Guide*. Available at: http://www.publications. doh.gov.uk/learningdisabilities/planning.htm (accessed 1 October 2007).

McNally, S. (2006). Person centred planning in intellectual disability nursing. In Gates, B. (ed.) *Care Planning and Delivery in Intellectual Disability Nursing*. Oxford: Blackwell Publishing; 68–84.

O'Brien, J., & O'Brien, C.L. (eds) (1998). *A Little Book about Person Centred Planning*. Toronto: Inclusion Press.

Reid, D., Everson, J., & Green, C. (1999). A systematic evaluation of preferences identified through person-centered planning for people with profound multiple disabilities. *Journal of Applied Behavior Analysis*, 32(4), 467–477.

Routledge, M., & Sanderson, H. (2001). *Planning with People – Towards Person Centred Approaches: Guidance for Implementation Groups*. Available at: http://www.dh.gov.uk/ assetRoot/04/05/96/00/04059600.pdf (accessed 1 October 2007).

Routledge, M., & Gitsham, N. (2004). Putting person-centred planning in its proper place? *Tizard Learning Disability Review*, 9(3), 21–26.

Sanderson, H. (2002). *A Plan Is Not Enough – Exploring the Development of Person Centred Teams*. Available at: http://www.nwtdt. com/Archive/pcp/docs/planne3.pdf (accessed 1 October 2007).

Sanderson, H. (2000). *Person Centred Planning: Key Features and Approaches*. Available at: http://www.paradigm-uk.org/pdf/Articles/helensandersonpaper.pdf (accessed 1 October 2007).

Sanderson, H., Jones, E., & Brown, K. (2002). Active support and person-centred planning: strange bedfellows or ideal partners? *Tizard Learning Disability Review*, 7(1), 31–38.

Smull, M., & Allen Shea & Associates (ASA) (2001). *Listen, Learn, Plan: A Guide for Developing Preliminary Essential Lifestyle Plans*. Available at: http://www.nwtdt. com/Archive/pcp/individual.pdf (accessed 1 November 2007).

Sweeney, C., & Helen Sanderson, H. (2002). *Factsheet – Person Centred Planning*. Available at: http://www.bild.org.uk/pdfs/05faqs/pcp.pdf (accessed 30 June 2008).

Thompson, J. (2004). Person centred planning and professional workshops. *Learning Disability Practice*, 7(1), 12–13.

Health action planning

DH (2004). *Health Action Plans*. Available at: http://www.dh.gov.uk/en/Policyandguidance/Healthandsocialcaretopics/Learningdisabilities/DH_4001807 (accessed 1 October 2007).

McCoubrie, M., Hollins, S., & Beckmann, R. (2006). *Health Action Plans: Some Guidelines for General Practitioners and Primary Care Teams*. Available at: http://www.intellectualdisability.info/how_to/HAPs.htm (accessed 1 October 2007).

Health profiling

Carey, J., & Smith, C. (1997). *Individual Health Profile*. Oxford: Oxfordshire Learning Disability NHS Trust.

Hutchinson, C. (1998). Positive health: a collective responsibility. In Lacey, P., & Ouvry, C. (eds) *People with Profound and Multiple Learning Disabilities: A Collaborative Approach to Meeting Complex Needs*. London: Fulton; 1–14.

Matthews, D., & Hegarty, J. (1997). The 'OK' health check: a health assessment checklist for people with learning disabilities. *British Journal of Learning Disabilities*, 25(4), 138–143.

Oxleas National Health Service Trust (2004). *Personal Health Profile*. Available at: http://91.186.163.216/patientinfo/php.html (accessed 1 October 2007).

Poxton, R., Greig, R., & Giraud Saunders, A. (2001). *Best Value Reviews of Learning Disability Services for Adults: A Framework for Applying Person Centred Principles*. Available at: http://www.dh.gov.uk/assetRoot/04/07/55/71/04075571.pdf (accessed 1 October 2007).

Health facilitation

Caan, W., Lutchmiah, J., Thomson, K., & Toocaram, J. (2005). Health facilitation in primary care. *Primary Health Care Research and Development*, 6(4), 348–355.

DH (2002). *Action for Health – Health Action Plans and Health Facilitation Detailed Good Practice Guidance on Implementation for Learning Disability Partnership Boards*. Available at: http://www.dh.gov.uk/assetRoot/04/07/96/50/04079650.pdf (accessed 1 October 2007).

Mir, G., Allgar, V., Cottrell, D., Heywood, P., Evans, J., & Marshall, J. (2007). *Health Facilitation and Learning Disability*. Available at: http://www.leeds.ac.uk/hsphr/hsc/documents/HF&LD.pdf (accessed 1 October 2007).

Thompson, J., & Pickering, S. (2001). (eds) *Meeting the Health Needs of People Who Have a Learning Disability*. Edinburgh: Baillière Tindall.

Useful websites

Essential Lifestyle Planning – http://www.allenshea. com/
ELP Learning Community – http://www.elpnet.net

Inclusion – http://www.inclusion. com/
Person Centered Planning – http://www.inclusive-solutions. com/pcplanning.asp
Social Role Valorization – http://www.diligio. com/srv_sites.htm

References

Blue-Banning, M., Turnbull, A., & Pereiara, L. (2000). Group action planning as a support strategy for Hispanic families: parent and professional perspectives. *Mental Retardation*, 38, 262–275.

Butterworth, J., Hagner, D., Heikkinen, B., DeMello, S., & McDonough, K. (1993). *Wholelife planning: A guide for organisers and facilitators*. Boston: Children's Hospital, Institute for Community Inclusion.

Circles Network (2005). *What Is Person Centred Planning?* Available at: http://www. circlesnetwork.org.uk/what_is_person_centred_planning.htm (accessed 27 June 2007).

Clark, J., & Gates, B. (2006). Care planning and delivery for people with profound intellectual disabilities and complex needs. In Gates, B. (ed.) *Care Planning and Delivery in Intellectual Disability Nursing*. Oxford: Blackwell Publishing; 277– 302.

DH (2001a). *Planning with People: Guidance for Implementation Groups*. London: Department of Health.

DH (2001b). *The Essence of Care: Patient-focused Benchmarking for Heath Care Practitioners*. London: HMSO.

DH (2001c). *Valuing People: A New Strategy for Learning Disability for the 21st Century CM5086*. London: HMSO.

DH (2002a). *Action for Health – Health Action Plans and Health Facilitation Detailed Good Practice Guidance on Implementation for Learning Disability Partnership Boards*. Available at: http://www.dh.gov.uk/assetRoot/04/07/96/50/04079650.pdf (accessed 1 October 2007).

DH (2002b). *Planning with People – Accessible Guide*. Available at: http://www.publications. doh.gov.uk/learningdisabilities/planning.htm#approaches (accessed 1 October 2007).

DH (2004). *Valuing People: Moving Forward Together HC507*. London: HMSO.

DH (2005). *Valuing People: Making Things Better cm6700*. London: HMSO.

DH (2006). *Our Health, Our Care, Our Say: A New Direction for Community Services. Cm 6737*. Available at: http://www.dh.gov.uk/assetRoot/04/12/74/76/04127476.pdf (accessed 12 September 2006).

Emerson, E., & Hatton, C. (1994). *Moving Out: The Effect of the Move from Hospital to Community on the Quality of Life for People with Learning Difficulties and Challenging Behaviour*. London: HMSO.

Emerson, E., Malam, S., Davies, I., & Spencer, K. (2005a). *Adults with Learning Difficulties in England 2003/4: Final and Summary Reports*. Available at: http://www.dh.gov.uk/en/ PublicationsAndStatistics/PublishedSurvey/ListOfSurveySince1990/GeneralSurveys/ DH_4081207 (accessed 1 October 2007).

Emerson, E., Routledge, R., Robertson, J., Sanderson, H., McIntosh, B., Swift, P., Joyce, T., Oakes, P., Towers, C., Hatton, C., Romeo, R., & Knapp, M.,(2005b). *The Impact of Person Centred Planning*. Available at: http://www.lancs.ac.uk/fass/ihr/publications/ ericemerson/the_impact_of_person_centred_planning_final_report.pdf (accessed 1 October 2007).

Fitton, P. (1994). *Listen to Me: Communicating the Needs of People with Profound Intellectual and Multiple Disabilities*. London: Jessica Kingsley Publishers.

Forest, M., & Pearpoint, J. (1992). MAPS: action planning. In: Pearpoint, J., Forest, M., & Snow, J. (eds) *The Inclusion Papers: Strategies to Make Inclusion Work*. Toronto: Inclusion Press; 52–56.

Grieg, R. (2005a). *Valuing People Review … The Story So Far*. Available at: *http:// valuingpeople.gov.uk/echo/filedownload.jsp?action = dFile&key = 3* (accessed 1 November 2007).

Grieg, R. (2005b). *Valuing People – What Do the Numbers Tell Us?* Available at: http:// valuingpeople.gov.uk/echo/filedownload.jsp?action = dFile&key = 6 (accessed 1 November 2007).

Howatson, J. (2005). Health action plans for people with learning disabilities. *Nursing Standard*, 19(43), 51–57.

Kendrick, M.J. (2004). Some predictable cautions concerning the over emphasis and over-reliance on person-centred planning. *BILD Bulletin*, 134/4.

Kerr, M., Felce, D., & Felce, J. (2005). *Equal Treatment: Closing the Gap: Final Report from the Welsh Centre for Learning Disabilities to the Disability Rights Commission.* Available at: http://www.leeds.ac.uk/disability-studies/archiveuk/kerr/Wales_learning_disability_study.pdf (accessed 1 November 2007).

Kinsella, P. (2000). *What Are the Barriers in Relation to Person Centred Planning?* Wirral: Paradigm.

Mansell, J., & Beadle-Brown, J. (2004). Person-centred planning or person-centred action? Policy and practice in intellectual disability services. *Journal of Applied Research in Intellectual Disabilities*, 17(1), 1–9.

Matthews, D.R. (1998). The OK way to keep track of clients' health needs. *Nursing Times*, 94(16), 52–53.

McNally, S. (2007). Helping to empower people. In Gates, B. (ed.) *Learning Disabilities: Towards Inclusion* (5th edition). Edinburgh: Elsevier; 599–617.

Meehan, S., Moore, G., & Barr, O. (1995). Specialist services for people with learning disabilities. *Nursing Times*, 91(13), 33–35.

Mount, B., & Zwernick, K. (1988). *It's Never too Early. It's Never too Late: A Booklet About Personal Futures Planning for Persons with Developmental Disabilities, Their Families and Friends, Case Managers, Service Providers, and Advocates*. St. Paul, MN: Metropolitan Council.

NHSE (1999). *Once a Day*. Available at: http://www.dh.gov.uk/assetRoot/04/04/27/79/ 04042779.pdf (accessed 1 October 2007).

O'Brien, J. (1987). A guide to life style planning: I'sing the activities catalog to integrate services and natural support systems. In Wilcox, B., & Bellamy, G.T. (eds) *A Comprehensive Guide to the Activities Catalog*. Baltimore: Brookes; 175–189.

O'Brien, J., & Towell, D. (2003). *Person Centred Planning in Its Strategic Context*. Available at: http://thechp.syr.edu/PCPStrategy.pdf (accessed 1 October 2007).

Office of the Strategic Health Authorities (OSHA) (2006). *The 'BETTER METRICS' Project Better Metrics Version 7*. Available at: http://www.osha.nhs.uk/infoexchange/ doc.aspx?id_Content = 713 (accessed 12 September 2006).

Pearpoint, J., Kahn, L., & Hollands, C. (undated). *Planning Tools*. Available at: http://www.inclusion. com/planningtools.html (accessed 1 October 2007).

Pearpoint, J., O'Brien, J., & Forest, M. (1993). *Path: A Workbook for Planning Possible Positive Futures: Planning Alternative Tomorrows with Hope for Schools, Organizations, Businesses, Families*. Toronto: Inclusion Press.

PMLD Network (2002). *Valuing People with Profound and Multiple learning Disabilities*. Available at: http://www.pmldnetwork.org/vppmldreport.pdf (accessed 1 October 2007).

PMLD Network (2006). *PMLD Network Questionnaire 2006 (on the Difference Valuing People Has Made to the Lives of Children and Adults with Profound and Multiple Learning Disabilities Since Its Launch in 2001)*. Paper presented at Learning Disability Today, London, 22 November.

Sanderson, H., Jones, E., & Brown, K. (2002). Active support and person centred planning: strange bedfellows or ideal partners? *Tizard Learning Disability Review*, 7(1), 31–38.

Sanderson, H., & Smull, M. (2005). *Person Centred Thinking and Planning*. Available at: http://elpnet.net/documents/pctandplanning.pdf (accessed 1 October 2007).

Smull, M.W., & Harrison, S. (1992). *Supporting People with Severe Reputations in the Community*. Alexandria, VA: National Association of State Mental Retardation Program Directors.

The Royal College of General Practitioners (2007). *Learning Disability Annual Health Check Audit*. Available at: http://www.rcgp.org.uk/continuing_the_gp_journey/circ/clinical_task_groups/learning_disabilities/work_and_projects/examples_of_annual_h_checks.aspx#LDHealthCheckAudit (accessed 1 October 2007).

Turk, V., & Burchell, S. (2003). Developing and evaluating personal health records for adults with learning disabilities. *Tizard Learning Disability Review*, 8(4), 33–41.

Turnbull, A., & Turnbull, H. (1996). Group action planning as a strategy for providing comprehensive family support. In Koegel, L.K., Koegel, R.L., & Dunlap, G., (eds) *Positive Behavior Support: Including People with Difficult Behavior in the Community*. Baltimore: Brookes; 99–114.

Turner, J., Gallop, J., Miller, R., Gray, G., & Chapman, S. (2003). *Access to Primary Health Care Project*. Oxford: Ridgeway Partnership (Oxfordshire Learning Disability NHS Trust).

Vandercook, T., York, J., & Forest, M. (1989). The McGill action planning system: a strategy for building a vision. *Journal of the Association for People with Severe Handicaps*, 14(3), 205–215.

Walton, S., Bedford, H., & Dezateux, C. (2006). Use of personal child health records in the UK: findings from the millennium cohort study. *British Medical Journal*, 332(7536), 269–270.

Webb, T., & Sanderson, H. (2002). What is person centred planning? *BILD Bulletin*, 134(1), 1–3.

Whitehead, G. (undated). *A Phenomenological Examination of the Role of Health Facilitation in Learning Disability Service*. Available at: http://www.hapresearch.cswebsites.org/default.aspx?page = 12942 (accessed 1 October 2007).

Wilkinson, J. (2001). *Nursing Process and Critical Thinking* (3rd edition). New Jersey: Prentice Hall Health.

Chapter 7

CLINICAL ASSESSMENT OF PEOPLE WITH PROFOUND INTELLECTUAL AND MULTIPLE DISABILITIES[1]

Steven Carnaby

Introduction

The task of assessing people with profound intellectual and multiple disabilities can be a daunting one, for experienced and newly qualified clinicians and practitioners alike. This chapter discusses a range of concerns and stresses the importance of collaborative working while also acknowledging that services can be ill-equipped to face the challenges presented by people with such complex and chronic support needs. Some recommendations are made for developing good practice in this crucial area of the support process.

Who are we talking about?

People with profound intellectual and multiple disabilities form a small but significant section of the wider population of people with intellectual disabilities. While *DSM-IV* (APA, 1994) states that *'the group with profound mental retardation* [sic] *constitutes approximately 1%–2% of people with mental retardation'*, in practice, prevalence is difficult to establish, as figures vary with the type of definitions adopted. The definitions of profound intellectual disability most often cited include having an IQ of below 20 (WHO, 1992), below 20–25 (*DSM-IV*, APA, 1994), or functioning with an IQ estimated to be five standard deviations from the norm (Hogg & Sebba, 1987). Ware (1996) suggests that people with a profound learning disability have a *'degree of learning difficulty so severe that they are functioning at a developmental level of two years or less (in practice well under a year)'*. Clinically, Ware's approach is potentially the most valuable.

---

[1] This chapter is based on Carnaby, S. (2007). Developing good practice in the clinical assessment of people with profound intellectual disabilities and multiple impairment. *Journal of Policy and Practice in Intellectual Disabilities*.

Profound intellectual and multiple disabilities can often be traced to extensive damage that results from what are often identifiable neurological conditions (APA, 1994). Individuals may experience any one or more of severe physical disability, severe visual impairment, severe hearing impairment, epilepsy and other complex health conditions for which medication is usually required, for example, chronic pulmonary disease (Hogg, 1992). There may also be impairments in the ability to detect touch, pressure, temperature and pain (e.g. Oberlander et al., 1999). It has become increasingly apparent that people with profound intellectual and multiple disabilities may also experience mental health problems (see Chapter 8), probably as a result of their lifestyles (e.g. Chaney, 1996; Matson , 1997).

For the practitioner, this results in the need for a highly individualised approach that relies heavily on reflective practice as a way of determining appropriate strategies for meeting needs. The potential range of clinical issues can be alarming for anybody initiating assessment. Unfortunately, this situation is likely to be compounded by dominant discourses in service culture. In Britain at least, the vagaries that still exist with regard to identifying people with profound intellectual and multiple disabilities have had a direct impact on the ways in which services approach the development of support for individuals and their families. Inconsistencies in both attitude and knowledge mean that services may not be willing to identify people with profound intellectual and multiple disabilities as a separate target group requiring specific attention or indeed be aware that such a distinction might be necessary (PMLD Network, 2002). Without a consistent strategy, staff providing direct support to individuals using services are unlikely to have the necessary skills or be able to access appropriate training for working with people with such complex needs. In addition, family members will not in turn have been supported to understand and appreciate their relative's disabilities, a phenomenon that has previously been supported by research (e.g. Hogg et al., 1990).

Given these uncertainties, the premise here is that effective clinical support demands careful assessment procedures, which need to be conducted with as much rigour as possible. The remainder of this chapter discusses the key issues relating to assessment as foundation for any provision, concluding with some recommendations for developing best practice in this challenging area.

The context of assessment

Cave (2002, p. 48), citing Kendall & Norton-Ford (1982), states that '*clinical assessment is the process of gathering information about a client in order to gain a better understanding of the person*'. She suggests that clinical assessment is carried out for three main reasons – diagnosis and screening, the evaluation of therapeutic interventions and for research purposes – and identifies the three main elements of the assessment process as clinical interview, observation and the use of standardised tests or measures.

However, Clements (2002) stresses the importance of setting an assessment 'agenda', and it is important to appreciate the context within which assessment is to be conducted. Here 'context' is discussed in terms of both service philosophy and service organisation.

Service philosophy

Normalisation and its emphasis on ordinary living and age appropriateness is clearly a powerful framework within which care staff and other supporters can work effectively to promote independence, respect and real choice in the lives of people with intellectual disabilities.

However, there are risks around using this approach without due care when working with people with profound and multiple intellectual disabilities. The need to treat people with respect and dignity can be solely interpreted as treating people of 18 years and over as adults, regardless of their level of cognitive development. Practitioners working with a focus on developmental functioning have challenged this approach. They argue that placing an emphasis on chronological age over and above an appreciation of an individual's developmental level of functioning can lead to an overestimation of their abilities – and the provision of inappropriate support as a consequence (Bartlett & Bunning, 1997). Indeed, other authors suggest that acknowledging and working with an individual's developmental level of functioning is the only way to work with respect and dignity (e.g. Nind & Hewett, 1996; see also Chapter 5).

Further weight is added to the argument for conceptualising the support needs of adults and young people with profound intellectual disabilities in this way by examining the scientific literature. Evidence presented by Hodapp (1995) suggests that everybody – regardless of any level of organic brain damage endured – progresses through the same sequence of developmental stages. Known as the 'similar-sequence' hypothesis, this conclusion is based on wide-ranging reviews of the literature (Weisz & Zigler, 1979; Weisz et al., 1982, cited in Hodapp et al., op cit.). Assessment, intervention and the overall approach to service provision surely then needs to progress in ways that acknowledge an individual's developmental level of functioning, 'joining' that person so that what is offered is meaningful, stimulating, personally relevant and designed to encourage development at that individual's pace.

Bunning (2003) highlights the importance of interpreting service philosophy carefully when working with people with profound intellectual disabilities, suggesting that inflexible adoption of O'Brien's (e.g. O'Brien & Tyne, 1981; Emerson, 1992) familiar five service accomplishments can lead to negative experiences for this population.

Organisational issues

In thinking about the demands placed upon organisations when faced with such breadth and depth of clinical issues, Orelove & Sobsey (1996) discuss three main models of discipline-based team organisation: multidisciplinary, interdisciplinary and transdisciplinary working. The main conclusion is that the challenge of working with people with multiple disabilities demands careful thought about the systemic nature of assessment and intervention and how it is organised.

Traditional assessment processes are likely to be discipline led. Relatives, carers or other supporters are likely to make a referral to a specialist team as a result of an observed 'problem' or issue. Whilst some services may take a more proactive approach and conduct assessment of people with complex disabilities as a matter of course, it is more likely that involvement of specialist health and social care services results from a specific concern or change in the individual's behaviour.

Community teams in Britain working with people with intellectual disabilities are required to provide a range of therapeutic services aimed at addressing difficulties faced by individuals in daily living or enhancing quality of life more generally. This is likely to be within a multidisciplinary approach. Depending on the nature of the issues in question, this input is provided by professionals trained in different disciplines including physiotherapy, occupational therapy, clinical psychology and speech and language therapy. Referrals to the team can be made by the individuals with intellectual disabilities themselves in some cases, but are more often made by carers and families, general practitioners or other professionals within statutory services.

However, any process of clinical assessment will rely heavily on a service's ability to recognise the 'case' in the first place (Moss, 1999). Where there exists both confusion over definition and lack of understanding with regard to the impact on functioning, people with profound intellectual disabilities may not always be visible (or regarded as 'high profile') within the clinical referral system. In addition, referrals for clinical input are more likely to concern 'challenging' behaviours, or for support with skills development. Anecdotal evidence from clinicians working with people with intellectual disabilities suggests that people with profound intellectual and multiple disabilities are more likely to be referred because they are presenting specific behaviours of concern such as self-injury, inappropriate masturbation or difficulties with eating and sleeping. Issues such as self-involvement (i.e. engaging in stereotype) or social isolation are unlikely to be deemed as warranting immediate attention.

Multidisciplinary teams may well discuss the referral together, and then determine the professional best placed to conduct assessment and design an appropriate intervention ('multidisciplinary' working). Contact and assessment with the individual may lead the professional concerned to consider that other specialist input is required, and thus another (intra-team) referral is made. This forms part of a linear chain of referrals and assessments, potentially taking considerable time to complete and produce enough information to inform tangible intervention.

An alternative approach might be for professionals from different disciplines (e.g. speech and language therapy and occupational therapy) to conduct a joint assessment. Orelove & Sobsey refer to this as 'interdisciplinary' working but suggest that while assessment may indeed involve joint working, it is still likely to lead to the design of discipline-led interventions. They go on to identify a third model, termed the transdisciplinary approach. Here the assessment is more collaborative in nature, and places the individual and family at the very heart of assessment, service planning and delivery. Table 7.1 summarises and compares the three models of team working, placing assessment within this context of collaboration and cooperation.

Table 7.1 Cooperation and collaboration in teams.

	Multidisciplinary	Interdisciplinary	Transdisciplinary
Assessment	Separate assessments by team members	Separate assessments by team members	Team members and family conduct a comprehensive developmental assessment together
Parent participation	Parents meet with individual team members	Parents meet with team or team representative	Parents are full, active and participating members of the team
Service plan development	Team members develop separate plans for their discipline	Team members share their separate plans with one another	Team members and the parents develop a service plan based on family priorities, needs and resources
Service plan responsibility	Team members are responsible for implementing their section of the plan	Team members are responsible for sharing information with one another as well as for implementing their section of the plan	Team members are responsible and accountable for how the primary service provider implements the plan
Service plan implementation	Team members implement the part of the service plan related to their discipline	Team members implement their section of the plan and incorporate other sections where possible	A primary service provider is assigned to implement the plan with the family
Line of communication	Informal lines	Periodic case-specific team meetings	Regular team meeting where continuous transfer of information, knowledge and skills are shared among team members
Guiding philosophy	Team members recognise the importance of contributions from other disciplines	Team members are willing and able to develop, share and be responsible for providing services that are a part of the total service plan	Team members make a commitment to teach, learn and work together across discipline boundaries to implement unified service plan
Staff development	Independent and within their discipline	Independent within as well as outside of their discipline	An integral component of team meetings for learning across disciplines and team building

Adapted from Orelove & Sobsey (1996, pp. 13–14).

Key elements of the assessment process

Given the potential breadth and range of issues, thorough assessment of individuals with profound intellectual disabilities and multiple impairment would need to cover the following core areas: overall developmental level of functioning; communication skills; engagement and activity; hearing and vision; physical health; emotional well-being; level of parent and carer stress. This list enhances that generally recommended for assessing the wider population of people with intellectual disabilities (e.g. see Emerson et al., 1998).

Much of the information will be gathered either through direct observation or through the use of an informant. The findings from direct observation are likely to be more valid if the observation itself has been carried out in a structured, methodical manner – for example, through the use of momentary or continuous time sampling (e.g. Beasley et al., 1993). Taking regular and measured 'snapshots' of the individual's experience enables conclusions to be drawn concerning how he or she spends time, how support is offered and the range of opportunities and activities that are made available. Similarly, using video recordings can enable supporters to reflect on their assumptions about the meaning of particular behaviours, or their approach to support and facilitation. Clearly, there are consent issues to be discussed here, and care is needed in deciding if and how video recording is appropriate for any individual at any given time. Similarly, discussion should take place about where the recordings are to be stored, how they are to be used, and perhaps most importantly, for whose use they are intended. It might be argued that any use of such material that cannot be directly traced to enhancing the individual's support needs to be robustly justified.

Using an informant is also likely to lead to the gathering of key information, but it is important that the choice of informant is made carefully. Assessors need to bear in mind a range of factors such as the role that the informant plays in the individual's life, and how this might colour perceptions about the individual's abilities, needs and lifestyle more generally. Family members may well have different perceptions of an individual's skills when compared to the perceptions of direct support staff or other professionals. They may also have different expectations about what an assessment can achieve and the potential for their input to shape any interventions or supports that arise from this involvement. For these reasons, it is essential that both the purpose of the assessment is made clear to informants from the outset, and that findings are fed back to them in ways that are meaningful and relevant. Parents and carers are likely to become frustrated and disillusioned if they are requested to participate in lengthy pieces of work with little explanation and no clear positive impact on the individual's life.

Practitioners are faced with a significant dilemma when selecting standardised tools for assessment, as there are very few that are directly relevant to the lives, abilities and developmental functioning of individuals with profound intellectual disabilities and multiple impairment. The Vineland Adaptive Behaviour Scales: 2nd edition (Sparrow et al., 2005) can be used to assess functioning in the four main areas of daily living, socialisation, communication and motor skills. Items are rated according to the individual's level of competence in each case, leading to raw scores that are then converted to age equivalents. The Developmental Assessment for Individuals with Severe Disabilities (DASH-2) (Dykes & Erin, 1999) can be used by the assessor as direct observer, or by using an informant, and unlike the Vineland is specifically designed for use with adults. Either tool can provide an estimate of an individual's level of developmental function, a useful starting point for any assessment process. Studies of utility for both of these tools can be found in the existing research literature (e.g. for Vinelands Scales, see Carter et al., 1998; Beail, 2003; for DASH-2, see Matson et al., 1996; Valdovinos et al., 2004).

This then enables further assessment of other domains of functioning. Communication is possibly the most important area to explore, where approaches that emphasise the role of the communication partnership (i.e. the quality of communication perceived dynamically between two people) are most helpful (e.g. Bartlett & Bunning, 1997; Bunning, 1997; Bradshaw, 2001) (see Chapter 4). Using tools such as the *See What I Mean* or SWIM guidelines (Grove, 1999) enable those supporting individuals with profound intellectual disabilities to both develop consistent approaches in their practice and identify areas for intervention and development. Findings from the assessment can establish the extent to which supporters are overestimating or underestimating an individual's expressive and receptive communication skills. This in turn leads to recommendations for interventions such as the use of personally relevant objects of reference or the development of interactive techniques such as Intensive Interaction (Nind & Hewett, 2001) (see Chapter 5).

Assessment of mobility and posture (see Chapter 17), as well as essential health screening (e.g. specific work relating to dysphagia and epilepsy, see Chapters 9 and 14), and assessment of pain, comfort and distress (Astor, 2001; University College, London/Institute of Child Health and Royal College of Nursing Institute, 2003; Zwakhalen et al., 2004; Regnard 2007) are equally important in ensuring a thorough approach. As well as having impact on the individual's well-being, this information can provide valuable insight into personal aspects such as tolerance of particular stimuli, attention, concentration and motivation.

Formulation

Once as much information has been gathered as possible, the process of formulation can begin. This makes links between elements of what has been discovered, in order to derive hypotheses and gain understanding about the individual and how she or her experiences the world. Box 7.1 and the resulting formulation presented in Figure 7.1 illustrate the ways in which both personal and environmental information can be drawn together to develop a clearer understanding of an individual's presentation, and help to identify key areas where intervention may be necessary. This systemic formulation draws on a cognitive behavioural model of behaviour at its centre (Greenberger & Padesky, 1995). In this case, it enables the clinical team to form hypotheses about Timothy's presentation using material from what can be observed and what has been discovered about his past experiences.

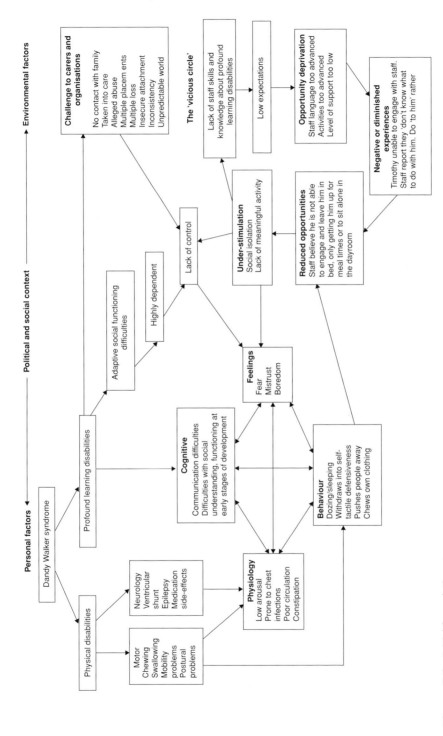

Figure 7.1 Initial formulation.

105

Box 7.1   Case study - Timothy

Timothy is a 26-year-old man with a diagnosis of Dandy-Walker syndrome. This predisposes Timothy to a range of physical disabilities and health issues, as well as profound intellectual disabilities. Timothy has moved to a semi-institutional setting, where staffing levels are low. Staff supporting Timothy have little experience in working with people with profound and multiple intellectual disabilities, and have requested input from the local community team. The issues of concern have been incidents where Timothy is pushing people away when they attempt to interact with him and a general feeling that people 'don't know what to do with him'.

   The community team has carried out a detailed assessment, beginning with Timothy's developmental level of functioning and moving on to his communication skills in more detail. A general health assessment has also been completed. A search of Timothy's file notes reveal information about his past and the settings in which he has lived, along with some of the experiences he has encountered along the way. The team compiled a diagrammatic formulation to help everybody make links between Timothy's current presentation, events from his past and the ways in which he is currently supported (see Figure 7.1). This approach enabled the community team and the direct support team to work together in getting to know Timothy on his terms, and in ways that were personally relevant and meaningful to him.

Recommendations for good practice in clinical assessment

Clinical assessment with people with profound intellectual and multiple disabilities can be an intimidating prospect, particularly for the less experienced clinician. However, clinical teams can arguably alleviate such anxieties by establishing best practice protocols and ensuring a consistent approach that fosters interdependence between clinicians from different disciplines. The following recommendations are suggested to facilitate this process.

Agree on terminology and inclusion criteria

This is an important first step, and its centrality to effective assessment cannot be overemphasised. Services need to publish their definitions and criteria for profound intellectual disability and multiple impairment, and ensure that all clinicians have a sound understanding of the agreed terms (see Chapter 1). It might also be beneficial to set up a working group, where multidisciplinary consensus can be attained through debate. Examples of this include the MDRT (multiple disability resource team) in Oxfordshire and the PMLD (profound and multiple learning disability) action group in Hackney, East London.

Take a transdisciplinary approach

The complexity of individuals' needs require an approach that is both holistic and person centred rather than discipline led. Only by developing work that transcends professional and disciplinary boundaries can clinicians be confident that the extent of the individual's strengths and needs have been properly identified. Working in this way also ensures collaboration between formal and informal carers, who together are more likely to provide the most powerful insights into the individual's daily living experience.

Use a developmental model

Finding a form of words to assist supporters to appreciate the importance of working with people developmentally can be both liberating and clinically effective, in that the development of support is not hindered by personal anxieties about age appropriateness and enables clear thinking about the issues to be addressed. Assessing an individual's developmental level of functioning is often crucial in assisting support staff to genuinely respect that individual – by 'joining' him or her in activities that are personally meaningful and relevant.

Consider the impact of neurological conditions

An individual's diagnosis needs to be thoroughly understood wherever possible (Howlin & Udwin, 2002), and regular assessment of the impact that a condition is having needs to take place. Obvious examples include syndromes that predispose individuals to chest infections, epilepsy or deterioration in function, but there may also be autistic traits or sensory impairment to consider as context for understanding a specific incident or aspect of behaviour.

Select measures and informants carefully

The relative paucity of appropriate standardised measures leaves the clinician with needing to make important decisions about the tools to be used, and often who might be best placed to act as informant. A combination of both quantitative and qualitative measures is likely to yield richer material, and where time and resources allow, a combination of informants will provide multiple perspectives on the individual's experience – a more interesting and often more reliable approach compared with relying on one person.

Assessment as an intervention

Clinicians may feel pressured to 'do' something, and hence be tempted to rush through the assessment in order to develop a tangible intervention. However, working with people with profound intellectual and multiple disabilities usually means needing to allocate a significant period of time to the assessment process, due to the breadth of material to be gathered, and this in itself might also be regarded as an intervention. Assessment often draws attention to an individual and provides focus for supporters and family members. This is turn can lead to reflection and re-evaluation of assumptions made about the individual, perhaps even shifts in thinking and understanding. The impact of this phenomenon should not be underestimated. At the very least, giving time to assessment is more likely to yield more reliable and valid data.

References

APA (1994). *Diagnostic and Statistical Manual* (4th edition). Washington, DC: American Psychiatric Association.

Astor, R. (2001). Detecting pain in people with profound learning disabilities. *Nursing Times*, 97(40), 38–39.

Bartlett, C., & Bunning, K. (1997). The importance of communication partnerships: a study to investigate the communicative exchanges between staff and adults with learning disabilities. *British Journal of Learning Disabilities*, 25, 148–152.

Beail, N. (2003). Utility of the Vineland Adaptive Behavior scales in diagnosis and research with adults who have mental retardation. *Mental Retardation*, 41(4), 286–289.

Beasley, F., Hewson, S., Mansell, J., Hughes, D., & Stein, J. (1993). *MTS Handbook for Observers*. Canterbury, Tizard Centre: University of Kent.

Bradshaw, J. (2001). Communication partnerships with people with profound and multiple learning disabilities. *Tizard Learning Disability Review*, 6(2), 6–15.

Bunning, K. (1997). The role of sensory reinforcement in developing interactions. In Fawcus, M. (ed.) *Children with Learning Difficulties: A Collaborative Approach to Their Education and Management*. London: Whurr.

Bunning, K. (2003). People with profound learning disabilities and multiple impairment. *Address to the British Psychological Society Division of Clinical Psychology Faculty for Learning Disabilities Conference*, 13th November. Voluntary Resource Centre, London.

Carter, A.S., Volkmar, F.R., Sparrow, S.S., Wang, J., Lord, C., Dawson, G., Fombonne, E., Loveland, K., Meisbov, G., & Schopler, E. (1998). The Vineland Adaptive Behavior Scales: supplementary norms for individuals with autism. *Journal of Autism and Developmental Disorders*, 28(4), 287–302.

Cave, S. (2002). Classification, assessment, diagnosis. In Cave, S. (ed.), *Classification and Diagnosis of Psychological Abnormality*. London: Routledge.

Chaney, R.H. (1996). Psychological stress in people with profound mental retardation. *Journal of Intellectual Disability Research*, 40(4), 305–310.

Clements, J. (2002). Establishing the assessment agenda. In Clements, J., & Martin, N. (eds) *Assessing Behaviours Regarded as Problematic*. London: Jessica Kingsley.

Dykes, M.K., & Erin, J. (1999). *DASH-2: An Assessment and Programming Instrument for Individuals with Severe Disabilities* (2nd edition). Austin, TX: Pro-Ed.

Emerson, E. (1992). What is normalisation? In Brown, H., & Smith, H. (eds), *Normalisation: A Reader for the Nineties*. London: Routledge.

Emerson, E., Hatton, C., Bromley, J., & Caine, A. (eds) (1998). *Clinical Psychology and People with Intellectual Disabilities*. Chichester: John Wiley & Sons.

Greenberger, K., & Padesky, C. (1995). *Mind over Mood*. New York: Guilford Press.

Grove, N. Bunning, K., Porter, J., & Olsson, C. (1999). See what I mean: interpreting the meaning of communication by people with severe and profound intellectual disabilities. *Journal of Applied Research in Intellectual Disabilities*, 12(3), 190–203.

Hodapp, R.M., Burack, J.A., & Zigler, E. (1995). The developmental perspective in the field of mental retardation. In Hodapp, R.M., Burack, J.A., & Zigler, E. (eds), *Issues in the Developmental Approach to Mental Retardation*. Cambridge: Cambridge University Press.

Hogg, J. (1992). The administration of psychotropic and anticonvulsant drugs to children with profound intellectual disability and multiple impairments. *Journal of Intellectual Disability Research*, 36, 473–488.

Hogg, J., & Sebba, J. (1987). *Profound Retardation and Multiple Impairment: Development and Learning*. London: Croom-Helm.

Hogg, J., Sebba, J., & Lambe, L., (1990). *Profound Mental Retardation and Multiple Impairment: Vol. 1 – Development and Learning*. London: Croom-Helm.

Howlin, P., & Udwin, O. (eds) (2002). *Preface to Outcomes in Neurodevelopmental and Genetic Disorders*. Cambridge: Cambridge University Press.

Kendall, P., & Norton-Ford, J. (1982). *Clinical Psychology*. London: John Wiley & Sons.

Matson, J.L., Baglio, C.S., Smiroldo, B.B., Hamilton, M., Packlowskyj, T., Williams, D., & Kirkpatrick-Sanchez, S. (1996). Characteristics of autism as assessed by the diagnostic assessment for the severely handicapped-II (DASH-II). *Research in Developmental Disabilities*, 17, 135–143.

Matson, J.L., Smiroldo, B.B., Hamilton, M., & Baglio, C.S. (1997). Do anxiety disorders exist in persons with severe and profound mental retardation? *Research in Developmental Disabilities*, 18(1), 39–44.

Moss, S. (1999). Assessment: conceptual issues. In Bouras, N. (ed.), *Psychiatric and Behavioural Disorders in Developmental Disabilities and Mental Retardation*. Cambridge: Cambridge University Press.

Nind, M., & Hewett, D. (1996). When age-appropriateness isn't appropriate. In Coupe O'Kane, J., & Goldbart, J. (eds) *Whose Choice? Contentious Issues for Those Working with People with Learning Difficulties*. London: David Fulton.

Nind, M., & Hewett, D. (2001). *A Practical Guide to Intensive Interaction*. Kidderminster: British Institute of Learning Disabilities.

Oberlander, T.F., O'Donell, M.E., & Montgomery, C.J. (1999). Pain in children with significant neurological impairment. *Journal of Developmental and Behavioural Paediatrics*, 20, 235–243.

O'Brien, J., & Tyne, A. (1981). *The Principle of Normalisation: A Foundation for Effective Services*. London: The Campaign for Mentally Handicapped People.

Orelove, F.P., & Sobsey, D. (eds) (1996). *Educating Children with Multiple Disabilities: A Transdisciplinary Approach*. Baltimore: Paul H. Brookes.

PMLD Network (2002). *Valuing People with Profound and Multiple Learning Disabilities (PMLD)*. Published by the PMLD Network through MENCAP, London.

Regnard, C., Reynolds, J., Watson, B., Matthews, D., Gibson, L., & Clarke, C. (2007). Understanding distress in people with severe communication difficulties: developing and assessing the disability distress assessment tool (DisDAT). *Journal of Intellectual Disability Research*, 51(4), 277–292.

Sparrow, S., Balla, D.A., & Cicchetti, D.V. (2005). *Vineland Adaptive Behaviour Scales (2nd edition). Interview Edition (expanded form)*. Circle Pines, MN: American Guidance Service.

University College, London/ Institute of Child Health and Royal College of Nursing Institute (2003). *Paediatric Pain Profile*. London: University College, London/ Institute of Child Health and Royal College of Nursing Institute.

Valdovinos, M.G., Zarcone, J.R., Hellings, J.A., Kim, G., & Schroeder, S.R. (2004). Using the diagnostic assessment of the severely handicapped-II (DASH-II) to measure the therapeutic effects of Risperidone. *Journal of Intellectual Disability Research*, 48(1), 53–59.

Ware, J. (1996). *Creating Responsive Environments for People with Profound Learning and Multiple Disabilities*. London: David Fulton.

Weisz, J., Yeates, K., & Zigler, E. (1982). Piagetian evidence and the developmental-difference controversy. In Zigler, E., & Balla, D. (eds) *Mental Retardation: The Developmental-Difference Controversy*. Hillsdale, NJ: Erlbaum.

Weisz, J., & Zigler, E. (1979). Cognitive development in retarded and non-retarded persons: piagetian tests of the similar sequence hypothesis. *Psychological Bulletin*, 86, 831–851.

WHO (1992). *The ICD-10 Classification of Mental and Behavioural Disorders: Clinical Descriptions and Diagnostic Guidelines*. Geneva: World Health Organisation.

Zwakhalen, S.M.G., van Dongen, K.A.J., Hamers, J.P.H., & Huijer Abu-Saad, H. (2004). Pain assessment in intellectually disabled people: non-verbal indicators. *Journal of Advanced Nursing*, 45(3), 236–245.

MEETING COMPLEX NEEDS

Chapter 8

MENTAL HEALTH PROBLEMS AND PEOPLE WITH PROFOUND INTELLECTUAL AND MULTIPLE DISABILITIES

Steven Carnaby

Introduction

The coexistence of intellectual disabilities and mental health problems, referred to as 'dual diagnosis' in the research literature, has attracted much interest in recent years (Sturmey et al., 2007) following a relatively late initial recognition around 1980 (Holden & Gitlesen, 2004). Studies exploring prevalence rates of psychiatric disorder in people with intellectual disabilities suggest an increased risk (e.g. Emerson, 2003), and much thought has been given to the vulnerability factors likely to be underpinning this phenomenon (Emerson, 2003; Hatton & Emerson, 2004). However, controversies about both the ways in which these conclusions have been reached (Whitaker & Read, 2006) as well as the conceptualisation of psychiatric disorder and its relationship with behaviour problems in people with severe and profound intellectual disabilities remains (e.g. Rojahn et al., 2004). The key ideas relevant to these controversies are discussed in this chapter as part of a brief overview of the literature on dual diagnosis and its relevance to people with profound intellectual disabilities. Implications for clinical practice and service provision are also considered.

Learning objectives

By the end of this chapter, readers will:

- understand the concepts of 'dual diagnosis' and 'diagnostic overshadowing' and the particular vulnerabilities of people with intellectual disabilities to poor mental health;
- be aware of the debate around assessment of poor mental health in people with intellectual disabilities;
- be more familiar with the presentation of mental health problems in people with intellectual disabilities; and

- be able to think about the implications of these concepts and phenomena for people with profound intellectual and multiple disabilities.

Mental health and mental health problems

According to the Health Education Authority (1997), mental health is the emotional and spiritual resilience which enables us to enjoy life and to survive pain, suffering and disappointment – a positive sense of well-being and an underlying belief in our own and others' dignity and worth. Being more than absence of illness, our mental health influences how we think and feel about ourselves and others, how we interpret events, our capacity to learn and communicate and to form and sustain relationships, and affects our ability to cope with change. People who have mental health problems experience changes in their thoughts, behaviours and emotions. Mental health is central to all health, because how we think and feel has a strong impact on our physical health (Holt et al., 2005).

Emerging 'mental health in intellectual disabilities' paradigm

The relatively late recognition of the importance of mental health in intellectual disabilities could be attributed to five main factors:

- Firstly, the separateness of mental health and intellectual disability services had resulted in service users in each directorate being seen as a discrete group, preventing an integrated model of training, assessment and treatment.
- This is perhaps linked to a second factor, the absence of adequate referral systems to mental health services. In the general population, people are referred to mental health services when they are having problems fulfilling social roles (Goldberg & Huxley, 1980); people with intellectual disabilities are more likely not to have such roles ascribed or available to them, and the onset of mental health problems can easily be ignored.

The other three factors all pertain to the assessment and diagnosis of mental health difficulties:

- People with intellectual disabilities are difficult to assess, as they are likely to find it more difficult to provide information about their internal mental state (see Moss, 1999).
- It is then of little surprise that 'diagnostic shadowing' occurs, where symptoms of mental illness are falsely attributed to intellectual disability itself (e.g. Mason & Scior, 2004).
- In addition, differential diagnosis between mental disorder and challenging behaviour is often poor (e.g. Bouras & Drummond, 1992).

Together, these observations have led to a 'mental health in intellectual disabilities' paradigm (Holt et al., 2005), which accepts and emphasises the emotional lives of people with intellectual disabilities and advocates that special attention is given to identifying support needs.

Prevalence of mental health problems in people with an intellectual disability

Research reported over the last few decades has led to a growing consensus that people with intellectual disabilities are more vulnerable to developing psychiatric disorders compared with the general population (e.g. Borthwick-Duffy, 1994; Moss, 2001; Chaplin, 2004; Mason & Scior, 2004). The literature contains a range of studies utilising many different methods of assessment, and their findings do not readily correspond to *Diagnostic and Statistical Manual* or ICD (International Statistical Classification of Diseases and Related Health Problems) criteria (Sturmey, 1993). Studies on unselected populations are more widely respected, but still appear fraught with methodological problems and inconsistencies. Rutter et al. (1970) studied the entire age group of 9- to 11-year-old children on the Isle of Wight, diagnosing psychiatric disorder in 7% of the total cohort, but in 30–42% of children with an IQ below 70. No measures of adaptive behaviour, as advocated in *DSM-IV*, were reported. Koller et al.(1983) conducted a longitudinal study of people with intellectual disabilities, collecting retrospective data to indicate that 60% had a behavioural disorder in childhood – but it is unclear whether these disorders met diagnostic criteria to be categorised as psychiatric disorders. Birch et al. (1970) established prevalence rates of 40% in those with severe intellectual disabilities compared with 10% in the non-intellectually disabled population. A review of prevalence studies by Borthwick-Duffy (1994) reports a rate of between 14 and 80% with the modal percentage at 45%.

Caine & Hatton (1998) have suggested that it can be expected that people with intellectual disabilities are more vulnerable to mental health difficulties, given their lifestyle trends and experiences. The trauma of birth itself through institutionalisation and stigmatisation, as well as poor social environments induced by unemployment, sparse social networks and a lack of intimate relationships are all recognised as potential stressors. In addition, the demands made by these impoverished lifestyles and experiences are likely to have more impact due to a reduced capacity in people with intellectual disabilities to deal with everyday life (Szymanski, 1994). The possible reasons for this higher prevalence have been categorised into four main domains: familial, social, biological and psychological factors (Holt et al., 2005). A summary of these factors is presented in Table 8.1.

However, a systematic review of the literature carried out by Whitaker & Read (2006) suggests that drawing firm conclusions about prevalence from the available empirical evidence is problematic. The epidemiological studies scrutinised as part of this review were compared to those determining prevalence in the general population, ensuring that the same sampling methods and diagnostic criteria were used

Table 8.1 Potential vulnerability factors for developing psychiatric disorder in people with intellectual disabilities.

Biological	Psychological
Brain damage	Personality development
Vision/hearing impairments	Deprivation/abuse
Physical illnesses/disabilities	Separation/losses
Genetic/familial conditions	Other life events
Drugs/alcohol abuse	Positive/negative learning experiences
Medication/physical treatments	Self-esteem/insight
Social	**Family**
Attitudes and expectations	Diagnostic/bereavement issues
Supports and relationships	Life-cycle transitions/crises
Inappropriate environments/services	'Letting go'
Under/overstimulation	Social/community networks
Valued/stigmatised roles/role models	Stress/adaptation to disabilities
Financial/legal disadvantage	Relationships/resources

From Holt et al. (2005).

throughout – for example, using community rather than pre-selected samples from psychiatric settings, and using the dual criterion of low IQ and impaired social functioning present in childhood. This thorough review concluded that while there is evidence that the prevalence of psychiatric disorder is greater in children *with* intellectual disabilities compared with children *without* intellectual disabilities, there is no reliable evidence that the prevalence of psychiatric disorders in adults with mild intellectual disabilities is greater than in the general population. The caution here is that this may be due to methodological shortcomings, as difficulties regarding the accuracy of data have been clearly and repeatedly identified (e.g. Kerker et al., 2004; Cooper et al., 2007).

Prevalence of mental health problems in people with severe and profound intellectual disabilities

Little is known about the mental health of people with profound intellectual disabilities, mainly because of studies using small and/or biased sample sizes as well as the limitations resulting from inconsistent classification or the approach to assessment (Cooper et al., 2007). There may well be an expectation of higher rates of mental health problems in people with more severe intellectual disabilities compared with people with mild intellectual disabilities or those without disabilities, considering that they often experience sensory loss, epilepsy and additional physical disabilities in addition to cognitive impairment (e.g. Cooper & Bailey, 2001). Whitaker & Read's review (2006) supports this assumption in that studies have reported higher prevalence of psychiatric disorder in both adults and children with severe intellectual disabilities.

Evidence to the contrary is also available. Holden & Gitlesen (2004) used the Mini PAS-ADD to compare symptomatology across a sample of participants with moderate, severe or profound intellectual disabilities and concluded that within their sample the prevalence of psychiatric disorder apparently decreased with severity of intellectual disability. The authors also comment that the usefulness of psychiatric illness models in explaining challenging and maladaptive behaviours also decreases with severity of disability. Other studies support their suggestion; Matson et al. (1997) found that some anxiety symptoms (e.g. unreasonable thoughts) cannot be assessed in people who are non-verbal, while Reid (1993) suggests that the verbal criteria for psychoses and mood disorder are difficult to apply to individual with an IQ less than 45. Findings derived from behavioural analysis suggest that verbal behaviour plays an important role in the development and maintenance of psychopathology, not only in anxiety and depression (Wilson et al., 2001).

A landmark study by Cooper et al. (2007) has attempted to establish both the prevalence of mental illness in people with profound intellectual disabilities and the most pertinent risk factors for its development (see later). The results have significant implications, with different rates being identified according to the criteria used: 52.2% using clinical criteria; 45.1% using DC-LD criteria (Royal College of Psychiatrists, 2001); 11.4% using DSM-IV-TR criteria (APA, 2000). The study highlights the problems inherent in using classification systems that differ in their emphases and setting of criteria, and helpfully provides summary findings that respectively include and exclude problem behaviours as symptoms psychological distress, to aid comparison of the findings with other studies. The overall conclusion is that both the incidence and prevalence of mental illness in people with profound intellectual disabilities is higher than that observed in both the general population and the population of people with intellectual disabilities.

Risk factors

Research into risk factors for mental health problems is greatly impeded by serious and fundamental difficulties within the process of assessment and diagnosis when working with people with intellectual disabilities. An initial question is whether criteria used for the diagnosis of psychiatric disorder in the general population can also be used with people with intellectual disabilities. A balance is needed between too rigidly or too loosely adhering to such criteria, leading to false negatives (underdiagnosing) and false positives (overdiagnosing), respectively. While DSM-IV and ICD-10 have increased reliability and validity of psychiatric diagnoses, there are clear problems when applying their criteria here, and some researchers call for their modification.

Risk factors for people with profound intellectual disabilities

Cooper et al. (2007) found that the predictive factors for the development of mental health problems in people with profound intellectual disabilities were both similar to the general population (e.g. preceding life events) and different (e.g. no apparent association with gender or level of deprivation in the area in which the individual was living). The authors emphasise issues relating to individuals' ability to make sense of changes and events in their lives, highlighting the importance of arranging and organising supports in ways that aid adjustment to these changes as much as possible. For people using services extensively, this is likely to include changes in personnel and the nature of regular activity, let alone the more stereotypical and significant changes associated with moving house, loss of a loved one or the adaptation to a new lifestyle that results from a serious illness.

Diagnostic overshadowing

People with intellectual disabilities face the risk of 'diagnostic overshadowing' – where clear signs of emotional disorder are inappropriately attributed to the person's intellectual disability *per se*. Conversely, an individual could potentially be diagnosed with psychotic illness when their developmental level has not been taken into account as an explanation for primitive behaviours, reduced social functioning, and disorganised thoughts and speech that can accompany periods of stress, confusion and change for adults with intellectual disabilities. A study by Spengler et al. (1990, cited in Mason & Scior, 2004) suggests that this phenomenon only appears to apply when the IQ of the individuals described in case vignettes was pronounced at under 58.

Presentation of mental illness in people with intellectual disabilities

Signs of mental illness in people with intellectual disabilities vary and depend on the following:

- Level of cognitive, communicative, physical and social functioning
- Usual behavioural repertoire
- Past and present interpersonal, cultural and environmental influences

Generally, signs and symptoms are less complex than those seen in the general population, but due to less well-developed cognitive and communication skills, people with intellectual disabilities are more likely to show disturbed and regressed behaviours and biological signs and complaints as presentations of emotional disorders (Gravestock, 1999).

Presentation of psychosis in people with intellectual disabilities

Symptoms of psychosis can include hearing voices when no one else can, seeing things that are not there, having odd ideas and beliefs, odd sensations or movements, muddled thinking and bizarre behaviour. In delusional disorders, people can feel persecuted, suspicious or hostile. The presentation of psychotic illness in people with mild intellectual disability is similar to people without intellectual disability; the content of delusions tends to be more bland and unremarkable. In people with more severe intellectual disability, there is less overt psychopathology (e.g. evidence of persecutory delusions and formal thought disorder – but then this is very difficult to assess), but there are usually increased displays of bizarre behaviour. Catatonia can become more prominent.

Other psychotic illnesses include psychotic depression – characterised by low mood, lack of interest, morbid thoughts, feelings of guilt, sleep and eating disturbance, lack of activity and energy, hearing voices – and bipolar disorder (episodes of depression and mania/hypomania). The features of the depressive phase are similar to those observed in psychotic depression, while in the 'manic' phase the individual experiences high and/or irritable mood, lack of sleep, overactivity, excessive, grandiose ideas, racing thoughts and a tendency to be talkative. In people with intellectual disabilities, grandiose delusions may seem less grandiose than in people without intellectual disabilities. Rapid cycling bipolar disorder (more than four episodes of either mania or depression in a year) is believed to be more common among people with intellectual disabilities.

Presentation of depression in people with intellectual disabilities

Clinical depression is often characterised by low mood, upsets in sleeping and eating patterns and social withdrawal. In people with intellectual disabilities, depressive illness may present atypically, for example, the individual may experience weight gain instead of weight loss, or hypersomnia instead of insomnia. Onset tends to be more insidious. In people with mild intellectual disability, there can be a general loss of confidence, tearfulness and deterioration in social and self-help skills. In people with more severe intellectual disability, increased dependence, psychomotor agitation, irritability, stereotypies, screaming and a worsening of existing behavioural problems such as self-injurious behaviour and temper tantrums can all be observed.

Presentation of anxiety in people with intellectual disabilities

People with intellectual disabilities can develop responses to stress and environmental changes. They may present with agitation, panic attacks, low mood, non-epileptic attacks, physical health concerns and 'overly-demanding' behaviours. Some individuals also have specific phobias (e.g. of dogs, heights and water), and these are common, particularly in adults with autistic spectrum disorder. The repetitive thoughts, ritualistic and obsessive behaviours which are resisted and cause anxiety to those with obsessive-compulsive disorder may be misdiagnosed as features of autism.

Eating disorders

Cases of anorexia nervosa and bulimia nervosa can occur in adults with mild to moderate intellectual disabilities. Other disorders include binge eating disorders and associated obesity. Pica and food regurgitation or rumination with being significantly underweight are most likely to occur in people with severe intellectual disabilities. Extreme food faddiness and refusal along with being significantly underweight are often associated with the eating and food-related rituals and obsessions seen in people with autistic spectrum disorder.

Personality disorders

Personality disorders are more likely to be diagnosed in adults with mild to moderate intellectual disabilities, and may present in adults with severe intellectual disabilities as challenging behaviour. As in general psychiatry, the diagnosis remains controversial.

Challenging behaviour and psychiatric disorder

Another key issue relating to assessment and diagnosis of mental health problems in people with profound disabilities concerns challenging behaviour; some studies are distorted by their inclusion of challenging behaviour as a psychiatric illness. When challenging behaviour is included, prevalence of psychiatric disorders can be cited as high as 35% (Reiss, 1990), but only 16% when challenging behaviour is excluded (Lund, 1985).

While not a clinical diagnosis, challenging behaviour can be a common reason for referral to a community intellectual disability team (Prosser, 1999), and is usually viewed as a long-term behaviour pattern, rather than as an illness with a particular time course (Moss, 1999). The prevalence of such behaviour depends largely on the definition used and how the behaviour is assessed, but it is generally agreed that it is commonly observed in the intellectual disabled population.

'Problem' or 'challenging' behaviours can be understood as learned responses to unhelpful environments and largely communicative in nature (see Chapters 4 and 5), as well as symptoms of underlying psychiatric disorder – for example, links have been made between self-injurious behaviour and obsessive-compulsive disorder (Bodfish et al., 1995).

Genetic disorders and behavioural phenotypes also need to be considered when attempting to formulate the underpinning causes of challenging behaviour. Table 8.2 lists some examples.

Accepting that the utility of psychiatric assessment decreases with severity of intellectual disability also leads one to the conclusion that mental illness as an explanation of challenging behaviour also decreases with severity of intellectual disability; this observation is unfortunate, particularly as rates of challenging

Table 8.2 Some genetic syndromes that can lead to severe or profound intellectual disability and their associated behavioural disorders.

Genetic syndrome	Associated 'problem' behaviours
Angelman's syndrome	Hyperactivity
Cri-du-Chat syndrome	Irritability
Fragile X syndrome	Hyperactivity; repetitive/autistic features
Lesch-Nyhan syndrome	Self-injury
Smith-Magenis syndrome	Self-injury; hyperactivity
Sotos syndrome	Aggression

From Gilbert (2000).

behaviour – particularly self-injurious behaviour – are reported to increase with severity of cognitive impairment (Holden & Gitlensen, 2004).

Assessment issues

One of the central issues faced when attempting to understand mental health in intellectual disabilities concerns the practical task of assessment. The nature of assessment is described by Bouras et al. (1995), who highlight six main principles (see Table 8.3).

All facets of the individual's life and experience need to be explored and held in mind when attempting to establish psychiatric disorder. This can be very complex. Moss (1999, p. 18) states:

It is often very difficult to determine the extent to which presenting behaviours are the result of an organic condition, a psychiatric disorder, environmental influences, or a combination of these.

Table 8.3 Main principles of assessment of mental health assessment for people with intellectual disabilities.

1. Information may need to be gathered from other informants as well as the individual being assessed
2. Mental disorders need to be differentiated from isolated challenging behaviour by way of the *pattern* of behaviours or experiences by which they are indicated
3. *Changes* in behaviour or experience are often important for diagnosis, but if a psychiatric problem has gone unnoticed, changes could be difficult to detect. Dementia is cited as particularly complex, and non-cognitive signs such as wandering or irritability might be more informative
4. Expression of symptoms is individual and likely to vary with degree of disability. People with more severe and profound disabilities will probably express their distress in behavioural rather than verbal ways
5. Gender, culture and individual life experience all influence both the expression of distress and its interpretation by professionals
6. Alternative explanations for unusual behaviours or experiences other than mental health problems need to be explored initially. These might include the expression of physical discomfort in people with limited communication skills or the side effects of medication.

From Bouras (1995).

Some elements can be addressed systematically; for example, when trying to understand an individual's behaviour that is causing concern, thorough multidisciplinary assessment (see Chapter 7) would hopefully enable the clinician or practitioner to rule out or establish the role played by physical health problems in the formulation of the challenging behaviour. Similarly, the potential role played by epilepsy needs to be considered (see Chapter 9), noting that while some studies have found an increased rate of problem behaviour in people with epilepsy, others have found the opposite (Smiley, 2005).

Once these possibilities have been explored – and either kept in mind as potential factors underpinning the individual's behaviour or eliminated from the formulation – clinicians need to think carefully about selecting the most appropriate tools available to gather the most reliable information.

Using a developmental perspective in assessment and diagnosis

Recent thinking has focused on the psychosocial development of individuals with intellectual disabilities as a framework for carrying out assessment and diagnosis. Dosen (2005a, b) suggests that a consideration of personality and emotional development can support a more traditional approach to psychiatric assessment. After cognitive assessment has been completed, an assessment of the individual's emotional development provides the clinician with a way of placing the individual's behaviour in a developmental context. Informed by research carried out by developmental psychologists (e.g. Piaget, 1953; Stern, 1985), this enables a bio-psycho-social-developmental model of behaviour to be applied in order to better understand what might be happening for the person.

Dosen (2005a) used the wider research literature to establish ten aspects of psychosocial development observed in children with intellectual disabilities (see Table 8.4). These aspects were found to be permanently present throughout life,

Table 8.4 Ten aspects of psychosocial development subject to changes during the different developmental phases.

1. How the person deals with his/her own body
2. Interaction with caregiver
3. Interaction with peers
4. Handling with material objects
5. Affect differentiation
6. Verbal communication
7. Anxiety
8. Object permanency
9. Experience of self
10. Aggression regulation

Adapted from Dosen (2005a).

Table 8.5 Basic emotional needs.

Developmental level	Emotional need
Phase 1	Regulation of physiological needs; integration of sensory input; structuring of space, time and people; social interaction
Phase 2	Bodily contact; attachment person; social stimulation; handling of material objects
Phase 3	Certain distance in contact; confirmation of autonomy; reward of social behaviour
Phase 4	Identification with important others; social acceptance and support; social competence

Adapted from Dosen (2005a).

and therefore subject to changes during the five different developmental phases (i.e. 0–6 months; 6–18 months; 18–36 months; 3–7 years; 7–12 years).

Dosen (1990, 1997) developed the *Schema of Appraisal of Emotional Development* (SAED), which maps these changes within each developmental phase. The SAED is completed by experienced clinicians who observe the individual and interview family members and/or carers. The questions are designed to help establish the level reached by the individual for each aspect. People with profound intellectual disabilities were found to regularly score under 18 months on all aspects. In cases of behavioural and psychiatric disorder, the individual's emotional development was found to be lower than their cognitive development.

Emotional needs are clearly an essential part of understanding an individual (see Table 8.5), and it is imperative that the person's emotional life is understood as much as possible before we are able to say with any confidence that we are supporting them appropriately (see Chapter 5). This recognition also 're-personalises' people who continue to be at significant risk of being dehumanised and seen only in terms of labels and behaviours. Taking a developmental approach to assessment in this way is hugely relevant for people with profound intellectual disabilities.

Assessment tools

Assessment tools used to identify mental health problems in people with intellectual disabilities are likely to fall within three main categories (Holland & Koot, 1998):

- *Assessments that characterise the nature and extent of the individual's intellectual disability and its effect on function.* Harris (1995) provides a useful review of standardised neurological and neuropsychological tests and rating scales.
- *Descriptive assessments that identify the nature and extent of problem behaviours*, including the Vineland Adaptive Behaviour Scales (Sparrow et al., 1984) and the Aberrant Behaviour Checklist (Aman et al., 1985).
- *Assessments that strive to establish aetiology*, including psychiatric diagnostic assessments and functional analyses.

Standardised tools

Mental health problems may be expressed in different ways, particularly in people with severe or profound disabilities (Moss, 1999). Furthermore, where individuals are unable to communicate their experiences or mental state in ways understood by the assessor, the validity of any diagnosis is highly questionable (Sturmey et al., 1991). Relatives and/or carers are usually consulted when the individual is unable to provide the relevant information. The difficulty is in establishing 'normality' for the individual according to his or her developmental stage, and considering whether current experiences are new and perhaps 'abnormal' to that person. Approaches include the use of the psychiatric assessment schedule for adults with a developmental disability (PAS-ADD; Moss et al., 1993) and the diagnostic assessment for the severely handicapped (DASH-2; Dykes & Erin, 1999). Independent studies of reliability and validity for these tools are still needed (Holland & Koot, 1998).

Given the complexities in the assessment of psychiatric symptomatology in profound disability, one strategy is to diagnose disorders on the basis of more limited behaviours (Clarke, 1999). Examples of this include screaming, self-injurious behaviour and aggression diagnosed as depression (Marston et al., 1997); cyclic self-injurious behaviour unresponsive to treatment diagnosed as rapid-cycling bipolar disorder (Osborne et al., 1992); repetitive, stereotyped and ritualistic self-injurious behaviour as obsessive-compulsive disorder (Emerson et al., 1999). While this approach may be problematic, there is evidence that it can succeed – though a positive response to medication does not necessarily imply the existence of a disorder prior to treatment (McBrien, 2003).

Moss (1999) suggests that assessment based upon diagnostic classification can only provide partial insight into the experience of people with intellectual disabilities who have mental health difficulties. He advocates a problem-based approach, as adopted with the general population, which is likely to assist with prevention and maximising quality of life as well as reduction of symptoms.

This model of assessment can be used to inform a range of psychological treatments, including individual therapy for anxiety and depression (Lindsay et al., 1997; Reed, 1997) and encompassing a range of techniques such as self-instructional training, role-play and anxiety management (Caine & Hatton, 1998). In addition, there is a clear lack of experienced practitioners to ensure the appropriate utilisation of any of the established treatments (Collins, 1999).

Formulation

Good formulations of an individual's difficulties (i.e. formulations that lend themselves fairly straightforwardly to the design of helpful interventions) are developed from thorough assessments, so time taken on gathering information is time well spent. Using the ideas outlined earlier to think about understanding mental health problems, the bio-psycho-social-developmental approach takes into account biological factors underpinning the difficulties; social and environmental factors that

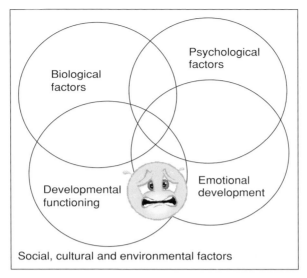

Figure 8.1   Formulating poor mental health in intellectual disabilities – a bio-psycho-social-developmental model in context.

might be contributing to the problem; psychological ('internal') issues and the person's level of disability, that is, their developmental and emotional functioning. Figure 8.1 illustrates how an individual's subjective distress can be understood by thinking about the potential contributions made by the respective influences and relationships between:

- the individual's level of cognitive impairment and resulting developmental functioning;
- his or her emotional development;
- biological and physical health; and
- psychological factors.

These complex interactions also need to be placed with a social and cultural context, both individual (e.g. the person's family, religious and cultural context) and within the wider world (i.e. the socio-economic climate). Careful thinking and drawing together these facets of the individual's experience hopefully leads to a diagnosis.

Intervention

Biological interventions

Medication is generally prescribed for mental illnesses such as schizophrenia, depression, mania, anxiety disorders, obsessive-compulsive disorder, bulimia nervosa (but not anorexia nervosa) and dementia, but can also be prescribed to treat behaviour problems such as self-injurious behaviour and aggression. When and what to prescribe will be influenced by:

- the type of illness (or disorder);
- the duration and severity of the illness;
- the prominence of particular symptoms (e.g. insomnia or overactivity);
- the level of risk the individuals pose to themselves or others;
- side effect profile;
- the ways in which the individual previously responded to medication; and
- a limited response or failure of psychosocial interventions.

The length of time that an individual needs to remain on medication depends on the clinical indication. For example, one or two doses may be sufficient for an acute episode of disturbed behaviour due to an environmental trigger which has since been removed, whereas medication can be administered for 6–9 months following recovery from a first episode of clinical depression to avoid relapse. With all medication, good practice would indicate starting with a low dose with monitoring for side effects. Regular medication reviews should address:

- the individual's mental state and behaviour since the last review;
- any side effects;
- impact on quality of life;
- ongoing need for medication; and
- capacity to consent.

Psychological interventions

These can be divided into *direct* and *indirect* interventions. Direct interventions involve working directly with the individual with intellectual disabilities and for this reason are used more commonly with people with moderate to mild intellectual disabilities. Behavioural treatment uses the collection of evidence using objective, scientific methods to look at the antecedents to incidences of behaviour causing concern and records the consequences to this behaviour (BPS, 2004). The clinician designs the manipulation of the environment – which here includes the reactions and behaviour of others – in order to influence the individual's responses.

Cognitive behaviour therapy supports people to make links between their thoughts, feelings and behaviour, usually in a structured, almost manualised way, aiming to establish with the individual, the meaning that they are given to key events, people and situations (see Stenfert Kroese et al., 1997). Systemic interventions (e.g. family therapy) work with the individuals in the context of their immediate social support network to review ways in which problems may be located between people as part of difficult interactions and/or are being maintained by unhelpful ways of relating (see Baum & Lynggard, 2006).

Indirect approaches are more commonly used with people with severe or profound intellectual disabilities and can involve working behaviourally through staff teams or families to systematically gather information about incidences of problem behaviour using functional analysis, or systemic consultative work that encourages reflection on challenging situations to enable systems to work more effectively together in supporting the individual. A useful technique is to look for patterns throughout the 'system' (e.g. mirroring of the individual's behaviour by the wider system) as a way of understanding how things are being maintained or have become 'stuck'.

These approaches are not mutually exclusive, and increasingly clinicians are using an integrative approach to working with individuals and their support networks to help contextualise and give meaning to very complex events. These methods aim to both acknowledge an individual's diagnoses and labels and move beyond them in order to think about how he or she seems to be perceiving and experiencing the world, and in turn, how this experience leads on to feelings and resultant behaviours or actions.

Whatever the theoretical orientation underpinning the intervention, it is important that it retains some key features. Ideally, it needs to be:

- holistic, encompassing all characteristics and elements of the individual's presentation, experience and lifestyle;
- reduce vulnerability and precipitating factors;
- use a person-centred approach (see Cambridge & Carnaby, 2005);
- increase social inclusion (i.e. use the least restricted approach when assessing and managing risk); and
- acknowledge and actively involve family carers and support staff in designing, implementing and evaluating the intervention.

Services and support for people with intellectual disabilities and psychiatric disorder

Difficulties in detecting mental health difficulties, as well as inadequacies in staff skills and training programmes, have led to a situation where it is possible that many individuals with intellectual disabilities are experiencing problems that remain undetected (Patel et al., 1993). This has led to inequalities within the mental health system for people with intellectual disabilities, not only in terms of the nature of provision but also regarding access to available services.

Service provision

The patchy nature of both local and national responses to the mental health needs of people with intellectual disabilities is likely to be ameliorated by research that provides clearer demographic and epidemiological data. More sophisticated understanding of mental health problems, more appropriate analyses and more effective interventions can only be created on the foundation of empirical evidence

(Gravestock, 1999). Specialist services are often necessary, but can still be provided in the community (Davidson et al., 1999). More research is needed to compare these local, interdisciplinary models of support with more traditional mental health services. While funding and its allocation are highly relevant to service develop- ment (Winterhalder, 1999), it is likely that local cooperation between stakeholders together with sensible interpretation of public policy is equally crucial to provid- ing effective service provision to such a vulnerable population. Acknowledging the difficulties faced by service providers has proved to be an important first step, but further integration of experience, sound evidence and interdisciplinary debate is still urgently needed

Training and knowledge of practitioners

Support for people with intellectual disabilities is often provided by direct care staff who have had very little training, particularly in mental health issues (Winterhalder, 1999). It is likely that this has significant impact when staff are supporting people with severe and profound disabilities. Behaviours resulting from mental disorders might be viewed negatively by staff with little mental health experience, leading to inappropriate responses and possibly detrimental effects upon the individual. The possibility that an individual with profound disabilities might be suffering from poor mental health might not even be considered.

Issues relating to the training of staff working with people with profound dis- abilities also apply to those working with people with milder disabilities. Where training in mental health issues is made available, it is often reactive with no re- gional or national coordination, although the Department of Health (Department of Health, 1999a, 2001) has acknowledged the need for more proactive strategies. Furthermore, the government publication *A Strategy for People with Intellectual Disabilities* (Department of Health, 1995) also stated that targeting mental health as outlined in the *Health of the Nation* policy equally applies to people with intel- lectual disabilities (Prosser, 1999). The other side of this situation concerns the ways in which mental health services need to adapt their practices in order to support people with intellectual disabilities. The National Service Framework for Mental Health (Department of Health, 1999b) advises that people with intellectual dis- abilities have the right to access mainstream mental health services, and this is also supported by the white paper *Valuing People* (Department of Health, 2001). In reality, there is a risk that individuals with intellectual disabilities bounce between intellectual disability specialist teams and mental health services, in the meantime potentially not receiving the care and support that they need.

Resources have appeared in recent years which both acknowledge and attempt to address shortfalls in provision (e.g. Holt et al., 2005). These materials place the responsibility across services, signifying the need for partnership between agencies and their commissioners. Much remains to be done before mental health services for people with intellectual disabilities are consistently and reliably person centred and effectively meeting needs.

Conclusion

Assessing and diagnosing psychiatric disorder in people with profound intellectual disabilities can be extremely challenging, not least because of the theoretical and conceptual dilemmas faced by the clinician. While services need to develop, the ways in which we conceptualise psychiatric disorder and subjective mental state in people with more severe intellectual disabilities also need to be revisited. Some authors suggest that while the principle of normalisation has done much for people with intellectual disabilities, it has failed to provide adequately for those with complex needs. Piachaud (1999, p. 47) writes:

> The five accomplishments of O'Brien have become a mantra, yet the heady social inclusion rebellion of the 1980's has faltered at the step of challenging behaviour and mental disorder.

It is important that those responsible for commissioning and delivering provision for people with profound disabilities are able to acknowledge that some individuals have 'extraordinary' needs that cannot be met straightforwardly by services designed to support 'ordinary' living (Smith, 1994), requiring concerted effort towards highly individualised provision. Elsewhere, the revised Mansell report (Department of Health, 2007) seems to be reiterating its original agenda published in 1993, also highlighting the need for local, competent provision built on collaboration and commitment to people requiring complex, individualised support.

The evidence presented here indicates that much is to be done in terms of how we think about assessment and how assessment outcomes lead to diagnosis and treatment. Indeed, perhaps the overarching issue is that along with developing our understanding in these areas, careful consideration needs to be given to the extent to which approaching mental health in people with profound leaning disabilities and complex needs in the same way as in the general population is helpful and valid.

References

Aman, M.G., Singh, N.N., Stewart, A.W., & Field, C.J. (1985). The aberrant behaviour checklist: a behaviour rating scale for the assessment of treatment effects. *American Journal of Mental Deficiency*, 89, 485–491.

APA (2000). *Diagnostic and Statistical Manual of Mental Disorders (4th edition) – Text revision*. Washington, DC: American Psychiatric Association.

Baum, S., & Lynggard, H. (2006). *Intellectual Disabilities: A Systemic Approach*. London: Karnac Books.

BPS (2004). *Psychological Interventions for Severely Challenging Behaviours Shown by People with Learning Disabilities: Clinical Practice Guidelines*. Leicester: British Psychological Society

Birch, H.G., Richardson, S.A., Baird, D., Horobin, G., & Illsley, R. (1970). *Mental Subnormality in the Community: A Clinical and Epidemiological Study*. Baltimore: Williams and Wilkins.

Bodfish, J.W., Crawford, T.W., Powell, S.B., Parker, D.E., Golden, R.N., & Lewis, M.H. (1995). Compulsions in adults with mental retardation: prevalence, phenomenology and comorbidity with stereotypy and self-injury. *American Journal on Mental Retardation*, 100, 183–192.

Borthwick-Duffy, S.A. (1994). Epidemiology and prevalence of psychopathology in people with mental retardation. *Journal of Consulting and Clinical Psychology*, 62, 172–177.

Bouras, N. (ed.) (1995). *Mental Health in Mental Retardation: Recent Advances and Practices*. Cambridge: Cambridge University Press.

Bouras, N., & Drummond, C. (1992). Behaviour and psychiatric disorders of people with mental handicaps living in the community. *Journal of Intellectual Disorders*, 36, 349–357.

Caine, A., & Hatton, C. (1998). Working with people with mental health problems. In Emerson, E., Hatton, C., Bromley, J., & Caine, A. (eds), *Clinical Psychology and People with Intellectual Disabilities*. Chichester: John Wiley & Sons.

Cambridge, P., & Carnaby, S. (eds) (2005). *Person Centred Planning and Care Management and People with Learning Disabilities*. London: Jessica Kingsley.

Chaplin, R. (2004). General psychiatry services for adults with intellectual disabilities and mental illness. *Journal of Intellectual Disability Research*, 48, 1–10.

Clarke, D. (1999). Functional psychosis in people with mental retardation. In Bouras, N. (ed.), *Psychiatric and Behavioural Disorders in Developmental Disabilities and Mental Retardation*. Cambridge: Cambridge University Press.

Collins, S. (1999). Treatment and therapeutic interventions: psychological approaches. *Tizard Learning Disability Review*, 4(2), 20–27.

Cooper, S.-A., & Bailey, N.M. (2001). Psychiatric disorders amongst adults with learning disabilities: prevalence and relationship to ability level. *Irish Journal of Psychological Medicine*, 18, 375–380.

Cooper, S.-A., Smiley, E., Finlayson, J., Jackson, A., Allan, L., Williamson, A., Mantry, D., & Morrison, J. (2007). The prevalence, incidence and factors predictive of mental ill-health in adults with profound intellectual disabilities. *Journal of Applied Research in Intellectual Disabilities*, 20, 6, 493–501.

Davidson, P.W., Morris, D., & Cain, N.N. (1999). Community services for people with developmental disabilities and psychiatric or severe behaviour disorders. In Bouras, N. (ed.), *Psychiatric and Behavioural Disorders in Developmental Disabilities and Mental Retardation*. Cambridge: Cambridge University Press.

Department of Health (1995). *The Health of the Nation: A Strategy for People with Learning Disabilities*. London: HMSO.

Department of Health (1999a). *Facing the Facts: Services for People with Learning Disabilities*. London: Department of Health Publications.

Department of Health (1999b). *A National Service Framework for Mental Health*. London: HMSO.

Department of Health (2001). *Valuing People: A New Strategy for Learning Disability for the 21st Century*. London: TSO.

Department of Health (2007). *Services for People with Learning Disabilities and Challenging Behaviour or Mental Health Needs*. London: TSO.

Dosen, A. (1990). *Psychische Stoornissen Bij Zwakzinnige Kindern*. Lisse, the Netherlands: Swets en Zeitlinger.

Dosen, A. (1997). *Psychische storungen bei geistig behinderten menschen*. Stuttgart: Gustav Fischer.

Dosen, A. (2005a). Applying the developmental perspective in the psychiatric assessment and diagnosis of persons with intellectual disability: part 1 – assessment. *Journal of Intellectual Disability Research*, 49(1), 1–8.

Dosen, A. (2005b). Applying the developmental perspective in the psychiatric assessment and diagnosis of persons with intellectual disability: part 2 – diagnosis. *Journal of Intellectual Disability Research*, 49(1), 9–15.

Dykes, M.K., & Erin, J.N. (1999). *Developmental Assessment for Individuals with Severe Disabilities (DASH-2)*. Austin, TX: Pro-Ed.

Emerson, E. (2003). Prevalence of psychiatric disorders in children and adolescents with and without intellectual disability. *Journal of Intellectual Disability Research*, 47, 51–58.

Emerson, E., Moss, S., & Kiernan, C. (1999). The relationship between challenging behaviour and psychiatric disorders in people with severe developmental disabilities. In Bouras, N. (ed.), *Psychiatric and Behavioural Disorders in Developmental Disabilities and Mental Retardation*. Cambridge: Cambridge University Press.

Gilbert, P. (2000). A-Z of *Syndromes and Inherited Disorders: A Manual for Health, Social and Education Workers* (3rd edition). Cheltenham: Nelson Thornes (Publishers) Ltd.

Goldberg, D.P., & Huxley, P. (1980). *Mental Illness in the Community: The Pathway to Psychiatric Care*. London: Tavistock.

Gravestock, S. (1999). Adults with learning disabilities and mental health needs: conceptual and service issues. *Tizard Learning Disability Review*, 4(2), 6–13.

Harris, J.C. (1995). *Developmental Neuropsychiatry: Assessment, Diagnosis and Treatment of Developmental Disorders*, Vol. II. Oxford: Oxford University Press.

Hatton, C., & Emerson, E. (2004). The relationship between life events and psychopathology amongst children with intellectual disabilities. *Journal of Applied Research in Intellectual Disabilities*, 17, 109–118.

Health Education Authority (1997). *Mental Health Promotion: A Quality Framework*. London: HEA.

Holden, B.I., & Gitlensen, J.P. (2004). The association between severity of intellectual disability and psychiatric symptomatology. *Journal of Intellectual Disability Research*, 48, 556–562.

Holland, A.J., & Koot, H.M. (1998). Mental health and intellectual disability: an international perspective. *Journal of Intellectual Disability Research*, 42(6), 505–512.

Holt, G., Hardy, S., & Bouras, N. (2005). *Mental Health in Learning Disabilities: A Training Resource*. Brighton: Pavilion Publishing.

Kerker, B.D., Owens, P.L., Zigler, P.I., & Horowitz, S.M. (2004). Mental health disorders among individuals with mental retardation: challenges to accurate prevalence estimates. *Public Health Reports*, 119, 409–417.

Koller, H., Richardson, S.A., Katz, M., & McLaren, J. (1983). Behaviour disturbance since childhood among a 5-year birth cohort of all mentally retarded young adults in a city. *American Journal of Mental Deficiency*, 87, 386–396.

Lindsay, W., Neilson, C., & Lawrenson, H. (1997). Cognitive-behaviour therapy for anxiety in people with learning disabilities. In Kroese, B.S., Dagnan, D., & Loumidis, K. (eds), *Cognitive-Behaviour Therapy for People with Learning Disabilities*. London: Routledge.

Lund, J. (1985). The prevalence of psychiatric morbidity in mentally retarded adults. *Acta Psychiatrica Scandinavia*, 72, 563–570.

Marston, G.M., Perry, D.W., & Roy, A. (1997). Manifestations of depression in people with intellectual disability. *Journal of Intellectual Disability Research*, 41, 476–480.

Mason, J., & Scior, K. (2004). 'Diagnostic overshadowing' amongst clinicians working with people with intellectual disabilities in the UK. *Journal of Applied Research in Intellectual Disabilities*, 17(2), 85–90.

Matson, J.L., Smiroldo, B.B., Hamilton, M., & Baglio, C.S. (1997). Do anxiety disorders exist in persons with severe and profound mental retardation? *Research in Developmental Disabilities*, 28, 39–44.

McBrien, J.A. (2003). Assessment and diagnosis of depression in people with intellectual disability. *Journal of Intellectual Disability Research*, 47, 1–13.

Moss, S. (1999). Assessment: conceptual issues. In Bouras, N. (ed.), *Psychiatric and Behavioural Disorders in Developmental Disabilities and Mental Retardation*. Cambridge: Cambridge University Press.

Moss, S. (2001). Psychiatric disorders in adults with mental retardation. In Glidden, L. (ed.), *International Review of Research in Mental Retardation*. New York: Academic Press.

Moss, S., Patel, P., Prosser, H., Goldberg, D.P., Simpson, N., Rose, S., & Lucchino, R. (1993). Psychiatric morbidity in older people with moderate and severe learning disability (mental retardation), Part I: development and reliability of the patient interview (the PAS-ADD). *British Journal of Psychiatry*, 163, 471–480.

Osborne, J.G., Baggs, A.W., Darvish, R., Blakelock, H., Peine, H., & Jenson, W. (1992). Cyclical self-injurious behaviour, contingent watermist treatment and the possibility of a rapid-cycling bipolar disorder. *Journal of Behaviour Therapy and Experimental Psychiatry*, 23, 325–334.

Patel, P., Goldberg, D.P., & Moss, S.C. (1993). Psychiatric morbidity in older people with moderate and severe learning disability (mental retardation), Part II: the prevalence study. *British Journal of Psychiatry*, 163, 481–491.

Piachaud, J. (1999). Issues for mental health in learning disabilities services. *Tizard Learning Disability Review*, 4(2), 47–48.

Piaget, J. (1953). *The Child's Construction of the Reality*. London: Routledge & Kegan.

Prosser, H. (1999). An invisible morbidity? *The Psychologist*, 12(5), 234–237.

Reed, J. (1997). Understanding and assessing depression in people with learning disabilities: a cognitive-behavioural approach. In Kroese, B.S., Dagnan, D., & Loumidis, K. (eds), *Cognitive-Behaviour Therapy for People with Learning Disabilities*. London: Routledge.

Reid, A. (1993). Schizophrenic and paranoid symptoms in persons with mental retardation: assessment and diagnosis. In Fletcher, R.J., & Dosen, A. (eds), *Mental Health Aspects of Mental Retardation*. New York: Lexington Books.

Reiss, S. (1990). Prevalence of dual diagnosis in community-based day programs in the Chicago metropolitan area. *American Journal on Mental Retardation*, 94, 578–585.

Rojahn, J., Matson, J., Naglieri, J., & Mayville, E. (2004). Relationships between psychiatric conditions and behaviour problems among adults with mental retardation. *American Journal on Mental Retardation*, 109, 21–33.

Royal College of Psychiatrists (2001). *DC–LD [Diagnostic Criteria for Psychiatric Disorders for Use with Adults with Learning Disabilities/Mental Retardation]* (Occasional Paper OP48). London: Gaskell.

Rutter, M., Graham, P., & Yule, W. (1970). *A Neuropsychiatric Study in Childhood*. London: Spastics International Medical Publication Smiley, 2005.

Smiley, E. (2005). Epidemiology of mental health problems in adults with learning disability: an update. *Advances in Psychiatric treatment*, 11, 214–222.

Smith, B. (1994). An ordinary life for people with a learning disability and sensory impairment? *British Journal of Learning Disabilities*, 22, 140–143.

Sparrow, S.S., Balla, D.A., & Cicchetti, D.V. (1984). *Vineland Adaptive Behaviour Scale.* Circle Pines, MN: American Guidance Service.

Spengler, P., Strohmer, D., & Thompson-Prout, H. (1990). Testing the robustness of the diagnostic overshadowing bias. *American Journal on Mental Retardation*, 95, 204–214.

Stenfert Kroese, B., Dagnan, D., & Loumidis. K. (eds.) (1997). *Cognitive Behaviour Therapy and People with Learning Disabilities.* London: Routledge.

Stern, D.N. (1985). *The Interpersonal World of the Infant.* New York: Basic Books.

Sturmey, P. (1993). The use of DSM and ICD diagnostic criteria in people with mental retardation: a review of empirical studies. *The Journal of Nervous and Mental Disease*, 181, 38–41.

Sturmey, P., Lindsay, W.R., & Didden, R. (2007). Editorial – special issue: dual diagnosis. *Journal of Applied Research in Intellectual Disability*, 20(5), 379–383.

Sturmey, P., Reed, J., & Corbett, J. (1991). Psychometric assessment of psychiatric disorders in people with learning difficulties (mental handicap): a review of measures. *Psychological Medicine*, 21, 143–155.

Szymanski, L.W. (1994). Mental retardation and mental health: concepts, aetiology and incidence. In Bouras, N. (ed.), *Mental Health in Mental Retardation: Recent Advances and Practices.* Cambridge: Cambridge University Press.

Whitaker, S., & Read, S. (2006). The prevalence of psychiatric disorders among people with intellectual disabilities: an analysis of the literature. *Journal of Applied Research in Intellectual Disabilities*, 19(4), 330–345.

Wilson, K.G., Hayes, S.C., Gregg, J., & Zettle, R.D. (2001). Psychopathology and psychotherapy. In Hayes, S.C., Barnes-Holmes, D., & Roche, B. (eds), *Relational Frame Theory. A Post-Skinnerian Account of Human Language and Cognition.* New York: Kluwer Academic/Plenum Publishers.

Winterhalder, R. (1999). Commentary – mental health needs of people with learning disabilities: assessment and therapeutic interventions. *Tizard Learning Disability Review*, 4(2), 33–35.

Chapter 9

EPILEPSY: IMPLICATIONS FOR PEOPLE WITH PROFOUND INTELLECTUAL AND MULTIPLE DISABILITIES

Mary Codling and Nicky MacDonald

Introduction

People with profound intellectual and multiple disabilities (PIMD) are a vulnerable group and are more likely to have a number of specific health needs. One such need is epilepsy. This chapter aims to further develop the readers' knowledge and understanding of epilepsy and the consequences for people with PIMD and will begin with a definition and description of epilepsy.

Also, in this chapter, we explore the implications of epilepsy not only for people with profound and multiple intellectual disabilities, but for carers and professionals who are responsible for meeting such needs. People with profound and complex intellectual disabilities are more often than not reliant on carers to meet their overall needs. Communication difficulties accompanied by physical disabilities in people with PIMD place them in a position of being cared for by others.

Finally, we will look at assessment and consider some of the aspects that created barriers to the identification and treatment of epilepsy amongst this group of people. This section is based on evidence from practice that was clinically driven from concerns raised by professionals and carers of the unmet needs of people with PIMD who have epilepsy.

Learning objectives

By the end of this chapter the reader will:

- have gained knowledge of the different seizure types and their impact on the lives of people with profound and multiple intellectual disabilities;
- understand some of the difficulties in diagnosing and treating epilepsy in people with profound and multiple intellectual disabilities;
- be able to consider their role in developing epilepsy services that meet the needs of both the individual with PIMD and their carer and develop an understanding

of the importance of the role of the carer in the diagnosis and treatment of epilepsy;

- gain knowledge of how care pathways can be developed to improve access to epilepsy provision and provide people with profound and multiple intellectual disabilities, their carers and professionals with a clear structure of the assessment process and appropriate services; and
- be able to recognise the benefits of practice-based evidence and how such evidence can influence service delivery that in turn can improve the delivery of care for people with epilepsy.

What is epilepsy?

The word 'epilepsy' is derived from the Greek word *epilamambanein* that means to possess, take hold of, to grab or to seize. In medical terms, epilepsy is defined as a condition for which the person is prone to experience recurrent epileptic seizures (Shorvon, 2000). By definition, a single occurrence is not epilepsy. Epilepsy is a common medical condition, but most people with the condition do not suffer from it throughout their lifetime.

Epilepsy is not an illness in its own right, but a symptom of many different diseases with varying causes. It can affect any person at any time of life, but incidence rates are highest amongst young people, the elderly and people with intellectual disabilities (Shorvon, 2000). An epileptic seizure is described as the manifestation of an abnormal and excessive synchronized discharge of a set of cerebral neurons (Sander & Thompson, 1989). The clinical presentation is usually a very brief stereotyped event whereby the individual's awareness of their surroundings is impaired and their behaviour may change. Attacks have a sudden onset, are short and cease spontaneously. Periods of drowsiness and confusion may follow.

There are many different types of seizures, but all are caused by a sudden disturbance of the normal functioning of the brain. People with PIMD may have more than one seizure type, and this has implications with regard to management and treatment. Seizures are classified by their symptoms, areas of the brain where the discharge starts or by the type of attack. Seizure types are classified into two main groups and relate to the area of the brain whereby the abnormal discharge occurs (ILAE, 1981).

For example, if the discharge starts in one area of the brain, they are termed partial seizures. If the discharge involves both sides of the brain, the seizures are termed generalised. Defining which group the seizure is aligned to is based on the signs and symptoms experienced by the person or a witness account. This is then followed with a series of medical investigations such as brain imaging, otherwise referred to as an MRI scan, and an electroencephalogram (EEG) that examines abnormal electrical discharges in the brain.

Generalised seizures, especially tonic clonic seizures, were previously referred to as *grand mal* seizures and this term is still used today, particularly by carers. With this seizure type there is no warning. The person suddenly goes stiff, falls down and their body will start to jerk. Breathing is laboured and the person salivates. They may be incontinent and during the seizure may bite their tongue. This type of seizure usually ceases after a few minutes and the person may experience confusion, drowsiness and headaches. It is not unusual for the person experiencing this type of seizure to want to sleep following recovery. The occurrence of this type of seizure is more widespread in people with profound and multiple disabilities due to the nature of damage to more than one area of the brain (Kerr, 1996).

Other types of generalised seizures are tonic seizure, in which there is a sudden increase in the muscle tone of the body whereby the person becomes rigid and if standing the person will fall to the ground. Recovery is quick from this type of seizure. Another form is atonic seizure or otherwise referred to as drop attack. In this form of seizure, there is a sudden loss of muscle tone and the person falls to the ground. There are no convulsions in this seizure and recovery is quick.

Two other types of seizures are absence seizure and myoclonic seizure. With absence seizures there is a period of blankness that may be accompanied by fluttering of the eyelids or nodding of the head. Such attacks usually only last for a few seconds, which is one of the reasons they tend to go unrecognised. This type of seizure usually occurs in childhood and early adolescence. The myoclonic seizure presents in an abrupt, very brief involuntary shock like jerks that may involve the arms, head or the whole body. This form of seizure usually happens in the morning, shortly after the person wakes up. Recovery from this form of seizure is immediate.

The second group of seizures are referred to as partial seizures, otherwise referred to as focal attacks are divided into three groups. The first is the simple partial seizure that occurs when the abnormal discharge to the brain remains localised and what happens in this form of seizure is dependent on the area of the brain where the discharge occurs. Presentation is in the form of localised jerking of one limb, twitching of one part of the body, numbness or abnormal sensation such as strange feelings, experiencing unusual smell or visual sensation. This stage is often referred to as an aura. This form of seizure may cease at this stage or it may progress into what is referred to as a complex partial seizure.

With complex partial, characteristics are similar to simple partial. However, in this form of seizure there is always an impairment of consciousness. The seizure may start off as simple and then progresses to present an alteration in the person's behaviour. This will present as the person fiddling with objects in a confused manner, plucking at their clothes, lip smacking, undressing and if mobile the person may wander around in what appears to be a drunken fashion. It is not uncommon for this type of seizure to be mistaken for a form of mental disorder. This type of seizures is often referred to as temporal lobe seizure, as most of the discharges that cause the seizure to start are in the temporal lobe area of the brain. Both these type of seizures can progress to all parts of the brain resulting in secondary generalised attacks that lead to a tonic clonic seizure that has the same characteristics as a generalised tonic clonic convulsion.

Most seizure types stop spontaneously but on some occasions the seizures may occur in quick succession, without any period of recovery in between seizures. This is referred to as status epilepticus and can occur with any type of seizure. It is particularly dangerous if it occurs in generalised tonic clonic seizures, and in this instance, the attack would be considered as an emergency.

Epilepsy: the impact on people with PIMD

The association between intellectual disability and epilepsy is reflected in the comparison of its incidence to the general population (Forsgren et al., 1996; Airaksinen et al., 2000; Patja et al., 2000). Twenty-five per cent of people with intellectual disabilities have epilepsy in comparison to 4% of the general population (Richardson et al., 1979; Cooper, 1998; Airaksinen et al., 2000). Epilepsy often presents as more complex in people with intellectual disabilities (Steffenburg et al., 1996). According to Espie & Paul (1997), there are few problems that present in people with intellectual disabilities as commonly and as persistently as epilepsy.

The prevalence of epilepsy in intellectual disability ranges from 6% amongst children with mild intellectual disability, to 24% in severe intellectual disability, and 50% in those with profound and multiple intellectual disability (Lhatoo & Sander, 2001). The association between the likelihood of having epilepsy if the individual has an additional impairment is strong. Hauser et al. (1987) showed an increase in the risk of epilepsy from 11 to 48% when a child with intellectual disability also has cerebral palsy. Others such as Sussova et al. (1990) and Steffenburgh et al. (1996) also confirm this association.

People with PIMD generally do not access healthcare in the same manner as people without disabilities. As a consequence, other needs pertaining to basic health needs are neglected, one of which is epilepsy. There is ample evidence to support this finding from studies such as Howells (1986), Beange et al. (1995), Kerr (1996), Welsh Office (1996), Branford et al. (1998a, b) and Scottish Executive (2004).

Yet despite these findings, epilepsy continues to present as a need that is unmet by services. Evidence of this can be obtained from the Clinical Standards Advisory Group (2000) who reported there was a lack of focus in services for people with epilepsy alongside the lack of coordination between primary and secondary care. Stuttaford (2003) suggests that epilepsy has a low political profile, as it is too often not socially accepted. In contrast, Hirst (2004) notes the reasons for poor service is that epilepsy is a poorly understood area and one that continues to be underfunded.

The implications of epilepsy for people with PIMD are enormous. Seizures alone are a frightening experience especially if the individuals have no awareness of what is happening to them. This in turn can cause great anxiety to carers who may have little knowledge of the condition. Carers' knowledge of epilepsy has generally been demonstrated to be inadequate (Branford et al., 1998a; Hannah & Brodie, 1998; Deb & Joyce, 1999).

Seizure can occur spontaneously, although in most cases there are often a number of triggers that can precipitate the occurrence of seizures. These include lack of sleep, too much sleep, tiredness, other illness, interaction of drugs that may be given for other conditions, incorrect medication, method of administration of medication (i.e. medication being administered via tube such as gastronomy), changes in medication and being prescribed more than one medication (Coughlan, 1997).

Epilepsy is also associated with an increased risk of mortality. It is estimated that mortality in people with intellectual disabilities is two to three times greater than that of the general population (Lhatoo & Sander, 2001). There is also developing evidence that sudden unexpected death is higher in people with intellectual disabilities than in the population of people with epilepsy generally (Nashef et al., 1995; Derby et al., 1996). Forsgren et al. (1996) found that standard mortality ratios in people with intellectual disabilities and epilepsy were substantially higher than those in patients with intellectual disability alone, and highest in people with intellectual disability, epilepsy and profound and multiple intellectual disabilities.

A number of formidable challenges arise in the identification, treatment and monitoring of epilepsy in people with profound and multiple intellectual disabilities. Jenkins & Brown (1992) identified one of the main difficulties in the assessment of people with intellectual disabilities is issues relating to diagnosis. This is further compounded for people with profound and multiple disabilities due to their inability to communicate as well as the lack of skills of medical professional in communicating with this population group (Lennox et al., 1997; Singh, 1997; Thornton, 1999).

Evidence from practice

As noted in the government's white paper *Valuing People* (Department of Health (DH) 2001) for people with intellectual disability, good quality services will ensure that people with additional and complex needs are appropriately cared for so that their needs are well managed and they can lead fulfilling lives. Nonetheless, good quality services can only be developed from evidence based on the assessment of need of a population group. Services can be aligned following this process to adequately meet identified need.

In Berkshire the needs of people with intellectual disabilities are assessed using a common assessment framework. This format seeks to assess need from a holistic approach, incorporating the social, health, and psychological, housing, spiritual and financial aspects. Although epilepsy is identified as a need within this format, it fails to amplify the characteristics of the condition or the extent to which this condition affects the person's life.

Health professionals and carers voiced their concerns that need pertaining to epilepsy were not being identified. Consequently, appropriate services could not be accessed. In order to investigate these concerns, we decided to explore the needs of people with intellectual disabilities who had epilepsy in our area, in order to provide evidence that in turn could influence practice-based assessment of epilepsy for people with profound and multiple intellectual disabilities.

Evidence-based practice is a term that has emerged as a major theme in National Health Service policy (DH, 1998, 1999, 2000). Previously, the perceived emphasis of this concept was reliant on randomised controlled trials to provide the most reliable source of evidence. Kitson (2002) reminds us that more recently recognition has been given to other sources such as clinical expertise and user and carer preferences.

The emergence of evidence-based practice prompted us to undertake some exploratory work to investigate the needs of people with intellectual disabilities and epilepsy living in the West of Berkshire. In exploring the best approach to adopt in seeking this information, we became aware of two important elements crucial to the identification of need amongst this population group. First, there was no database that specifically identified individuals with epilepsy.

Alongside, evidence from the literature suggests that carers lack appropriate knowledge relating to epilepsy. Yet, carers are the most frequent observers of seizure occurrence amongst people with intellectual disabilities especially those with profound and complex needs (Espie et al., 1998). In doing so, we sought to use a valid questionnaire that was used in previous research to extract similar data. The questionnaire located was Branford et al. (1998a) who sought information in five areas. These are as follows:

1. The number of people with epilepsy
2. Current treatment
3. Type of seizures
4. Services accessed
5. Frequency of contact with services

The questionnaire was sent to all people with intellectual disabilities living in the West of Berkshire. This was distributed via schools, day centres, residential care homes, respite centres and further educational colleges. Details of the survey were advertised in local newspapers in attempting to reach people who had little or no contact with services. In total 600 questionnaires were distributed for which 487 were returned; of these, carers completed the questionnaire in 67%, 24% by relatives and 8% by others.

The findings confirm the concerns expressed by carers and professionals that need pertaining to epilepsy in people with intellectual disabilities were not being met. For example, a number of people were taking two or more anticonvulsant medication, a large proportion had not seen a neurologist, many seizures occurred at night-time and few people had seen their general practitioner (GP) within the last year for their epilepsy.

The survey was followed up with semi-structured interviews offered to all carers who wished to discuss in more detail, the needs of the person being cared for. The findings revealed a key theme that is consistent with the literature. This is the lack of knowledge and awareness of carers on issues relating to epilepsy such as identification of seizures, current treatments, what to do in an emergency and services available locally (Hannah & Brodie, 1998; Deb & Joyce, 1999).

Meeting identified need

This compelling evidence was published to enable other services to replicate what proved to be a useful study (Codling, 2001). These findings also prompted services in our own area to develop a new vision surrounding the assessment of people with epilepsy and adopt a change to current practice. In making sense of the findings, a number of workshops were organised with health colleagues to explore their perception of current services and their role in meeting the needs arising from the survey.

Evaluation of feedback from these workshops revealed that arrays of professionals were duplicating interventions, with poor communication between all involved. The lack of a cohesive structure prompted professionals to develop a system that focused first and foremost on the presenting need, followed by delivery of care in a structured and coordinated manner. In contrast, evidence from the survey indicated that no clear process or structure existed for mapping the care of people with intellectual disabilities and epilepsy. Developing a framework would provide potential to work together on case-related activity that in turn would offer a structured approach to meeting the needs of people with epilepsy.

The integrated care pathway concepts seemed the most suitable as evidence of their use is reported as most effective in people who have a predictable course of care, such as a specific health condition (Campbell et al., 1998). Integrated care pathways bring together the separate elements from a multidisciplinary, towards a coordinated approach, resulting in a more effective delivery of care. In other words, integrated care pathways are a means of promoting change in practice by creating opportunities for the systematic delivery of care between professionals and services.

A number of professionals were selected to form a working group for the purpose of discussing current care provided and explore areas that would improve the process of care for people with epilepsy. Although patterns of care may be evident among professionals, it can cause immense confusion to service users and carers especially, if all professionals are offering a service for the same condition. Mapping this process of care enables users and carers to have a clearer understanding of services and be more focused in their understanding of the care they expect to receive.

After much collaborative, multidisciplinary discussion as well as incorporating evidence arising from the survey (Codling, 2001), the integrated care pathway was developed (Codling et al., 2005). A number of authors describe the process of professionals getting together to agree a consensus view of care as being of major benefit (Riches et al., 1994; Nelson, 1995; Cheater, 1996). We found the process enabled a range of professionals to share their skills and create a better understanding of when and where their input would be required in the pathway of care.

The pathway was formulated to contain six stages. The first stage commences with the initial referral and proceeds through the stages in mapping the process of care from referral to completion. The care pathway process map can be found in Figure 9.1. The group identified that the key coordinator of the pathway should be the intellectual disability nurse. The rationale for this is that intellectual disability nurses have both the skill and the knowledge of epilepsy and are therefore best placed to conduct this process and coordinate other professionals' involvement as and when required.

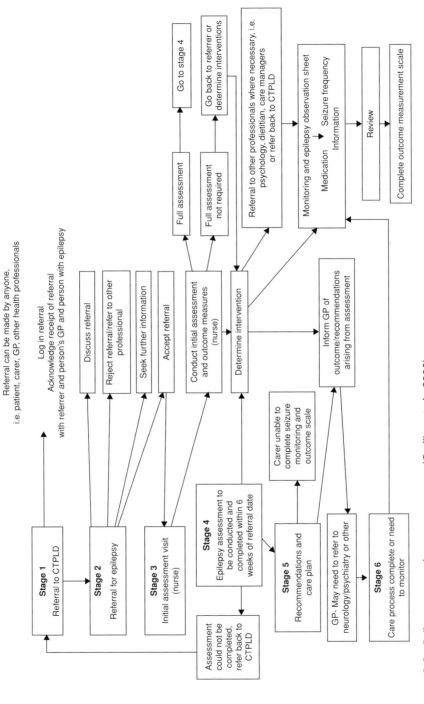

Figure 9.1 Epilepsy care pathway process map (Codling et al., 2005).

As a result, the pathway has provided a gateway for involving carers and professionals in the plan of care of people with PIMD with epilepsy. This in turn has enabled need to be assessed holistically, refreshing the vision and setting the direction for the needs of people with PIMD and their carers to be met in a structured and needs-led format.

This process entails the intellectual disability nurse conducting an initial assessment and deciding at this point whether there is a need for a more detailed assessment. This detailed assessment was complied by the integrated care pathway group and encapsulates need from a multidimensional perspective. The nurse on completion of the assessment will recommend a number of interventions and will act as the key person in ensuring these interventions are delivered. Some examples of these interventions are as follows:

- Referral to a neurologist for further neurological investigations
- Referral to the GP for ill health that may be impacting on seizure frequency or for review of medication
- Referral to dietitian for advise on nutrition and diet
- Input from psychology for stress- or anxiety-related conditions that may be responsible for increase in seizure frequency

Following on, the nurse will review the pathway to ensure that the needs of the person with epilepsy and their carers are met. Following this, there may be further interventions that are required such as monitoring of seizures or changes to medication. In this instance the pathway will continue until the interventions are met. Once the pathway is completed, a copy is sent to all relevant people involved in the individuals care alongside their GP. A review date is set at this point to ensure that the person's epilepsy continues to be monitored on a regular basis.

In evaluating the effectiveness of the care pathway, we used the Epilepsy Outcome Scale develop by Espie & Paul (1998) to measure the knowledge of carers and users where applicable. This format consists of a set of questions that seeks to explore concerns held about epilepsy. This was completed prior to the introduction of the pathway and again on completion. The findings indicated that a change in knowledge particularly of carers was evident following intervention.

This also highlighted the vulnerability of carers in their role of caring for an individual with complex needs with little knowledge or guidance. This is consistent with findings from Mencap (2003) who reported there is a lack of trained carers to care for people with profound and complex needs. The evidence arising from our intervention enabled us to recognise that knowledge and support for carers is of utmost importance, especially where healthcare is being delivered.

Carers' needs

Carers of people with profound and multiple needs are often neglected. In terms of research, we know surprisingly little about the precise impact of epilepsy on carers.

Thompson & Upton (1992) inform us that levels of stress and dissatisfaction are high amongst carers of people without intellectual disabilities who have epilepsy.

Evidence arising from our own study (Codling, 2001) suggested that carers' disaffection was attributed to the lack of information they received from services and professionals about epilepsy. Although epilepsy is well described in text, carers poorly understand it. In view of this we decided to address this issue by delivering training to carers'. The intellectual disability nurse initially delivered this to individual carers' in their homes or in residential homes where a number of people with intellectual disabilities resided.

However, in time this method of delivery became very time-consuming and exhaustive. We conducted an analysis of the number of people delivering this training, the number of hours per week spent in this role and the knowledge imparted to carers. Following analysis, we presented the findings along with a proposal for a more structured approach for delivery of training to the education and training department of our local Primary Care Trust.

The Primary Care Trust agreed to finance and deliver the proposed outline for training. This involved organising a set programme that would be delivered on a monthly basis and could be accessed by carers. The Primary Care Trust was keen to utilise the skills of the intellectual disability nurse as the core trainer. A number of intellectual disability nurses who had undertaken the epilepsy specialist nurses training agreed to be trainers for this programme. The training programme is distributed to all carers' and organisations across Berkshire. The content of the training is as follows:

- What is epilepsy
- What is a seizure
- Recognising and identifying a seizure
- Description of different seizure types
- What causes and triggers seizure occurrence
- Medical investigations
- Treatment for epilepsy
- What to do in the event of a seizure
- What to do in an emergency
- The recovery position
- Administration of medication and rectal diazepam
- Care plans, policies and protocols
- Recording and monitoring of seizure occurrence
- Services available and how to access them

Summary

This project proved to be beneficial to people with intellectual disabilities, including those with profound and multiple intellectual disabilities, as well as those professionals working with this population group. Obtaining evidence from carers surrounding the needs of people with profound and complex needs has in turn enabled services to respond in meeting such needs. Redesigning and developing services such as the care pathway and the epilepsy training has reaped its benefits. Designing and implementing the care pathway has provided a clear outline to meeting the needs of people with epilepsy. Carers, professionals, GPs and neurologists welcomed this as it informs everyone involved in the person' care of the expected interventions and outcomes. The availability of training on epilepsy has injected confidence and skills in carers in managing seizures and being prepared in the event of an emergency.

As a result, the needs of people with PIMD and epilepsy are now being given the attention they need, aiding better healthcare and improved quality of life. Carers' feel more in tune with the needs of the person they care for and are more aware of services available to them in meeting such needs.

References

Airaksinen, E.M., Matilainen, R., Mononen, T., Mustonen, K., Partanen, J., Jokela, V., & Halonen, P. (2000). A population based study on epilepsy in mentally retarded children. *Epilepsia*, 41(9), 1214–1220.

Beange, H., McElduff, A., & Baker, W. (1995). Medical disorders of adults with mental retardation: a population based study. *American Journal of Mental Retardation*, 99(6), 595–604.

Branford, D., Bhaumik, F., Duncan, F., & Collacott, A. (1998b). A follow up study of adults with learning disabilities and epilepsy. *Seizure*, 7(6), 469–472.

Branford, D., Bhaumik, S., & Duncan, F. (1998a). Epilepsy in adults with learning disabilities. *Seizure*, 7(6), 473–477.

Campbell, H., Hotchkiss, R., Bradshaw, N., & Porteous, M. (1998). Integrated care pathways. *British Medical Journal*, 316(7125), 133–137.

Cheater, F. (1996). Care pathways: good tools for clinical audit? *Audit Trends*, 4(2), 73–75.

Clinical Standards Advisory Group (2000). *Services for Patients with Epilepsy*. London: HMSO.

Codling, M. (2001). Compelling evidence. *Learning Disability Practice*, 4(4), 22–25.

Codling, M., Macdonald, N., & Chandler, B. (2005). Integrated care pathway for people with epilepsy. *Learning Disability Practice*, 8(3), 32–37.

Cooper, S.A. (1998). Clinical study of the effects of age on the physical health of adults with mental retardation. *American Journal of Mental Retardation*, 102(6), 582–589.

Coughlan, B.J. (1997). Epilepsy, learning disability and anti-convulsant drug status. *Mental Health Care*, 1(1), 25–28.

Deb, S., & Joyce, J. (1999). Characteristics of epilepsy in a population based cohort of adults with learning disabilities. *Irish Journal of Psychological Medicine*, 16(1), 5–9.

Derby, L.E., Tennis, P., & Jick, H. (1996). Sudden death among subjects with refractory epilepsy. *Epilepsia*, 37(10), 931–935.

DH (1998). *A First Class Service: Quality in the New NHS*. London: Department of Health.

DH (1999). *Making a Difference: Strengthening the Nursing, Midwifery and Health Visiting Contribution to Health and Health Care*. London: Department of Health.

DH (2000). *The NHS Plan: A Plan for Investment, a Plan for Reform*. London: HMSO.

DH. (2001). *Valuing People. A New Strategy for Learning Disability for the 21st Century. CM: 5086.* London: HMSO.

Espie, C.A., & Paul, A. (1997). In Cull, C., & Goldstein, L.H. (eds), *The Clinical Psychologists Handbook of Epilepsy.* London: Routledge.

Espie, C.A., Paul, A., Graham, M., Starrick, M., Foley, J., & McGarvey, C. (1998). The epilepsy outcome scale: the development of a measure for use with carers of people with epilepsy plus intellectual disability. *Journal of Intellectual Disability Research*, 42(1), 90–96.

Forsgren, L., Edvinsson, S., Nystroim, L., & Blomguist, H.K. (1996). Influence of epilepsy on mortality in mental retardation: an epidemiological study. *Epilepsia*, 37(10), 956–963.

Hannah, J.A., & Brodie, M.J. (1998). Epilepsy and learning disabilities – a challenge for the millennium? *Seizure*, 7(1), 3–13.

Hauser, W.A., Shinnard, S., Cohen, H., Inbar, D., & Benedeth, M.D. (1987). Clinical predictors of epilepsy amongst children with cerebral palsy and/or mental retardation. *Neurology*, 37(Supplement 1), 150.

Hirst, J. (2004). Message from our chairman. *Epilepsy News: The Newsletter of the Fund for Epilepsy.* Available at: http://www.epilepsyfund.org.uk/autumn04/epnews19.pdf (accessed 28 September 2007).

Howells, G. (1986). Are the medical needs of the mentally handicapped being met? *Journal of the Royal College of General Practitioners*, 36(291), 449–453.

ILAE (1981). International league against epilepsy. Proposal for revised clinical and electroencephalographic classification of epileptic seizures. *Epilepsia*, 22, 489–501.

Jenkins, L.K., & Brown, S.W. (1992). Some issues in the assessment of epilepsy occurring in the context of disability in adults. *Seizure*, 1, 49–55.

Kerr, M. (1996). Epilepsy in patients with learning disabilities. *Aspects of Epilepsy*, 3, 1–6.

Kitson, A. (2002). Recognising relationships: reflections on evidence-based practice. *Nursing Inquiry*, 9(3), 179–186.

Lennox, N.G., Diggens, J., & Ugoni, A. (1997). The general practice care of people with intellectual disability: barriers and solutions. *Journal of Intellectual Disability Research*, 41(5), 380–390.

Lhatoo, S.D., & Sander, J.W.A.S. (2001). The epidemiology of epilepsy and learning disability. *Epilepsia*, 42(Supplement 1), 6–9.

Mencap (2003) *Treat Me Right. Better Health Care for People with a Learning Disability.* London: Mencap.

Nashef, L., Fish, D.R., Garner, S., Sander, J.W., & Shorvon, S.D. (1995). Sudden death in epilepsy. A study of incidence in a young cohort with epilepsy and learning difficulties. *Epilepsia*, 36(12), 1187–1194.

Nelson, S. (1995). Following pathways in pursuit of excellence. *International Journal of Health Care Quality Assurance*, 8(7), 19–21.

Patja, K., Iivanainen, M., Vesala, H., Oksanen, H., & Ruoppila, I. (2000). Life expectancy of people with intellectual disability: a 35-year follow up study. *Journal of Intellectual Disability Research*, 44(5), 591–599.

Richardson, S.A., Katz, M., Koller, H., McLaren, J., & Rubenstine, B. (1979). Some characteristics of a population of mentally retarded young adults in a British city. *Journal of Mental Deficiency Research*, 23(4), 275–285.

Riches, T., Stead, L., & Espie, C.A. (1994). Introducing anticipated recovery pathways: a teaching hospital experience. *International Journal of Health Care Quality Assurance*, 7(5), 21–24.

Sander, L., & Thompson, P. (1989). *Epilepsy. A Practical Guide to Coping.* Wiltshire: The Crowood Press.

Scottish Executive (2004) *The Same as You? A Review of Services for People with Learning Disabilities.* Edinburgh: The Scottish Office.

Shorvon, S. (2000). *Handbook of Epilepsy Treatment.* Oxford: Blackwell Science.

Singh, P. (1997). *Prescription for Change: A Mencap Report of GP's and Carers' in the Provision of Primary Care for People with Learning Disabilities.* London: Mencap.

Steffenburgh, U., Hagberg, G., & Kyllerman, M. (1996). Characteristics of seizures in a population-based series of mentally retarded children with active epilepsy. *Epilepsia*, 37(9), 850–856.

Stuttaford, T. (2003). The hidden disease. *Epilepsy*, Autumn, 37–38.

Sussova, J., Seidl, Z., & Faber, J. (1990). Hemiparetic forms of cerebral palsy in relation to epilepsy and mental retardation. *Developmental Medicine and Child Neurology*, 32, 792–795.

Thompson, P.J., & Upton, D. (1992). The impact of chronic epilepsy on the family. *Seizure*, 1, 43–48.

Thornton, C. (1999). Effective healthcare for people with learning disabilities: a formal carers' perspective. *Journal of Psychiatric and Mental Health Nursing*, 6(5), 383–390.

Welsh Office (1996). *Welsh Health Survey 1995.* London: HMSO.

Chapter 10

'SIGHT IS MIGHT'[1]: VISION AND VISION IMPAIRMENT IN PEOPLE WITH PROFOUND INTELLECTUAL AND MULTIPLE DISABILITIES

Gill Levy

Introduction

Vision and hearing are the key ways to understand the world. 'Information received through the senses can be considered as the basis for an individual's learning about and acquiring a conceptual understanding of the properties of the physical world' (Warren, 1984).

There are some particular issues that are important when considering people with sensory impairments and profound intellectual and multiple disabilities (PIMD). Many have conditions that have not been fully assessed; these unidentified health problems and impairments can so reduce people's quality of life and their ability to participate that others may underestimate their potential (DH, 2002).

There is prejudice against people with PIMD accessing services (DRC, 2006) but there are also real difficulties – such as small optometry practices being inaccessible to people using large wheelchairs (College of Optometrists, 2000).

Approximately 30% of people with intellectual disabilities have a significant impairment of sight and 40% have significant hearing problems. There is a high rate of underdetection of sensory impairments, most of which can be treated (NHS Executive, 1998). This means that there are two 'groups' of people with sight problems:

- People who are blind/severely sight impaired or partially sighted/sight impaired and need appropriate help.
- People who have difficulty seeing because they need glasses, eye surgery or other treatment to improve their sight.

Mencap found that 53% of people with intellectual disabilities had not had a sight test in the last 2 years (Mencap, 1998). While anecdotal evidence suggests that there

---

[1] 'Sight is might'– saying of pupils in a school for blind children.

has been a marked improvement in the number of 'able' people with intellectual disabilities having sight tests, people with PIMD may still be considered too disabled to test by their carers and supporters.

Staff working in eye care services may lack experience and may provide inferior assessments, they may not know about:

- the special tests available, or how to adapt techniques;
- people whose visual impairment is caused by unidentified damage in the brain; and
- routine problems, such as an eye infection, causing additional difficulties for a person with PIMD and their supporters.

Learning objectives

By the end of this chapter, readers should be able to:

- acknowledge the prevalence of sight problems in people with intellectual disabilities and the lack of identification of visual impairment in people with PIMD;
- appreciate the potential difficulties for individuals, carers, supporters and services;
- have a critical understanding of formal ways to assess vision and how these may be adapted for individuals with PIMD; and
- gain an appreciation of the many ways to help people maximise their vision.

Sight problems

It is a scandal that so many people have unidentified eye problems which may cause pain and lower potential and which undermine successful participation in a range of activities (Levy, 2007a).

Eye problems in people with profound disabilities are so common that supporters actively need to look for them (see Appendix 10.1 for the checklist to identify possible signs of sight problems).

There are many ways to help people once their visual impairment is diagnosed and its implications for the individual understood. People need this help. They have a right to it.

People with PIMD, those with 'ordinary vision' and people who are visually impaired – may need glasses. This may be because they are:

- short sighted;
- long sighted; and
- astigmatic (when the eye is shaped more like a rugby ball than a football, affecting the vision).

People with astigmatism are usually short sighted or long sighted too.

Whilst total blindness is rare, many people with PIMD have sufficiently poor sight to be registerable as blind/severely visually impaired or partially sighted/severely visually impaired. (Information about registration is available on the RNIB[2] website.)

People may be born with sight problems or acquire them in infancy. They may have a single visual impairment or several. They may have:

- blurred vision;
- patchy vision;
- reduced visual field (all-round vision);
- tunnel vision;
- sight on one side only;
- sight in the upper part of their visual field;
- sight in the lower part of their visual field; and
- nystagmus – involuntary eye movements.

Many people with severe/profound disability (especially people with cerebral palsy) have cerebral visual impairment. This results from damage to the visual systems in the brain that deal with processing and integrating visual information. Their eyes may be 'normal' so this condition may not be diagnosed by a routine eye test.

People with PIMD are now living long enough to acquire the eye problems associated with ageing, especially cataracts. Sight loss is a disturbing experience for people of all levels of ability, and may cause depression, anxiety and/or behaviour that challenges.

Some people with intellectual disabilities damage their sight by eye poking. Supporters need to establish if a person's eye poking is a harmless self-stimulatory habit, or sight-threatening. It is important to ensure that a person does not damage their eyes by keeping their hands clean wherever possible and ensuring that their fingernails do not have 'square corners'.

Potential difficulties for individuals and their supporters

Minimising or underestimating the social effects of sensory impairment may condemn people to unnecessarily impoverished lives.

Many people with intellectual disabilities have poor sight and urgently need help to use their vision more effectively. If this help is denied, they are likely to experience problems.

Social exclusion

People with visual impairments and severe disabilities may be isolated and afraid. Their lives may be a series of random events because no one has tried to help them understand their world. People need involvement in activities that are meaningful to

---

[2] http://www.rnib.org.uk

them – otherwise they may withdraw into themselves or develop behaviours which others may find hard to understand.

Communication

People with visual impairment may have poor communication skills. Eye contact helps in 'taking turns' to talk. Sight enables people to understand facial expressions, body language and individual gestures. Vision and hearing problems may mean the person is not aware of efforts to communicate with them.

The inability to see can affect the early bonding process between blind children with severe disabilities and their parents. In the past, blind children were at particular risk of being admitted to long-stay hospital (Oswin, 1978; Ellis, 1982). Families reported difficulty understanding their blind child's body language or early attempts to respond to them. Blind babies may move their hands when another child's response would be a change of facial expression (Fraiberg, 1977).

People with sight problems often find it hard to learn sign language, which may need to be adapted to the individual's eye condition. Visually impaired people may not be able to see some signs at all. They may only see part of other signs (Waite & Levy, 2007).

A visual impairment may make it hard for people to express their needs, resulting in people developing 'behaviour that challenges' in unresponsive environments.

> *People with more severe disabilities and people with additional disabilities (e.g. sensory impairments, receptive and expressive communication disorders) are at increased risk of showing challenging behaviour* (Emerson et al., 2001, p. 36).

Whilst a visual impairment may make it hard for people with PIMD to express their needs; many people are in settings which do not respond to their attempts to communicate. It is important to adopt communication methods, such as objects of reference, to help people make sense of their world (Bradley, 2007).

Motivation

Sight helps to create motivation – blind children often need to be encouraged to reach out for things. If they are unable to see desirable objects across the room, they may not be motivated to discover and touch things. They may not be bothered about learning to walk, and may lack the confidence to move in an unknown environment. Visually impaired adults with intellectual disabilities often seem to be lacking in 'drive'. A common complaint is that 'they just wait for things to happen – they don't do anything' (Thomas & Levy, 1998).

People who have not learned that they have the power to control their environment may appear compliant or passive. However, their whole personalities may appear to change when they receive appropriate help to develop communication, mobility and self-help skills. Finding ways to motivate blind people with intellectual disabilities may not be easy – particularly when they have discovered that staff and family carers expect them to fail. While different people are motivated by different things, many blind people with severe disabilities are most likely to need rewards other than just visual ones. It is, therefore important to break tasks down into tiny steps and to make activities fun and rewarding for an individual, giving him/her plenty of encouragement and praise. (*Further information available in the Look Up*[3] *Factsheets: Hints on teaching skills to people with visual and learning disabilities and understanding and using sight: issues for work with people with learning disabilities.*)

Coordination

Sight coordinates information from other senses – hearing, touch, taste, smell, and so on; vision helps integrate the mass of sensory information. . . . When faced with a situation where accurate vision information is not readily available it is still possible for us to structure the situation, and make use of particular 'compensatory strategies' (Brown et al., 1998, p. 32). Sight is a permanent sense. It tells us what is there, even when we can no longer hear, touch, smell or taste something.

Learning and development

Sight plays an important part in learning and personal development – both through planned structured teaching in schools and individual programmes, and informal learning from watching television and copying others.

Children and adults who have visual impairment and intellectual disabilities usually need extra help to discover about their world. They may learn little by chance. Often staff and families have been overprotective, so the person's natural curiosity has been stifled. It is not uncommon to find relatives or staff so anxious about an individual hurting him/herself, that s/he has actually been stopped from moving about alone.

To help learning and personal development, blind people with intellectual disabilities constantly need the world explained to them; every possible opportunity should be exploited to give people information and ways of learning so that they are not deprived of 'visual things'.

Assessing people, places and situations

A sighted person may enter a room and instantly be aware of who is present, what is going on, and, without thinking may be conscious of details such as carpets, furniture and lighting. A blind person may gather this information – but it would probably take him or her very much longer, and the information might be incomplete. This can be remedied by providing clear explanations, perhaps supported by clues – such as noises and floor textures.

People with severe/profound disabilities need plenty of time to discover things for themselves so that they can make their own decisions based on knowledge they

---

[3] http://www.lookupinfo.org

have gained. They need to learn to assess if situations are safe or if risks are worth taking.

Memory

Sight provides the memory with useful prompts and reminders. Memory is based on the previous receipt of information, and the ability to 'file' knowledge. People with visual impairments may need specially created 'prompts' to jog their memory.

Knowledge of self and self-image

Without visual feedback, it may be difficult to develop a true picture of oneself. People need to know where they begin and end, how much space their body occupies, and how they look.

Space, size and abstract concepts

Young sighted children have no difficulty in grasping quite abstract concepts such as size, direction, distance and space – even when they cannot touch the objects concerned. Many blind people with intellectual disabilities find the concept of 'object permanence' difficult – that an object is still there, when it cannot be seen, heard, touched, smelled or tasted. When someone leaves the room, are they gone forever, or will they return (Levy, 2007b)?

Balance, movement and mobility

Sight helps people maintain their balance. Good balance allows people to move independently and safely without fear of falling. People with little or no sight may be apprehensive about textures underfoot – for example, carpets, grass and sand on the beach. They may experience hills and slopes or changes in surface level more dramatically than people with 'ordinary vision'. However, different surfaces provide people with useful clues about where they are.

Sight plays a key role in finding one's way around, travelling and learning routes and recognising one's destination when it has been reached.

Trust

Trust is based on previous knowledge of people, places and situations and an assessment of personal security – so sight plays an important part in the development of trust. People, whose visual impairment has never been acknowledged, may never have learned to trust others. They may not have received help to understand what is going on around them, so they experience their lives as a series of random events which make them feel insecure.

Concentration and attention span

Most people find it easier to concentrate on an activity for long periods if they can see clearly and focus their attention on the process. People with little or no sight may require help to develop their powers of concentration with verbal feedback to tell them of their successes. In this way, they know it is worth concentrating and finishing a task. They may not feel motivated to persevere unless they are told about their progress and achievements.

Many tasks may seem to have little relevance or interest to them. People happily concentrate on the things they find rewarding – sometimes to the point of obsession. Staff need to see what an individual enjoys, and try to incorporate this into other things.

Autonomy and independence

Sight helps people to be more independent when they want to be, enabling them to make a whole range of choices, based on firsthand knowledge. Visually impaired people with intellectual disabilities may need special help to become assertive and autonomous. They may often be in situations where their special needs are over-looked, so they are forced to be dependent upon other people for basic informa-tion, explanations and interpretations of their surroundings. Supporters need to help them to develop positive feelings about themselves.

Visually impaired people may need help to use their hearing

Blind and partially sighted people are particularly dependent upon their hearing to make sense of the world. However, significant proportions also have hearing problems or wax in their ears, which may be unidentified. It is therefore important that people have regular ear examinations and hearing tests. People need help to make the best possible use of their hearing.

Deafblindness

There is no statutory definition of deafblindness but a person should be regarded as deafblind if she or he has a severe degree of combined visual and auditory impair-ment, resulting in problems of communication, information and mobility. Such a description applies to those with dual sensory impairment whose resultant handicap is separate and distinct from a single sensory impairment (DH & SSI, 1989).

Deafblindness is now seen as a separate disability in its own right. The inter-play between sight and hearing is complex. Sight assists hearing. Equally, hearing supports and complements sight (Levy & McKelvie, 1993 cited in Stevens, 1993, p. 148). Those supporting people with PIMD, who have both sight and hearing problems, need to carefully consider the 'meaning' of the dual loss, its impact upon the individual and seek expert help.

Eye care

As with the general population, people with intellectual disabilities should have regular eye tests – once every 2 years, or more frequently if the optometrist recom-mends.

There are several components to an eye test and all should be included:

- The optometrist should take a medical history and ask about symptoms.
- They should also enquire if the person or their family has a history of eye problems.
- An eye health check is vital to look for eye diseases or damage (inside and outside the eye), to ensure that both eyes are working together, and to test the pressure inside the eye.
- 'Visual field' tests should be carried out to make sure someone has 'all round vision'.
- Tests to establish level of vision ('visual acuity'), at distance and near and contrast sensitivity: how much something stands out from its background, need to be conducted.
- 'Refraction' is a test to assess if a person is short sighted, long sighted or astigmatic, and whether he/she can focus accurately at near, and to determine the need for glasses or contact lenses for distance or near vision (Levy & Woodhouse, 2007a).

Most people with PIMD in the UK qualify for a free NHS sight test. For information on entitlement refer to form (DH, 2005) *HC11: Help with health costs.*

The role of the health facilitator/health supporter

Before planning a sight test, it is worth to have the health supporter visit the optometrist to discover any potential problems – such as transport, parking and whether the practice is accessible for wheelchair users (including toilets) (refer to Chapter 16 for details regarding accessible toilets). It provides an opportunity to assess the practice and look at the equipment to be used.

People with intellectual disabilities need to be prepared for the full range of tests that the optometrist will undertake. A plan of action is required for a successful sight test and eye examination. It is important to prepare the receptionist, optometrist and individual and also to ensure that appropriate support is available.

The health supporter accompanying the person to their eye test appointment needs to be able to provide the optometrist with relevant, accurate and up-to-date information about the level of support the person receives. It is also helpful if the health supporter has already made some notes about what the individual can see. Rather than taking the whole Person Centred Plan to the appointment it is important to collate the relevant information about the person's medical history in relation to their visual health. A Personal Health Profile is ideally suited for this as it is designed to contain health information in a portable format (see Chapter 6).

It is crucial that the Personal Health Profile contains the person's date of birth and home address and telephone number. It is also important that the person or their health supporter can also inform the optometrist about any benefits. (The optometrist or receptionist must see evidence of benefits for the person to qualify for a free test and voucher for glasses.)

The health supporter can influence the outcome of a sight test with prior thought and planning. For example, shifts may need reorganisation so that a person is supported by someone who knows them well.

The supporter needs to know about that person's method of communication. He/she may need to act as an interpreter or advise the optometrist that a person has poor hearing and so needs words spoken slowly and clearly.

It is important to consider the timing of the appointment. Some people function better in the afternoon, others are on medication which may make them sleepy. If possible a visit to the optometrist should be done when the person is alert and healthy.

Waiting around should be avoided wherever possible. It is important to plan appointments at a time which reduces the risk of having to wait.

It is important to ensure that the person brings their most recent pair (or pairs) of glasses with them when they visit the optometrist.

- A standard pre-test form, 'Telling the optometrists about me' is available for download from the Look Up website.

Preparing the optometrist's receptionist

To increase the likelihood of a positive experience at the optometrist it is helpful to contact the receptionist in advance of the appointment to advise the optometrist of a person's individual needs and discuss any potential problems, sharing the results of the pre-test form. If possible provide them with a copy of this document.

Often people with PIMD respond better to eye tests appointments if they are given the opportunity to familiarise with the new environment. The receptionist's help is often crucial when planning to familiarise the individual with the practice. This may consist of frequent visits to the practice while the optometrist is not busy.

Most people with PIMD will require an extended appointment. Depending on the person concerned either try and negotiate an extended appointment or alternatively, arrange multiple short appointments to complete all separate components of an eye test.

Preparing the optometrist

Optometrists need information about the person before his/her eye test. Supporters may wish to download the 'Telling the optometrist about me' form from the Look Up website.

Sometimes optometrists want to obtain information on the individual and family history before starting the eye examination but this information may not be available. It may be preferable to leave some individuals in the waiting room while this takes place, especially if there is something there to entertain them.

The optometrist will need to know before the appointment that their patient has intellectual disabilities and may need a different approach from other patients. It is important that both the sight test and eye health check are carried out in an unhurried way.

The optometrist will need to be informed of the following:

- How the person communicates
- Whether the person is deaf or hard of hearing
- Whether the person needs tests for people who cannot cooperate with an ordinary eye test ('preferential looking')
- Whether the person has any special likes or dislikes, such as bright lights
- Whether the person needs to be approached slowly, or from one particular side to avoid alarming him/her
- Whether the person has a tendency to respond 'yes' to questions and requests

Information given to the optometrist may influence the way tests are carried out, or in what order.

People who are deaf and hard of hearing are often dependent upon their sight to make sense of what is going on. Whilst the eye health checks need to be done in the dark, much of the test can be carried out with normal lighting. This may make people less anxious.

Preparing the individual

There are parts of the eye examination and sight test which may present particular problems. However, people can have full eye examinations even if they cannot cooperate.

The individual needs to get used to several aspects of the setting in advance of the eye examination:

- The waiting room
- Reduced light levels
- Raised or special seats
- Small enclosed consulting room
- Unknown area and new people
- Strange equipment

Working through the *Telling the Optometrist about me* form, available from the Look Up website, enables supporters to gather information in a structured way about the individual in advance of the test.

Frequent visits to the optometry practice may help the person to get used to certain procedures and assist to reduce anxiety levels. Time should be allowed to practise some of the procedures at home or in the optometry practice. The following procedures are valuable if applied as part of 'systematic desensitisation':

- Having light shone into the eye
- The optometrist getting very close (physical proximity)
- The test lens frame (large and heavy) being placed on the face
- Covering one eye in turn (disorienting/sensitivity to touch)

- Putting the chin on a piece of equipment
- Having eye drops put into the eye (disorienting)
- Trying to focus on something in the distance

Most people can have an eye test if adequate preparation has been done. However, some optometrists may find it hard to complete certain tests with some people, especially people with a short concentration span. The optometrist needs information about the individual in advance.

Measuring acuity (sharpness)

The Snellen letter chart is the best-known way of measuring acuity and there are simplified versions. Picture tests (most commonly the Kay Picture Test) may be used when the person can match pictures or shapes. Staff have often been surprised that people have learned matching skills.

Preferential looking tests, including the Cardiff Acuity Test, were designed for people who were 'hard to test'. Using this technique, the person being tested does not have to cooperate. A picture is presented either at the top or the bottom of a card held at eye level, and the tester watches for the person's involuntary eye movements towards where the picture is on the card.

Testing each eye

Each eye needs to be tested in turn. The tester has to move very close and put something in front of the eye, such as an adhesive eye patch or an occluder. The person may be willing to put their own hand over their eye, or have this done by a familiar person, such as the health supporter.

Sometimes the vision is tested with both eyes open – especially for people with nystagmus (rapid involuntary eye movements). The optometrist may hold a 'blurring lens' in front of one eye to test the other, avoiding these problems.

Eye drops

Some people, especially those who have difficulty cooperating during the eye examination, may be given drops to relax their eyes and make the pupil bigger. Optometrists may carry out an initial vision check, and possibly the test for visual acuity (level of vision), before inserting drops.

Drops help the optometrist to examine the back of the eye for disease and treatable conditions using an ophthalmoscope (a modified torch).

The person undertaking this examination has to get very close to the person as this instrument can only examine a very small area of the eye at a time. The optometrist may need to hold their eyelids open gently for a few seconds which is another strange experience which may provoke a reaction.

It is important to find out if drops are to be used and to find out what type and strength. Some eye drops sting and make the person light sensitive (photophobic), so dark glasses, a hat or eyeshade may help out of doors. Drops may blur vision, making it harder to occupy people in waiting rooms. It is important to find out how long the person's vision may be affected.

Testing eye pressure

The methods to measure pressure within the eye are very different so it is important to obtain information from the optometrist before the test.

Testing visual fields (all-round vision)

A sight test should be able to establish if a person cannot see on one side or the other, or has lost his/her central vision, or has tunnel or patchy vision.

It is important that the optometrist/optician tests a person's visual field, the extent to which a person can see around him/her without moving either his/her eyes or head. There are different ways of completing this test, so it is important to obtain information in advance.

Feedback from the eye test

It is important to know what the optometrist has found. Some will provide a written report. The optometrist may be willing to complete the report *Feedback from the optometrist about my eye test*[4]. However, it is important to note that some optometrists may ask for a fee for this service.

- How good is the person's vision?
- Why are there difficulties seeing?
- Are the person's eyes, eyelashes and eyelids healthy?
- Was a full eye examination possible? Were the results limited to the person's difficulty in cooperating, anxiety or boredom?
- Why have glasses been prescribed? When should they be worn?

If the person has poor sight, even when glasses have been prescribed, it is important to establish the following:

- What is the reason for the sight problem?
- How is the person affected?
  - Generally blurred?
  - Patchy?
  - Loss of vision – on the left or right side?
  - Tunnel vision

---

[4] http://www.lookupinfo.org

- Loss of central vision
- Mixed loss (all the above)
- Unusual eye movements
- Problems with glare

When people understand what has been found, they need to share this information with others who are important in the person's life so they can help the person make the best possible use of their sight.

This information should also be included in:

- an educational programme and/or care plan;
- health action plan;
- medical notes; and
- person-centred plan.

Glasses

Newly prescribed glasses may change the way people see their world – things may seem bigger and frightening. People need to be introduced to glasses gently. They need to wear their glasses for short periods of time for activities that they find motivating – such as seeing food, watching TV and so on – and then 'wearing time' can be built up.

Glasses are more likely to be rejected if:

- supporters do not know if the glasses are for 'near' or 'distance';
- they do not fit comfortably;
- they are so dirty that people cannot see through them;
- they are heavy on the face; and
- people have spots or sores behind their ears.
- (Levy & Woodhouse, 2007b)

Eye surgery

Sight loss is stressful and can cause severe depression and/or behaviour which challenges.

Eye operations (especially cataract operations) are increasingly available to adults with PIMD, including people who eye poke or self injure. People need careful preparation before and after eye surgery (Levy & Harris, 2007).

When surgery is refused, it is important to discover if this is in the person's best interests. There may be ways to ensure that surgery does take place, perhaps involving a psychologist to reduce a person's eye poking. Alternatively, discussion may be required about how to tackle key components of the recovery process, such as inserting eye drops.

When surgery is not considered appropriate, people must be referred to local services for visually impaired people.

Low-vision services

Low vision is when a person has poor sight, even when they are wearing the correct glasses or contact lenses. A vision assessment is needed for everyone who has poor sight.

Low-vision clinics (in eye hospitals or clinics) may be the best suited to provide it. People can often be trained to see better; it is important that individuals are offered this help so that their supporters can understand what can be achieved and do not have unrealistic expectations. However, few clinics have experience of working with people with PIMD because most low-vision work is directed at helping people to read. An orthoptist may feel more confident in providing this service. (Note: Orthoptists are qualified to diagnose and treat eye coordination problems. They work closely with members of the 'eye care team'. They work mostly with children. They work in hospitals or in the community, some needing a GP (general practitioner) referral.) Local services operate in different ways, so supporters should find out whom to approach.

Before any appointment for a person with PIMD is made it is worth contacting the health care professional to ensure that he/she is aware that the person may need a different approach from their typical patients.

Supporters should aim for the person to have both a low-vision assessment and a functional assessment of vision – although it may be hard to obtain both.

Functional assessment of vision

A 'functional assessment of vision' is a way of observing how the person uses their vision throughout the day. It is often carried out by rehabilitation officers for the visually impaired – 'ROVIs' (usually employed by social services/social work departments or the local voluntary society for blind and partially sighted people) or someone trained in this technique. People with PIMD should be referred to ROVIs for assessment. However, with Fair Access to Care (DH, 2003) (in England) they may be deemed 'not at risk' and be viewed as low priority for assistance.

Using information from the optometrist, supporters will find that observing some-one in several settings at different times of the day can provide helpful information to help people see better – such as:

- the best way to approach someone so as not to startle them;
- the best position in a room – such as sitting with the light behind them;
- the type of lighting which will help them most, including 'task lighting';
- times of day best avoided for activities – such as when people are tired and see less well; and
- ways to decorate a building to promote independence.

Low-vision services can also offer advice on lighting and colour contrast (Ryan et al., 2007).

A functional assessment can also record that someone needs to have their wheelchair 'parked' in the right position for them to join in. It can highlight how someone might take time to turn their head to see, and to make sense of what they are seeing.

Helping people with poor sight

Many people with PIMD have poor sight – even when wearing the correct glasses – and are eligible for registration as blind/severely sight impaired or partially sighted/sight impaired.

Registration is voluntary, but there are certain benefits and concessions. Ophthalmologists (eye doctors) do not always consider registration for people with PIMD – but it is one way of alerting services to a need. Registration is often a 'passport' to services for visually impaired people, although people do not need to be registered to get help.

Only a consultant ophthalmologist can certify a person as sight impaired/partially sighted or severely sight impaired/blind. (There are slightly different systems of registration in the four countries of the UK.)

People who are registered usually are visited by a rehabilitation officer for the visually impaired. They may:

- assess functional vision;
- provide advice on environmental issues and guiding people;
- provide training – for independent movement, daily living skills;
- offer advice on benefits, concessions and resources; and
- recommending equipment and teaching people how to use it.

(Willetts & Perry, 2007).

However, there is a great deal supporters can do to help people with poor sight. The basic 'rules' for helping people are described below:

- *Big*: Most people see big things more easily than small objects. People often make things bigger for themselves – they sit very near to the television or bring an object close to their eyes.
- *Bold*: Objects need to stand out clearly from their background. It is hard to see a white plate on a white tablecloth because it does not contrast with the background. It would be easier to see a white plate on a green cloth. Many people with poor sight find it hard to see things that are poorly contrasted with the background. Cluttered backgrounds make it impossible for people to see objects.
- *Bright*: Lighting is very important to people with poor sight. Most people need even clear lighting while others prefer dim settings. It is important to avoid 'glare', which literally 'blinds' people and causes pain. Visually impaired people may experience glare when people with 'ordinary vision' do not consider the light to be particularly bright. Glare can be caused by shiny surfaces, metal objects, etc.

Two additional factors need to be considered for people with profound and multiple intellectual disabilities:

- *Position*: People need to be in the right position to make the best use of what sight they have. They may have adopted unusual head positions to make the best use of their vision or supporters need to ensure that a person's wheelchair is positioned to enable people to take part in activities.
- *Time*: When the brain receives unclear messages it takes time for people to work out what they are seeing and how they should respond. The person may experience their world as a series of blurred images which may be confusing and hard to interpret – especially if they do not have a 'visual memory' and remember how things used to look. If a person sees only part of the whole, it may take them time to move their eyes or turn their head to 'scan' an area. But even having searched, they may still find it hard for them to piece the sections together and interpret a complete visual picture of a large object, such as a house.

Variations in sight

Sighted people watching visually impaired people are often confused because they wrongly believe that an individual's sight is static and unchanging. They may believe, quite incorrectly, 'she can see when she wants to'. Each person's sight and the way they use it is unique to that person. They will not always see the same things in the same way. A person's sight may alter considerably throughout a single day. Indeed some people's sight can vary over very short periods being influenced by both environmental factors and personal issues. These influences include their current health state, effects of medication, time of day, lighting, level of engagement and motivation. Given these multiple influences it is important not to make judgements about the ability of the person with PIMD but to conduct a thorough assessment which includes observing visual behaviour over time. This will provide more reliable information about their sight and how they use it.

Conclusion

People with PIMD need their sight as much – if not more – than the rest of us. They may be unable to tell anyone that their sight is deteriorating. Even a small reduction in vision may cause distress. It is therefore important that people with PIMD have regular eye tests, for which they are prepared and supported by a familiar person.

People with PIMD usually need assistance to adapt to wearing glasses which may change the way they see their world.

Eye surgery is increasingly available to people with profound and multiple intellectual disabilities. Careful planning can ensure positive outcomes. Every avenue should be explored if surgery is refused.

Where people are found to be blind or partially sighted, they need to be referred to low-vision clinics and rehabilitation officers for the visually impaired.

Whilst people with PIMD and poor sight have a right to specialist input, supporters can help considerably by remembering the basic rules of low vision:

- big
- bold
- bright

and the two special considerations for people with severe disabilities:

- position
- time

Life can be so much easier for everyone when we have a better understanding of how a person sees and experiences their world. There are so many things we can do to help people use their existing vision better and get more out of life!

Appendix 10.1

Eye problems – what to look for

These checklists provide possible signs of sight problems. However, it is important to note that some people may have no outward signs of their visual impairment, while other people display various clues.

One major problem in looking for eye problems in people is that they may have considerable variations in their vision throughout their day – according to their environment, health, medication, and so on. Staff may find that the checklists give different results on different days – or even at different times on the same day. These variations in vision are an indication that an eye examination is needed.

Appearance of eyes

- No eyes at all
- Very small eyes
- Closed or partially closed eyes
- In-growing eyelashes
- Red eyes
- Yellow eyes
- Eyes without a pupil – the round black central part
- Pupils which are 'off centre'
- Pupils that seem distorted or incomplete
- Eyes which look 'milky'
- Eyes which appear to 'rove' or constantly move
- Eyes which bulge, seem pointed or have an unusual shape
- Eyes which seem scarred or damaged

- Frequent eye infections or sticky eyes
- Frequent cysts or sties on the eyelids
- One eye turning in or out – squinting
- Very fast eye movements – side to side, up or down
- 'Unusual' eye movements
- Watery eyes

Behaviour

- Frequent touching of eyes – such as poking, rubbing, and so on
- 'Light gazing' – appears fascinated by light
- 'Finger flapping' – enjoys flapping hand in front of eyes
- 'Unusual' head positions
- Moves head to look at things – but eyes do not move much
- Unusual head movements – for example, frequent head shaking
- 'Head rolling' – circular movement of head
- Puts hand over one eye
- Constant frowning
- Constant blinking
- Blinks at bright lights
- Avoids bright lights
- Avoids close work
- Draws very small pictures
- Draws very large pictures
- Seems to see some colours better than others
- Obvious problems in focusing – for example, distant to close objects and large to small objects
- Short attention span
- Poor self-care skills
- Poor communication skills – difficulty learning sign language
- Dramatic changes in behaviour – may become upset or anxious for no apparent reason
- Body rigidity – seldom seems relaxed
- Startled by noises

Responses to other people

- Does not seem to recognise people – unless spoken to
- Does not make eye contact with other people
- Peers at people
- Jumpy when approached without being warned
- Lack of regard for other people, environment, etc.
- Sees people wearing bright colours better
- Sees people some of the time – for example, when they wear certain colours

Responses to objects

- Close examination of objects
- Peers at objects
- Moves objects towards light
- Prefers object to be placed in a particular position, for example, on one side or the other, near and far
- Preference for bright objects
- Sees bright objects on colour-contrasting backgrounds better, for example, a red plate on a white tablecloth
- Appears to see moving objects better than things that stay still

Movement

- Crashes into objects – such as doors and furniture
- Is anxious or unwilling to walk alone
- Finds it difficult to judge distances
- Seems clumsy and uncoordinated, for example, problems with balance
- Copes better in well-lit areas
- Copes better in twilight-type lighting
- Finds it difficult to cope with changes in the environment – walks confidently indoors but reluctant to walk out of doors
- Walks confidently in well-lit rooms, but has difficulties in dimly lit corridors or stairwells
- Constant looking down – for example, for steps
- Feels way around, not obviously using sight, for example, sliding feet to find steps
- Becomes confused/disorientated
- Gets lost when moving about

Useful resources

Look Up – an information service on eye care and vision for people with learning disabilities and their supporters – http://www.lookupinfo.org. Helpline 0800 121 8900
Peripatetic teachers for visually impaired children – employed by local authorities.
Rehabilitation officers for visually impaired people – employed by social services/social work departments (RNIB has contact details) – http://info.rnib.org.uk/Agencies/allagencies.htm

Further reading

Department of Health (DH) (2002). *Action for Health – Health Action Plans and Health Facilitation. Detailed good practice guidance on implementation for learning disability partnership boards.* London: DH.
DH (2007). *HC12: charges and optical voucher values.* Available at: http://www.ppa.org.uk/pdfs/ppc/HC12.pdf (accessed 1 October 2007).

Lacey, P., & Ouvry, C. (eds). (1998). *People with Profound and Multiple Learning Disabilities: A Collaborative Approach to Meeting Complex Needs*. London: David Fulton.

McLinden, M., & McCall, S. (2002). *Supporting Children with Visual Impairment and Additional Disabilities*, London: David Fulton.
An excellent book, with ideas that can easily be adapted for adults

Ockelford, A. (2002). *Objects of Reference; Promoting Early Symbolic Communication*. London: RNIB.
A helpful illustrated book, which considers how to introduce objects of reference and ways of moving from objects to other forms of communication.

Sonsken, P., Levitt, S., & Kitzinger, M. (1984). Identification of constraints acting on motor development in young visually disabled children and principles of remediation. *Child Care, Health and Development*, 10(5), 273–286.

References

Bradley, H. (2007). *Encouraging and Developing Early Communication Skills in Adults with Multiple Disabilities*. Epsom: Look Up Info.

Brown, N., McLinden, M., & Porter, J. (1998). Sensory needs. In Lacey, P., & Ouvry, C. (eds), *People with Profound and Multiple Learning Disabilities: A Collaborative Approach to Meeting Complex Needs*. London: David Fulton; 29–38.

College of Optometrists (2000). *The Care and Management of Patients with Learning Disabilities*. London: DOCET.

Department of Health (2002). *Action for Health: Health Action Plans and Health Facilitation, Detailed Good Practice Guidance on Implementation for Learning Disability Partnership Boards*. London: Department of Health.

Department of Health (2003). *Fair Access to Care Services – Guidance on Eligibility Criteria for Adult Social Care*. London: Department of Health.

DH (2005). *HC11: help with health costs*. Available from the Department of Health. Available at: http://www.dh.gov.uk/.

DH & SSI (1989). *Sign Posts – Leading to Better Social Services for Deaf-Blind People*. London: Department of Health (DH) & Social Services Inspectorate (SSI).

DRC (2006). *Equal Treatment: Closing the Gap. A Formal Investigation into Physical Health Inequalities Experienced by People with Learning Disabilities and/or Mental Health Problems*. Stratford upon Avon: Disability Rights Commission (DRC).

Ellis, D. (1982). Visually and mentally handicapped people in institutions. Part 1: their numbers and needs. *Mental Handicap*, 10(4), 135–137.

Emerson, E., Hatton, C., Felce, D., & Murphy, G. (2001). *Learning Disabilities, the Fundamental Facts*. London: The Foundation for People with Learning Disabilities.

Fraiberg, S. (1977). *Insights from the Blind: Comparative Studies of Blind and Sighted Infants*. New York: Basic Books.

Levy, G. (2007a). *Access to Eye Care for Adults with Learning Disabilities*. Epsom: Look Up Info.

Levy, G. (2007b). *Understanding and Using Sight: Issues for Work with People with Learning Disabilities*. Epsom: Look Up Info.

Levy, G., & Harris, L. (2007). *Minimising Problems in Eye Surgery for Adults with Learning Disabilities*. Epsom: Look Up Info.

Levy, G., & McKelvie, D. (1993). Care management and assessment of people with multiple impairments. In Stevens, A. (ed.), *Back from the Wellhouse: Discussion Papers on*

Sensory Impairment and Training in Community Care, CCETSW Paper 32. London: Central Council for Education and Training in Social Work (CCETSW); 148.

Levy, G., & Woodhouse, M. (2007a). *Eye Tests for Adults with Learning Disabilities*. Epsom: Look Up Info.

Levy, G., & Woodhouse, M. (2007b). *Glasses for Adults with Learning Disabilities*. Epsom: Look Up Info.

Mencap (1998). *The NHS – Health for all? People with Learning Disabilities and Health Care*. London: Mencap

NHS Executive (1998). *Signposts for Success in Commissioning and Providing Health Services for People with Learning Disabilities*. London: HMSO.

Oswin, M. (1978). *Children Living in Long-Stay Hospitals*. Lavenham: Spastics International Medical Publications.

Ryan, B., Levy, G., & Karas, M. (2007). *Low Vision Services for People with Learning Disabilities*. Epsom: Look Up Info.

Thomas, M., & Levy, G. (1998). *Focus 23, You'll Never Walk Alone!* London: RNIB's Information Service on Multiple Disability.

Waite, L., & Levy, G. (2007). *Using Sign with People Who Have Learning Disabilities and Sight Problems*. Epsom: Look Up Info.

Warren, D. (1984). *Blindness and Children: An Individual Differences Approach*. Cambridge: Cambridge University Press.

Willetts, G., & Perry, C. (2007). *Obtaining Specialist Support for People with Sight Problems and Learning Disabilities*. Epsom: Look Up Info.

Chapter 11

HEARING AND AURAL HEALTH

Laura Waite

Introduction

It has long been recognised that there is a higher than average prevalence of hearing impairment in individuals with intellectual disabilities (McCracken, 2002; Picard, 2004); however, people with profound intellectual and multiple disabilities are much more likely to experience 'diagnostic overshadowing' (Ouellette-Kuntz et al., 2005) with symptoms frequently being ascribed to the severity of their intellectual impairment. Alborz et al. (2003) apportion blame to family members and professional carers for either missing or misinterpreting symptoms in the individual they were supporting, while Band (1998), following a health survey, suggested that GPs (general practitioners) were at fault in failing to refer people with intellectual disabilities to audiological services as hearing impairments were 'to be expected and therefore tolerate' (p. 11). However, the evidence is contested, it remains that the impact of hearing impairment on the lives of people with profound intellectual and multiple disabilities demands serious attention.

It is important to note that this chapter does not address 'communication' as something which can be studied *apart* from the experiences, practices and issues of learning difficulty and sensory impairment. Indeed, communication is here seen as the fundamental ground of any professional practice or research activity which seeks to prevent or minimise the exclusive effects on communicative and hence cultural competence of being a hearing-impaired person with profound and multiple learning difficulties. Whilst readers are referred to Chapter 4 for a more conceptually focused treatment of communication issues, those issues permeate all discussion of experiences and practices in this chapter.

Finally, readers who wish to explore further some of the material encountered in this chapter are referred to Appendix 11.1 for details of supplementary reading.

Learning objectives

By the end of this chapter readers should:

- have an understanding of the main categories of hearing impairment;
- be familiar with a range of causes of hearing impairment;
- show critical understanding of the impact of hearing impairment on individuals with profound intellectual and multiple disabilities;

- be able to describe a series of tests that are relevant to those with profound intellectual and multiple disabilities; and
- be able to describe a range of interventions appropriate to the needs of individuals with profound intellectual and multiple disabilities.

What is hearing impairment?

Hearing impairment can be categorised in four ways, and is largely related to the specific location within the hearing system that is not working as it typically should:

- *Conductive deafness*: Where sound cannot pass freely through the outer or middle ear (see Figure 11.1).
- *Sensorineural deafness*: Where there has been damage to the cochlea in the inner ear or auditory nerve.
- *Mixed deafness*: Where there is sensorineural and conductive deafness present.
- *Auditory processing disorder*: Where there is damage to the part of the brain responsible for processing auditory information.

Common causes of hearing impairment

We have seen a significant shift in the causes of hearing impairment with particular reference to sensorineural deafness. Widespread vaccine programmes have done much to decrease some of the childhood infectious diseases which are well known for their effects on hearing, for example, mumps, measles and rubella (Picard, 2004).

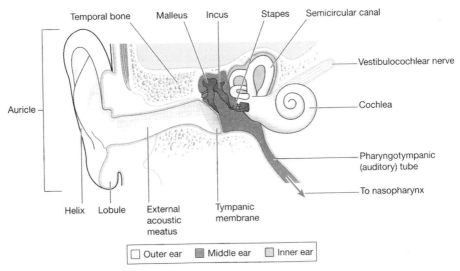

Figure 11.1 A cross section of the ear showing the outer ear, middle ear and inner ear. (Reprinted from Waugh & Grant (2006) with permission from Elsevier.)

However, a new concern is for those born prematurely; Cone-Wesson et al. (2000) rank extreme prematurity as the 'fifth most prevalent cause of hearing loss in infants' (in Picard, 2004, p. 226). The following are some of the main causes of hearing impairment in people with profound intellectual and multiple disabilities.

Outer ear – conductive deafness

Blockages in the external ear canal can have a significant effect on hearing as well as increasing the risk of infection, causing dizziness, a feeling of fullness and sometimes pain. The main offender is wax which the ear produces naturally to clean itself. Different individuals vary considerably in the quantity and consistency of their ear wax (Fransman, 2006) but it will normally migrate out of the ear on its own. Wax only really becomes problematic when it becomes impacted and obstructs the ear drum. In the USA, Roeser & Ballachanda (1997) estimated the incidence of impacted wax in the general population at 5–17% but studies (e.g. Wilson & Haire, 1990; Fransman, 1996, 1998) have consistently shown that people with intellectual disabilities are far more likely to experience impacted wax with an incidence ranging from 59 to 64%. A recent study by Fransman (2006) provides one explanation for such an increase. She highlights that a crucial factor in normal wax migration is jaw movement and in particular the movement involved in chewing, and she concludes that the absence of back teeth can significantly affect this process. With this evidence in mind it is worth considering that (a) dental disease is very prevalent amongst people with intellectual disabilities (Chapter 13) and (b) an increasing number of individuals with profound intellectual and multiple disabilities are using alternative and often safer methods of nutrition that do not involve chewing; both of these factors could potentially inhibit normal wax migration in the individual.

Middle ear – conductive deafness: otitis media with effusion

This is an infection or inflammation of the middle ear which is usually caused by a viral or bacterial infection. The Eustachian tube becomes blocked, preventing air from reaching the middle ear. When air is unable to circulate sufficiently the middle ear fills up with fluid that can become thick, like glue, hence the condition's more frequently used name 'glue ear'. The fluid affects the mobility of the eardrum and ossicles causing hearing loss and can sometimes be painful. Although it is usually only prevalent in young children as their middle ear cavity develops and their Eustachian tube grows, individuals with Down's syndrome may be troubled by it into adulthood due to their shorter and narrower Eustachian tubes.

There are generally four approaches to tackling glue ear:

1. 'wait and see' – glue ear can clear up on its own accord;
2. medical intervention – with antibiotics and decongestants;
3. surgical intervention – the fluid can be drained and tiny ventilation tubes (grommets) inserted to allow air to circulate more freely; and

4. amplification – this is sometimes the preferred treatment if individuals are experiencing reoccurring glue ear, for example, individuals with Down's syndrome.

Cholesteatoma

Cholesteatomas are slow growing, non-malignant growths behind the ear drum which if left untreated, can result in erosion to the mastoid bone and serious damage to the middle and inner ear. A common cause of a cholesteatoma is severe or reoccurring episodes of glue ear; Fransman (1998) suggests that this can be more common in people with intellectual disabilities, particularly those who have spent much of their life living in hospital. It is usually treated with antibiotics providing it has been identified at an early enough stage after which surgery may be necessary.

Perforated eardrums

The most frequent causes of a perforated eardrum include being poked, ear infections including untreated glue ear and injury to the head. They generally heal by themselves but if not they can be surgically treated.

Damaged ossicles

The tiny bones in the middle ear can either be malformed from birth or damaged through infection or head injury. Surgical intervention can repair or replace the bones.

Inner ear – sensorineural deafness

This is most often the result of damage to the hair cells in the cochlea. Causes that may be relevant to people with profound intellectual and multiple disabilities include:

- ageing (presbyacusis);
- head injury;
- illness (e.g. meningitis); and
- heredity.

Additionally, we have seen an increase in the numbers of 'unknown causes' of hearing impairment with some researchers speculating genetic origins (Picard, 2004).

As with visual impairment there are certain 'groups' within the profound and multiply disabled population who are at greater risk of experiencing either congenital or acquired hearing impairment. These include people with:

- cerebral palsy;
- Down's syndrome;
- fetal Rubella syndrome;
- CHARGE syndrome;
- fragile X syndrome;

- kernicterus (bilirubin encephalopathy);
- congenital cytomegalovirus;
- individuals whose impairments are as a result of meningitis; and
- people over the age of 40.

Why hearing impairment is a concern for people with profound intellectual and multiple disabilities?

Whilst the impact of hearing impairment has been researched widely for many years, only a limited amount of studies relate directly to people with profound intellectual and multiple disabilities. Of course the impact of hearing impairment on the individual is influenced by many factors some of which are psychosocial, others of which are audiological; Morgan-Jones (2001) believes that of the audiological factors, time of onset and degree of impairment are the most significant. However, sadly, a substantial proportion of people with profound intellectual and multiple disabilities will not have had their hearing impairment even identified so will not have received the appropriate support needed. Indeed Evenhuis & Nagtzaam (1998) suggest that delayed identification of hearing impairment is likely to have harmful effects on the social, cognitive, emotional and communicative development of an already disabled group. Furthermore, they point out that if an individual is not supported to manage their hearing impairment appropriately then their experience of intellectual impairment may be magnified or they may be at risk of developing behaviour difficulties. Roberts (2005, p. 254) similarly warns that individuals may well miss out on essential learning experiences which impact on 'how they know themselves and the environment'. She expands on this by suggesting that this is further compounded by environments not being manipulated to meet the sensory needs of individuals.

Recognition as to the increased incidence of mental health and emotional difficulties amongst people with hearing impairment has increased in the last decade (see Hindle & Kitson, 2000; McKenna, 2001), and in parallel there is a growing, if recent acknowledgement that people with profound intellectual and multiple disabilities can experience mental health difficulties – a phenomenon deemed highly unlikely until very recently (see Chapter 8). Although this may be an under-researched conjecture, it is extremely likely that there will be a coincidence of these conditions in some individuals with consequent difficulties in identification, assessment and remediation.

Multidimensional nature of the experience of hearing impairment

It is important to note that many people who are born with hearing impairment and identify themselves as culturally Deaf (i.e. those for whom sign languages and Deaf communities represent their primary allegiance) do not perceive their experience as an 'audiological' one, but feel more akin to other language minorities (Ladd, 2003). Interestingly, few people with profound intellectual and multiple disabilities ever grow up culturally Deaf. If a parent has a child who has a severe hearing impairment then they might be advised (as one option) to introduce sign language as the child's primary language and perhaps to attend a school for Deaf children. However, if the child has hearing impairment and other complex needs it would be unlikely that this would be suggested, with physical or health needs being deemed more pressing and therefore addressed first. This child is then usually raised in an oralist environment where they have difficulty hearing language. This leads to the vital question of whether the child is disadvantaged by not being raised in an environment that is rich in visual language.

Evidence-based practice

A number of documents relating to the health needs of people with profound intellectual and multiple disabilities provide a key baseline of relevant evidence in the identification of audiological and/or other health needs. These include the following:

- DH (2001): Valuing People, Chapter 6: Improving health for people with learning disabilities.
- NHS Quality Improvement Scotland (2006): Promoting access to healthcare for people with a learning disability – a guide for frontline staff.
- Northway et al. (2006) Shaping the future: a vision for learning disability nursing.
- Royal College of Nursing (2006): Meeting the health needs of people with learning disabilities.
- Scottish Executive (2002): Promoting health, supporting inclusion – the national review of the contribution of all nurses and midwives to the care and support of people with learning disabilities.

There are, however, a number of documents relating to audiological services that – while not specifically aimed at people with profound intellectual and multiple disabilities – are of general use; these include the following:

- ADSS, BDA, LGA, NDCS, NCB, RNID (2002): Deaf children: positive practice standards in social services.
- ADSS, BDA, LGA, RNID (1999): Best practice standards: social services for deaf and hard of hearing people.
- Department of Health (2007): Improving access to audiology services in England.
- Down's syndrome Medical Interest Group (2001) Surveillance guidelines – hearing impairment.
- National Deaf Children's Society (2005): Quality standards and good practice guidelines: transition from child to adult services.
- Royal National Institute for Deaf People (2002): Best practice standards for adult audiology.
- Sense (2000): Standards for services for adults who are deafblind or have a dual sensory impairment.

Assessment

As noted previously (see Chapter 10), seven out of ten people with intellectual disabilities were found to have never had their hearing tested (Band, 1998) and there has been much speculation as to why this is. One explanation lay in the misconception that people with intellectual disabilities and in particular people with profound intellectual and multiple disabilities would not be able to comply with a hearing test. Of course, while people with profound intellectual and multiple disabilities present audiology services with some challenges, testing is not impossible (and indeed, neonatal screening provides evidence to offset this argument). The National Newborn Hearing Screening Programme (NHSP) was introduced in 2001 and it is hoped that its implementation will lead to individuals with profound intellectual and multiple disabilities having any congenital hearing impairment identified early. The tools used in this screening process (BSER (brainstem evoked response test) and OAE (otoacoustic emissions)) are invaluable in the assessment of people with profound intellectual and multiple disabilities and are detailed further on in this chapter.

Before outlining the type and function of a range tests it is necessary to identify some of the barriers that individuals with profound intellectual and multiple disabilities frequently face in obtaining hearing care. The guidance offered by Royal National Institute for Deaf People (2002), National Deaf Children's Society (2000) and Royal College of Nurses (2006) goes some way to address these barriers, but they are by no means eliminated! The Scottish Executive (2002) divides barriers to healthcare into five areas: physical, administrative, communication, attitudinal and knowledge. By using these categories we can highlight some examples of barriers that might be found in audiology services.

> *Physical barriers*: Examples of such barriers include the doorways to sound proofed rooms may not be able to accommodate a wheelchair; waiting areas can be cramped and cluttered, both visually and acoustically.
>
> *Administrative barriers*: Examples of such barriers include appointments which are insufficient in length; clinics at a time when the individual is 'not at their best'; overrunning clinics resulting in individuals having to wait for long periods.
>
> *Communication barriers*: Examples of such barriers include hospital staff may be unsure of the communication needs of people with profound intellectual and multiple disabilities and therefore neglect to obtain useful information such as: 'How might this person tell me that it is ok for me to look in their ears?'
>
> *Attitudinal barriers*: Examples of such barriers include hospital staff may have negative assumptions and attitudes about people with profound intellectual and multiple disabilities which reduce the likelihood of individuals being referred for sedation, for testing or for interventions such as hearing aids, cochlea implants or others surgical procedures; after all – as a not uncommon attitude might have it – 'why would *these people* need to hear?' Adults with profound intellectual and multiple disabilities are also frequently seen in paediatric clinics because of course they have the same needs as children!

Knowledge barriers: Examples of such barriers include hospital staff may have limited knowledge and practice experience of the audiological needs of people with profound intellectual and multiple disabilities resulting in some of the attitudes highlighted above but also increasing the risk of diagnostic overshadowing because of not being aware of facts such as the high prevalence of presbyacusis (age-related hearing impairment) in middle-aged people with Down's syndrome (Buchanan, 1990; Evenhuis et al., 1992).

Finally, it should be noted that in many instances there will be a complex presence of several – if not all – of these barriers, continuing to create a daunting inhibition to effective identification and intervention. As the role of the intellectual disability nurse develops and expands, with a greater emphasis on partnership working with mainstream healthcare (Northway et al., 2006) it is hoped that their expertise will have considerable impact on breaking down some of the above barriers.

Testing, testing . . .

Following a routine recording of medical history, an investigation and diagnosis might typically be informed by some or all of the following:

- Otoscopy
- OAE
- Evoked response audiometry
- Tympanometry
- Behavioural response audiometry
- Functional hearing assessment

Otoscopy

Otoscopy is an examination of the ear with an instrument called an otoscope (or auriscope). It is performed to examine the ear canal and ear drum and problems such as blockages, perforations and fluid in the middle ear can be identified. While otoscopy is normally carried out by practitioners involved in hearing care, it is possible for other professionals with some knowledge of audiology to receive training using the British Society of Audiology Guidelines on Minimum Training Standards for Otoscopy and Impression Taking (BSA Education Committee, 2004).

If otoscopy reveals impacted wax then this will obviously need to be removed if an individual is to have their hearing levels assessed. This can be achieved with drops, water jets (irrigation), suction and surgical instruments by a trained practitioner. Fransman (2006) points out that many people with intellectual disabilities have a limited audiological history available and advises us to be cautious when removing impacted wax. It is not always clear what lurks beneath and if a perforation is present then the frequently favoured method of irrigation is likely to create further complications not to mention considerable pain for the individual during the procedure.

Of course, having one's ears examined can be an intrusive experience, especially if intellectual impairment affects the individual's capacity to understand why a stranger is invading their space and poking things down their ears! For some people, particularly those who favour not being touched too much, a short spell of preparatory conditioning is likely to be beneficial; providing the individual with the opportunity to experience someone being close to their face and touching their ears should help to prepare them for the process. Furthermore, a cue could be introduced to assist the individual in understanding when someone is going to examine their ears, for example, an object of reference, a sign or a touch cue.

Once the ears have been checked then people with profound intellectual and multiple disabilities are likely to require a series of objective hearing tests. These are tests which do not require the individual to make a behavioural response, but they do need to be able to cooperate with the procedures (which again is why a spell of conditioning might be necessary).

Otoacoustic emissions

If the cochlea in the inner ear is functioning normally then it creates an internal echo as it processes sound. This echo can be measured using a small probe which is inserted into the ear. The test is painless, relatively quick and can provide information on the functioning of the cochlea and middle ear.

Evoked response audiometry

There are a series of tests which involve recording the electrical activity that is induced by a sound signal at varying points along the auditory pathway. One of these tests which is applicable for people with profound intellectual and multiple disabilities is the BSER, this involves the application of electrodes to the head. It is necessary for the individual to be resting for this test, so sedation is often recommended. Through clinical experience it has been found that this is often the sticking point for using this test with people with profound intellectual and multiple disabilities as professionals can fear that sedating an individual who may already have complex health needs and take other medications may be risky. Whilst undoubtedly consideration should be given to this, the potential impact of undiagnosed hearing impairment on an individual who is already significantly compromised should equally be recognised. Additionally, if in a supportive hospital environment it can be possible to coordinate a series of health checks or treatments to be carried out at the same time, for example, dental treatment. This way the risk of having to be sedated on several occasions can be reduced.

Tympanometry

A tympanometer is used to provide information about the status of the middle ear. In a similar way to OAE (see p. x), a probe is inserted into the ear and acoustic signals are presented. The instrument measures the mobility or 'compliance' of the eardrum and middle ear and can identify problems such as glue ear and damaged ossicles.

Behavioural observation audiometry (BOA)

BOA is when a sound is presented to the individual being tested and a behaviour is observed, for example, increased movement, stilling, eye widening, glancing at sound source. The sounds presented may include speech, warble tones or pre-measured sound making toys (Maltby & Knight, 2000).

Functional hearing assessment

A functional hearing assessment is used to determine how the individual uses their hearing. Initially the tester should carry out a number of observations to ascertain how the individual typically responds to sensory information before moving on to examine how they respond specifically to auditory information. This should involve the people who best know the individual in making observations and recording data. Next, the tester will probably carry out more structured assessment to establish the types of responses that the individual is making to acoustic signals. This will typically employ sounds that are relevant, interesting and known to the individual and could be generated by human, object or environment. Durkel & Moss (2005) usefully outline some of the responses that might be looked for under the following headings:

- A *reflexive, awareness level*: For example, a startle
- A *regulating level*: For example, the use of sound to enter and maintain a quiet and alert state, or an agitated state
- A *motor level*: For example, the ability to turn towards or reach for an object or person making a sound, even if they cannot see or touch its source
- A *play level*: For example, the enjoyment of making noises, either with their mouth, by activating switches, hitting two objects together, playing musical instruments
- An *associative level*: For example, the capacity to associate a particular sound with a particular event
- A *communication level*: For example, the recognition of common words, such as their name, the use of sounds consistently to communicate

Unfortunately very little published work has come out of the UK about functional hearing assessments for people with profound intellectual and multiple disabilities, although at the time of writing the National Special Interest Group for Hearing Impairment in People with Intellectual disabilities (see Appendix 11.2) is trying to remedy this by developing a 'toolkit' of resources. Again, the lack of published material available is probably a telling reflection of the attitudes towards this population of people, but it may also stem from an unease frequently seen in audiological professionals when something lacks 'science'. Indeed it may well be a role for the intellectual disability nurse to reassure their fellow health colleagues that it is nevertheless very useful to obtain results that have no numerical value. Undeniably, a functional hearing assessment will not provide us with information about each ear separately and this could make the fitting of a hearing aid experimental. However, if the information from a functional hearing assessment is combined with that from the objective tests outlined above, then we may obtain a reasonably comprehensive – subjectively as well as objectively informed – picture of how someone is hearing.

Another advantage of the functional hearing assessment is that it normally involves those who know the individual well. Murdoch (1994) suggests that the assessment of people with profound intellectual and multiple disabilities relies on an expert knowledge of the individual being assessed rather than expert knowledge of the process of hearing. The family member or supporter must therefore be an integral part of the assessment.

Intervention

Hearing aids

Following a Department of Health programme to modernise NHS hearing aid services in England in 2000, digital hearing aids are now available on the NHS. This is an exciting development although throws up some issues for people with profound intellectual and multiple disabilities or more accurately the health professionals involved in their hearing care. One of the virtues of digital aids is that they can be programmed to meet the recipient's specific hearing needs more closely because the mechanism that processes sound is essentially a mini-computer. Typically, the non-learning disabled patient would have their hearing assessed using Pure Tone Audiometry (Graham & Martin, 2001). This requires the patient to wear headphones and give a response to single frequency tones being presented at varying pitches and intensities to each ear in turn. The results of this test are then plotted onto a graph which in turn allows the audiologist to tune the digital aid to match the pattern of hearing loss. For the individual with profound intellectual and multiple disabilities that graph may not be so clear and is likely to contain gaps. Some audiologists may be reluctant to fit a hearing aid on a patient who does not have that full graph of information. However, as stated earlier, use of all the data from the tests that *are* appropriate to people with profound intellectual and multiple disabilities, plus those from a functional hearing assessment, will generate a reliable understanding of what the individual is hearing, and this could form the basis from which to fit a hearing aid. It might mean experimenting, for example, starting with a small amount of amplification to the frequencies which the results suggest are most impaired and gradually increasing it over time whilst carefully monitoring its effects. Given the potential impact that hearing impairment can have on the lives of people with profound intellectual and multiple disabilities, practitioners should be encouraged to undertake such intervention – albeit informed with caution as to the possible risks involved (such as the individual rejecting the aid).

We should also be cautious in our interpretation of incomplete evidence of the efficacy of digital aids; such evidence is at best anecdotal and there is a clear need for a research base critically to evaluate emerging technologies in the lives of hearing impaired people with intellectual disabilities.

Typology of hearing aids

Broadly speaking, most services will draw from a range of aids according not only to recipient's perceived needs but also to their own professional preferences and, indeed, budgetary considerations. The following outlines the different variations of hearing aids:

Behind the ear (BTE): This is the most commonly prescribed hearing aid which is made up of a mould that fits into the ear and a plastic shell containing microphone, receiver, battery and amplifier that sits at the back of the ear. They can vary in size and colour depending on the person's needs.

Body worn (BW): These aids can be very powerful and are made up of a box that can be placed in a top pocket or attached to clothing, connected by a lead to an earphone and ear mould. They are generally easier to use by people with limited dexterity, as the controls are larger than other hearing aids.

In the ear (ITE), *In the canal (ITC)* and *Completely in the canal (CIC)*: These aids sit inside the ear and have no tubes or wires. They are only suitable for people with mild/moderate hearing impairments.

Bone anchored (BAHA): These aids are made up of a small receiver that is surgically implanted into the mastoid bone behind the ear which then transports acoustic signals directly to the cochlea for transmission to the brain. They are offered to people who suffer with chronic infection of the ear canal, people who are allergic to the materials used in ear moulds or those whose outer ears are not typical in shape.

Bone conduction (BC): These aids work in a similar way to the bone anchored aids except they do not require surgery as the receiver is clamped against the mastoid bone with a headband. It is usual that a person who is being considered for a BAHA would have a trial with a BC aid first.

Cochlea implants

The criteria for obtaining a cochlea implant are fairly complex, as is the pre- and post-surgery therapy and as a result of this most recipients tend to be post-lingually deafened adults. However, in more recent years people with profound intellectual and multiple disabilities have been offered them.

One of the issues around people with profound intellectual and multiple disabilities not being offered the range of medical interventions open to non-disabled people is that health professionals frequently fail to see how something would benefit the individual. This is largely as a consequence of criteria being designed without their needs being considered. For example, when considering whether someone should have cataract surgery, the quality of life assessment which would be carried out contains questions such as: 'Can this person no longer read? Can they no longer drive?' which are manifestly inappropriate if not absurd. There is however, an abundance of people who would be devastated if they could not see their mum's face clearly, for example, or the piece of coloured plastic that they enjoy twiddling! And for cochlea implants, the decision-making process involves factors such as the individual's ability to recognise speech or to lip read and the ability to have realistic expectations of how the implant might work, again none of which are necessarily relevant to people with profound intellectual and multiple disabilities. There is thus a clear and well-indicated role for the intellectual disability nurse as the coordinating professional who could help their fellow health colleagues adapt criteria so that they took into account a more diverse range of lives than those who merely speak, read and drive!

It is also important to note that another factor that influences the decision-making process is the evidence. Consequently, there has been very little research carried out as to the qualitative benefits of cochlea implants for this group but in time it is hoped that this will be addressed.

Vibrotactile aid

Finally, although as yet little used, recent developments in vibrotactile aids point to possible applications for people with profound intellectual and multiple disabilities. These aids are usually worn on the wrist and transmit information about sounds to the skin. They are generally offered to people for whom hearing aids are of minimal benefit and for whom cochlea implants are unsuitable or undesirable. Maltby & Knight (2000, p. 50) describe the information that is received from a vibrotactile aid as 'limited' but it would include the absence or presence of sound, its rhythm, duration, intensity and speed. They can be single, dual or multi-channelled, the last of which provides the most information. They are often worn in addition to hearing aids and introduced using a detailed programme to teach the person how to interpret the vibrations. While the latter is not appropriate for people with profound intellectual and multiple disabilities, there could be a strong argument that they could be helpful for people with little or no useful hearing in providing signals for environmental sounds, and reassurances that they are 'in the world'.

Acoustic environment

While the use of amplification can be valuable for many individuals, even more so are a consideration for and/or modification of the acoustic environment that they are in. It is therefore essential that supporters take into account the following factors.

Background noise

Background noise can be problematic for anyone but it can sometimes be especially troublesome for individuals with profound intellectual and multiple disabilities when their ability to filter out sound is compromised. Quiet environments are more likely to help people concentrate and use any residual hearing more effectively. From personal experience it has been observed that people with profound intellectual and multiple disabilities frequently find themselves in environments that have lots of background noise such as day services, further education colleges and residential services. It is paramount that such services are encouraged to do what they can to reduce noise from internal and external sources. It should also be noted that some people with hearing impairment may find excessive sound difficult to tolerate and even experience pain.

Lighting

When people experience hearing impairment they will be much more reliant on their vision. Therefore it is essential that there is good lighting so that people can pick up on visual clues.

Surfaces

Sound waves reflect off hard surfaces. Therefore, places like dining rooms with hard tables, plates and clanking cutlery can be a difficult environment for a person who has a hearing impairment, especially if they are hearing aid users. Soft furnishings absorb sound waves and can help, for example, tablecloths, cushions and curtains.

Distractions and 'visual clutter'

Trying to interact with someone with a hearing impairment in a room with lots of distractions can be problematic. The person may find it difficult to concentrate on the conversation if there is too much going on around. If it is not possible to reduce the distractions, move somewhere else to continue the interaction.

Environmental equipment

Some might consider the employment of environmental equipment around the home (such as amplified doorbells, vibrating alarm clocks and flashing smoke detectors) to be of little benefit to people with profound intellectual and multiple disabilities who have hearing impairment. After all – the argument might go – they will not be answering the door independently, getting up independently or evacuating the building independently! Then again, that depends on your definition of being independent. With the emergence of the Independent Living Movement we have been provided with more useful insights into what disabled people themselves mean by being 'independent'. The Disability Rights Commission (2003) states, 'The term independent living refers to all disabled people having the same choice, control and freedom as any other citizen – at home, at work and as members of the community. This does not necessarily mean disabled people 'doing everything for themselves', but it does mean that any practical assistance people need should be based on their own choices and aspirations'. I would therefore suggest that people with profound intellectual and multiple disabilities have a fundamental right to be alerted to there being someone at their door!

Conclusion

Whilst there are some exceptional examples of good practice to be found across the UK, it remains that many audiology services are failing to meet the complex needs of all their patients with profound intellectual and multiple disabilities (and they become yet another example of arbitrary 'postcode lottery' quality and distribution of service). So what makes a service successful? At this point I should probably be emphasising the importance of a systemic commitment to people with profound intellectual and multiple disabilities or stressing the need for effective multi-agency working. However, in my professional experience, while these are indeed essential there is another element that goes deeper than this: services need creative practitioners – those who do not believe that 'these people' can only be tested if they have the appropriate resources; those practitioners who will sit and ponder over ideas on how to adapt a test to meet an individual's needs; those practitioners who will keep on making appointments with the individual until they have as much information as they need; and those who will take the risk and fit a hearing aid because they believe it will make a difference. And I remain convinced that creativity comes to those practitioners who see the humanity within the clinical and are prepared to uphold the right of every patient to be seen as an individual with their own horizon.

Appendix 11.1

There is a series of factsheets that are available to download free of charge from www.lookupinfo.org which will expand on some of the material covered throughout this chapter. Titles include:

- identifying hearing impairment in people with learning disabilities;
- supporting people with learning disabilities with hearing assessment;
- the effects of hearing impairment on people with learning disabilities;
- ways to help people with learning disabilities who have hearing impairment; and
- hearing aids and environmental equipment for people with learning disabilities.

Further resources are also available form the RNID at: http://www.rnid.org.uk.

Appendix 11.2

The National Special Interest Group on Hearing Impairment in People with Learning Disabilities is a group of professionals from across the UK who meets biannually.

The professional backgrounds of the members vary but include intellectual disability nurses, audiologists, speech and language therapists and hearing therapists. Over the last decade, the group has made a significant contribution to improving hearing care for people with learning disabilities/intellectual disabilities by carrying out research, contributing to publications and developing resources. The group is an open forum and welcomes new members.

Further information can be sought from Laura Waite – waitel@hope.ac.uk.

References

ADSS, BDA, LGA, NDCS, NCB, RNID (2002). *Deaf Children: Positive Practice Standards in Social Services*. London: RNID.

ADSS, BDA, LGA, RNID (1999). *Best Practice Standards: Social Services for Deaf and Hard of Hearing People*. London: RNID.

Alborz, A., McNally, R., Swallow, A., & Glendinning, C. (2003). *From the Cradle to the Grave: A Literature Review of Access to Health Care for People with Learning Disabilities Across the Lifespan*. Available at: http://www.sdo.nihr.ac.uk/files/project/23-final-report.pdf (accessed 1 July 2008).

Band, R. (1998). *The NHS – Health for all? People with Learning Disabilities and Health Care*. London: Mencap.

British Society of Audiology (2004). *Guidelines on Minimum Training Standards for Otoscopy and Impression Taking*. Available at: http://www.thebsa.org.uk/docs/otoscopytrainingstandardsfinalversionoct2004.doc (accessed 2 August 2006).

Buchanan, L.H. (1990). Early onset of presbyacusis in down syndrome. *Scandinavian Audiology*, 19(2), 103–110.

Cone-Wesson, B., Vohr, B., Sininger, Y., Widen, J., Folsom, R., Gorga, M., & Norton, S. (2000). Identification of neonatal hearing impairment: infants with hearing loss. *Ear & Hearing*, 21(5), 488–507.

Department of Health (2001). *Valuing People: A New Strategy for Learning Disability in the 21st Century*. London: HMSO.

Department of Health (2007). *Improving Access to Audiology Services in England*. London: HMSO.

Disability Rights Commission (2003). *Policy Statement on Social Care and Independent Living*. Available at: http://www.drc-gb.org/library/policy/health_and_independent_living/drc_policy_statement_on_social.aspx (accessed 9 July 2006).

Down's Syndrome Medical Interest Group (2001). *Surveillance Guidelines – Hearing Impairment*. Available at: http://www.dsmig.org.uk/library/articles/guideline-hear-8.pdf (accessed 2 August 2006).

Durkel, J., & Moss, K. (2005). *Formal Versus Informal Hearing Tests: What Is Functional Hearing?* Available at: http://www.tsbvi.edu/Outreach/seehear/summer05/functional.htm (accessed 1 October 2007).

Evenhuis, H.M., & Nagtzaam, L.M.D. (eds) (1998). *Early Identification of Hearing and Visual Impairment in Children and Adults with an Intellectual Disability*. IASSID International Consensus Statement. SIRG Health Issues.

Evenhuis, H.M., Van Zanten, J.A., Brocaar, M.P., & Roerdinkholder, W.H.M. (1992). Hearing loss in middle aged persons with down syndrome. *American Journal on Mental Retardation*, 97(1), 47–56.

Fransman, D.L. (1996). Special needs need a specialist service. *Therapy Weekly*, 23 May, 6.

Fransman, D.L. (1998). *Cerumen Screening Programme in an NHS Hospital for People with Learning Disabilities*. Unpublished audit report. Derbyshire: Southern Derbyshire Community Health Services NHS Trust.

Fransman, D.L. (2006). Can removal of back teeth contribute to chronic earwax obstruction? *British Journal of Learning Disabilities*, 34(1), 36–41.

Graham, J., & Martin, M. (2001) *Ballantyne's Deafness* (6th edition). London: Whurr.

Hindle, P., & Kitson, N. (2000). *Mental Health and Deafness*. London: Whurr.

Ladd, P. (2003). *Understanding Deaf Culture: In Search of Deafhood*. Clevedon: Multilingual Matters.

Maltby, M.A., & Knight, P. (2000). *Audiology*. London: David Fulton.

McCracken, W. (2002). *Deafness and Other Disabilities*. Available at: http://www.deafnessatbirth.org.uk/content2/deafness/disab/01/content.pdf (accessed 1 October 2007).

McKenna, L. (2001). Psychological aspects of acquired hearing loss. In Graham, J., & Martin, M. (eds), *Ballantyne's Deafness* (6th edition). London: Whurr; 258–271.

Morgan-Jones, R.A. (2001). *Hearing Differently: The Impact of Hearing Impairment on Family Life*. London: Whurr.

Murdoch, H. (1994) 'He can hear when he wants to!' Assessment of hearing function for people with learning difficulties. *British Journal of Learning Disabilities*, 22, 85–89.

National Deaf Children's Society (2000). *Quality Standards in Paediatric Audiology: Guidelines for the Early Identification and Audiological Management of Children with Hearing Loss*. London: NDCS.

National Deaf Children's Society (2005). *Quality Standards and Good Practice Guidelines: Transition from Child to Adult Services*. London: NDCS.

NHS Quality Improvement Scotland (2006). *Promoting Access to Healthcare for People with a Learning Disability – A Guide for Frontline Staff*. Edinburgh: NHS QIS.

Northway, R., Hutchinson, C., & Kingdon, A. (eds). (2006). *Shaping the Future: A Vision for Learning Disability Nursing*. Available at: http://www.lnnm.co.uk/publications/shapingthefuture.pdf (accessed 1 July 2008).

Ouellette-Kuntz, H., Garcin, N., Lewis, M.E., Minnes, P., Martin, C., & Holden, J.J. (2005). Addressing health disparities through promoting equity for individuals with intellectual disability. *Canadian Journal of Public Health*, 96(2), S8–22.

Picard, M. (2004). Children with permanent hearing loss and associated disabilities: revisiting current epidemiological data and causes of deafness. *VOLTA Review*, 104(4), 1221–1236.

Roberts, B. (2005). Promoting healthy lifestyles. In Grant, G., Goward, P., Richardson, M., & Ramcharan, P. (eds), *Learning Disability: A Life Cycle Approach to Valuing People*. Maidenhead: OU Press.

Roeser, R.J., & Ballachanda, B.B. (1997). Physiology, pathophysiology, and anthropology/epidemiology of human earcanal secretions. *Journal of the American Academy of Audiology*, 8(6), 391–400.

Royal College of Nursing (2006). *Meeting the Health Needs of People with Learning Disabilities*. London: RCN.

Royal National Institute for Deaf People (2002). *Best Practice Standards for Adult Audiology*. London: RNID.

Scottish Executive (2002). *Promoting Health, Supporting Inclusion – The National Review of the Contribution of all Nurses and Midwives to the Care and Support of*

People with Learning Disabilities. Available at: http://www.scotland.gov.uk/Publications/2002/07/15072/8572 (accessed 7 September 2007).

Sense (2000). *Standards for Services for Adults who are Deafblind or have a Dual Sensory Impairment*. London, Sense.

Waugh, A., & Grant, A. (2006). Anatomy and Physiology in Health and Illness (10th edition). UK: Churchill Livingstone; p. 190.

Wilson, D.N., & Haire, A. (1990). Health care screening for people with mental handicap living in the community. *British Medical Journal*, 301, 1379–1381.

Chapter 12

RESPIRATORY HEALTH OF PEOPLE WITH PROFOUND INTELLECTUAL AND MULTIPLE DISABILITIES

Colin Wallis

Introduction

Many individuals with profound intellectual and multiple disabilities (PIMD) experience health problems related to the chest or airways. There are a number of precipitating factors and contributing features that increase this propensity to chest pathology. Sometimes the impact is short-lived and requires an acute intervention with a subsequent return to full lung functioning. Other times there is a chronic element requiring lifelong attention and prevention to maintain health. There are also some patients with PIMD who require long-term ventilatory support as part of their respiratory care.

This chapter looks at the factors that predispose to lung injury in those with profound intellectual disabilities, discusses the interventions available to prevent or limit lung damage and discusses the role of long-term ventilation in management.

The information and techniques presented in this chapter are developed from the highly specialist work of the author. Colin Wallis is a consultant paediatrician in the respiratory unit at Great Ormond Street Hospital for Children; he works within the guidelines of the General Medical Council. Sources of further reading are provided at the end of the chapter.

Learning objectives

- To recognise the importance of lung health in individuals with PIMD for survival and reduced morbidity;
- To recognise the role of aspiration as a cause of lung damage;
- To recognise and limit the impact of predisposing factors for chest infection;
- To reduce, where possible, the implications of weakness and chest wall deformities on respiratory insufficiency; and
- To consider the option of long-term ventilatory support in selected individuals, recognising the ethical implications that such interventions may carry.

Aspiration into the lungs: aspiration 'over the top'

We are all equipped with a highly sophisticated swallowing mechanism to ensure that our swallow is safe and that ingested food and oral secretions do not penetrate through the vocal chords and enter the airways. We have neurologically controlled stages of swallowing that are both volitional and involuntary, ensuring that the food bolus moves from the front of the oral cavity into the pharynx using coordinated tongue movements (see Chapter 14). Closure of the epiglottis, in the post-pharyngeal stage, allows safe propulsion of the food bolus or fluid into the oesophagus. Even in full health, minor aspiration episodes can occur. In these instances, a strong cough reflex will ensure that the accidental penetration of foreign material through the vocal chords is rapidly and forcefully expelled.

In children and adults with PIMD, especially those with associated neurological compromise, the complex swallowing mechanisms can fail and aspiration 'over the top' occurs. A disorganised swallowing mechanism, with failure of epiglottic and vocal chord closure, combined with a weak or ineffective cough, results in penetration of food or secretions into the airways. The clinical features of aspiration in the presence of severe or profound intellectual disabilities can also be masked and 'silent aspiration' may occur. In this instance the carer or parent may not even be aware that aspiration is occurring and lung damage may occur without warning.

The impact of aspiration – either over the top or secondary to refluxing of abdominal contents (see later) – can have a very variable effect on the lungs. In some children and adults, there is very little evidence of bronchial damage even in the presence of known aspiration. In others, damage rapidly ensues and bronchiectasis (irreversible widening of medium-sized airways (bronchi) in the lung), pneumonia, collapse and consolidation result. The reasons for this variability in impact on the lung's structure are not fully understood.

Investigation

If aspiration over the top is suspected, the individual will require a clinical and possibly radiological assessment by a speech and language therapist with experience in this area. The therapist will take a careful history and observe normal feeding and swallowing mechanisms looking out for possible signs of aspiration as indicated in Table 12.1. A videofluoroscopic study is a useful technique to evaluate the safety of the swallowing mechanism. For this investigation, the person is monitored in the radiology department and imaging of the swallow is recorded – often with a variety of textures and consistencies. The stages of deglutition are evaluated and the presence of undercoating of the epiglottis, penetration of small amounts of contrast medium through the vocal chords and frank aspiration into the airways is recorded. The ability of the person to handle different consistencies such as fluids, purees and solids can also be assessed as can different feeding techniques and positions.

An example of severe aspiration is indicated in Figure 12.1. This child represents an extreme form of 'silent' aspiration that is not uncommon in the person with PIMD – aspiration occurring with no, or very limited, clinical evidence.

Table 12.1 Possible signs of aspiration.

Coughing and choking with feeds
Difficulty with mealtimes and food refusal
Excessive tearing
Prolonged feeding times
Gagging with certain consistencies/inability to cope with lumps
Wheezing episodes following a bottle or fluid feed
Repeated chest infections
Repeated episodes of lung or lobar collapse
Blue episodes or desaturation during bottle feeding
Silent aspiration with diffuse changes on chest imaging

Management

The management of the person with aspiration over the top can be very challenging. Occasionally, with the advice of the speech and language therapist, feeding conditions can be created that minimise the aspiration risk. Attention to the thickening of fluids, careful choices of purees and avoidance of lumpy textured foodstuffs (see Chapter 14), when combined with an optimal seating position (see Chapter 17) and skilled feeding techniques by carers who know the individual well, will help keep aspiration episodes to a minimum and may facilitate safe oral feeding.

In other children and adults, the risk of aspiration is too high no matter what precautions are introduced and non-oral feeding is indicated to protect the lungs from damage. A gastrostomy is inserted directly into the stomach and it provides a safe alternative for nutrition – especially fluids (see Chapter 15). Often there is some parental or carer resistance to the insertion of the gastrostomy tube as it is seen as a highly invasive procedure. This can be especially difficult when the carer is having to act in the best interests of the child providing consent on their behalf or when supporting an adult with PIMD to reach a decision in their 'best interest' (Department for Constitutional Affairs, 2007). The advantages however can be significant and parents and carers will comment on the life-changing benefits it has given the person and the family once the surgery has been performed (Rollins, 2006). Mealtimes can still be enjoyed as a social occasion and safe tastes may still be permitted, but the pressure to achieve sufficient caloric intake and a balanced diet is relieved and chest infections are reduced.

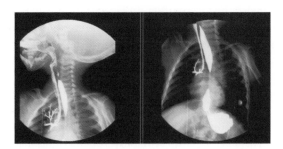

Figure 12.1 Child presenting with an extreme form of 'silent' aspiration.

Occasionally, health professionals will encounter a family who cannot accept non-oral feeding. There is a strong natural drive to feed one's offspring, and some parents will argue that eating and tasting food is the one small enjoyment in the child's day. These situations have to be handled with care and diplomacy. Sometimes compromises can be found – for example, the majority of the nutrition goes down the gastrostomy tube with just tastes and small purees allowed orally. Due to the associated risks, this intervention would be monitored by a speech and language therapist, paediatrician or physician.

If consent for a gastrostomy tube is refused by the consenting adult then ongoing careful surveillance of the chest is required by a paediatrician or physician with experience in this area to ensure that irreversible lung damage does not ensue.

It is useful to reiterate the three chief principles of feeding:

- mealtimes must be enjoyable for both the feeder and the child/adult;
- intake must be sufficient to ensure adequate nutrition and growth;
- feeding must be safe and not result in lung damage from aspiration.

If these three tenets are achieved then it may be safe to continue to observe with regular follow-up and review.

Aspiration of oral secretions

Those individuals with swallowing abnormalities, who have moved to non-oral nutrition, may also experience difficulties in dealing with normal oral secretions. This commonly manifests as drooling. In others, secretions pool in the pharynx and lead to upper airway obstructive sounds that can be transmitted throughout the chest and mimic infection on auscultation. The mucus can become thick and tenacious and lead to distressing coughing and choking episodes and aspiration. Although, theoretically, accidental aspiration of salivary contents is less destructive to the lung than food particles, some people can have frequent episodes of chest infection which, in the absence of any oral intake, is attributed to the aspiration of oral secretions.

Management

Drying agents such as glycopyrrolate given orally or the use of hyoscine patches placed on areas of thin skin (commonly placed behind the ear) can be helpful in reducing the volume and hydration of the oral secretions (Dreyfuss et al., 1991). There is some anecdotal evidence that antibiotic prophylaxis with agents such as azithromycin can be helpful in controlling repeated episodes of chest infection.

Surgical interventions are reserved for the most refractory cases that are not responding to medical management. Duct diversion of the submaxillary ducts is sometimes recommended to reduce the social and nursing impact of excessive drooling. Care must be taken not to convert a 'drooler' into an 'aspirator'. Parotid nerve or duct ablation using agents such as botulinum toxin or surgical ligation is reserved for the most refractory cases. In some instances, when aspiration of saliva is compounded by distressing and life-threatening choking episodes, a tracheostomy is offered. This is an important decision in the life of the person with PIMD and needs a carefully considered multidisciplinary approach with all those involved in the individual's care. The practice of surgically sewing down the epiglottis over the laryngeal opening (laryngeal epiglottoplasty) is used less frequently as the complications of this radical procedure often outweigh any benefits at preventing aspiration.

Gastro-oesophageal reflux

Up to 50% of individuals with an intellectual disability could be suffering from GERD (gastro-oesophageal reflux disease) (Böhmer et al., 2000). In individuals with PIMD, the presence of gastro-oesophageal reflux can be missed and is probably underdiagnosed (Böhmer et al., 1997, 1999). An inability to report accurately the symptoms of heart burn or epigastric discomfort, together with the contributing impact of postural abnormalities, convulsions and gastrostomy feeding, all contribute to a predisposition for reflux.

Gastro-oesophageal reflux can lead to aspiration of regurgitated stomach contents. Symptoms and signs include recurrent wheezing episodes, repeated pneumonias, intermittent tachypnoea and lobar or subsegmental areas of pulmonary collapse. Gastro-oesophageal reflux can sometimes be mistakenly diagnosed as asthma.

Investigations

There is unfortunately no gold standard test for reflux-associated aspiration. The pH study is considered by many as a useful investigation. Here a pH-sensitive probe is inserted into the oesophagus and left to hang in the lower two-thirds of the oesophagus. Over a 24-hour period, changes in the intra-oesophageal acidity are recorded and analysed to establish the percentage of time that the probe is bathed in acid. All antacid reflux therapy needs to be stopped prior to the study and normal feeding should be maintained. For the person with severe reflux disease, these provisos may not be clinically possible.

Contrast studies for reflux with a radio-opaque dye placed in the stomach and then observed over a short period can often show free return of the contrast material up into the oesophagus. Milk scans using radioisotope-labelled milk can demonstrate a similar effect.

Management

Medical therapies using a combination of prokinetic agents (to enhance gut motility and gastric emptying) in combination with anti-acid therapy to reduce the acidity of the gastric secretions are commonly prescribed as medical management for reflux. Thickeners can be added to the milk of infants and the fluids of older patients.

Surgical procedures to reduce the propensity for reflux are undertaken commonly in persons with PIMD and severe gastro-oesophageal reflux. The Nissen fundoplication uses a technique where the top of the stomach is wrapped around the lower oesophagus, tightening the gastro-oesophageal junction and significantly limiting the ability of gastric contents to reflux. In many people with swallowing abnormalities, this procedure is combined with the insertion of a gastrostomy. Complications include gas bloating and difficulties with wind, an inability to vomit, and failure of the procedure with an unwrapping of the fundoplication requiring redo surgery.

Foreign-body aspiration

The risk of foreign-body aspiration is ever present in young children especially toddlers. Older cognitively aware children will usually alert their carers to the possibility of this occurrence. In patients with profound intellectual disabilities, the aspiration of a foreign body may go unnoticed or unrecorded. Foreign-body aspiration should receive special consideration in individuals with PIMD who have a persistent area of infection, consolidation or collapse that is not responding to routine therapy. A rigid bronchoscope is used to identify and remove the object.

Recurrent chest infections

Even in the absence of aspiration, there are a number of additional reasons why individuals with PIMD are susceptible to repeated episodes of chest infection and pneumonia. Examples are listed in Table 12.2.

Two factors would appear to render a child or adult with PMID particularly vulnerable to recurrent pneumonias: the absence of an effective cough and limited expansion to fully inflate the lungs.

An effective cough requires the ability to sense the presence of foreign material in the pharynx or upper airway, the coordination to close the glottis while building up intra-thoracic pressure following inspiration, the capacity to generate power to forcefully expel the air using abdominal and intercostals muscles with simultaneous opening of the vocal chords. This highly effective protective mechanism against foreign material is often compromised in PIMD.

Table 12.2 Additional reasons why individuals with PIMD are susceptible to repeated episodes of chest infection and pneumonia.

Poor cough reflex
Aspiration
Concomitant medical conditions
Cardiac disease
Epilepsy
Neuromuscular weakness
Cerebral palsy
Lung disease of prematurity
Hypotonia with decreased lung expansion
Decreased physical activity with associated obesity
Limited chest wall excursion with lung atelectasis
Poor dental hygiene
Altered immunity
As a syndromic feature, e.g. di George association
Accelerated immunological ageing, e.g. Down's syndrome
Institutionalisation with congregate living arrangements

A normally shaped thorax with good inspiratory musculature and diaphragmatic function is required to ensure full inspiration of the lung bed especially during exercise or intermittently during the day and night as a 'sigh' breath. This prevents areas of microatelectasis and a propensity to infection. The ability to achieve this functional residual capacity may be diminished for a number of reasons in those people with PIMD.

Management

An individualised approach is required to address those areas of compromise that may predispose to infection. This may involve assessment by a physiotherapist to ensure good posture, maximal activity and fitness and structured chest physiotherapy techniques for those who are unable to self-achieve respiratory airway clearance.

Routine vaccinations in addition to the 'flu vaccine' are required. In some children and adults with refractory or frequent episodes of chest infection, the use of prophylactic antibiotics is recommended although there are currently no well-constructed trials to support this practice.

Thoracic cage abnormalities

Respiratory health is heavily dependent on a symmetrical thoracic cage of adequate volume and good musculature for both inspiration (diaphragms, intercostal muscles, accessory muscles of ventilation such as the sternocleidomastoid) and expiration (intercostals, abdominal muscles).

Deformations and malformations of the thoracic skeleton

Changes in the shape of the thoracic cage are not uncommonly found in children and adults with PIMD especially those with a syndromic component. Frequently, there is little that can be done medically or surgically to correct these abnormalities.

Spinal deformities need to be monitored closely. This can be particularly important during the growth spurt of adolescence. A curvature of the thoracic spine can have significant impact on the functioning of the thoracic cage and the optimal expansion of the lungs. Correction may be required if impact on lung functioning is demonstrated or suspected – either by attention to seating, bracing, or by surgical procedures to fix, fuse or straighten the deformity (Figure 12.2).

Neuromuscular weakness

Physiotherapy and occupational therapy are mainstays in the treatment of children and adults with weakness and PIMD. Therapists will give attention to posture (see Chapter 17), seating, movement, airway clearance techniques and the use of specialised devices to assist with chest physiotherapy. Examples of such devices include the cough-assist device (to aid the expulsion of secretions through a mechanically simulated cough), the inflatable vest (which provides a vibrating decompression of the chest after inspiration to help with removal of secretions) or intermittent artificial

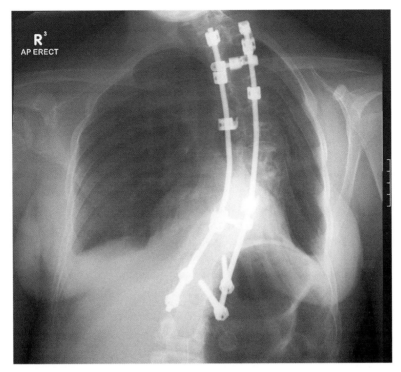

Figure 12.2 Image showing curvature of the thoracic spine.

lung inflations with the use of a bi-level non-invasive ventilator – all contributing in differing ways to maintaining lung health and lessen the risk of infection and atelectasis.

Care must be taken to avoid obesity. Dietetic advice with attention to calorie intake can be important especially in sedentary or weak children and adults (see Chapter 15).

Compliance issues in the management of lung disorders

The management of common respiratory illnesses such as asthma or pneumonia can be further complicated and less effective in those who have, in addition, PIMD.

Delays in the diagnosis of chest infections are common. There are a number of reasons for this: symptoms can be poorly communicated or missed in the non-verbal person and signs can be masked by the underlying disabilities. Investigations such as lung function testing may not be possible. The administration of physiotherapy may be complicated by poor compliance or an inability to cooperate with the required techniques.

Drug administration in respiratory medicine can include the use of inhalers and spacers for conditions such as asthma. Such devices can be difficult to use and require alternative delivery routes such as nebulisation.

Long-term ventilatory support

Respiratory failure can be acute (short-term, needing respiratory support in an intensive care with the potential for full recovery) or chronic (permanent changes to respiratory functioning that require long-term ventilatory support to sustain life – preferably in a home environment).

Ventilatory failure can be broadly divided into four categories:

- Obstruction of the upper airways
- Acute or chronic alteration to lung parenchyma with a failure to transfer gases across the alveolar–capillary membrane
- Failure of the bellows action of ventilation due to thoracic cage abnormalities or weakness of the muscles of ventilation
- Failure of a central drive to maintain breathing (especially during sleep) or to compensate during periods of increased demand such as exercise or infection

Upper airway obstruction

A sophisticated (and mostly involuntary) system of neurological coordination is required to maintain a patent upper airway for effective breathing. This is particularly relevant during periods of dream or rapid eye movement (REM) sleep, when loss of tone to the muscles of the pharynx leads to potential for upper airway obstruction.

Children and adults with PIMD can have significant problems with upper airway obstruction, occasionally whilst awake but more commonly during sleep. This can lead to oxygen desaturation and sleep disruption with frequent disturbances of the normal sleep architecture occurring when the oxygen levels drop and the sleeping individual must arouse to regain airway patency. If not addressed, significant hypoxia can, in turn, lead to right ventricular heart strain and eventually to irreversible pulmonary hypertension.

The cause of the upper airway obstruction may be related to the underlying syndrome of Intellectual Disability – Trisomy 21, for example, may have a large tongue with propensity to posterior pharyngeal obstruction; craniofacial syndromes such as Crouzon disorder can have small mid-facies; individuals with cerebral palsy can have malformation of facial bones with narrowed nasopharyngeal structures.

Management

Many children and adults with PIMD and upper airway obstruction will present with snoring or a history of obstructed breathing efforts during REM sleep. An overnight oximetry recording is useful to determine the degree and extent of the desaturation that is occurring (Figure 12.3). More detailed sleep studies looking at chest wall movement, sleep staging and degrees of airway flow obstruction may also be required.

The management of individuals with PIMD and associated upper airway obstruction can be fraught with difficulties. An assessment by an ENT surgeon is required to ensure that there is no residual tonsillar or adenoidal tissue that can be usefully

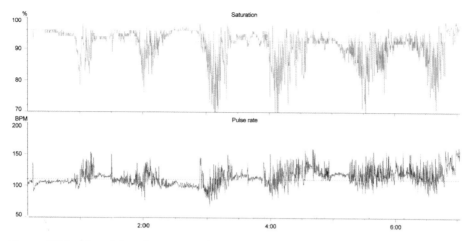

Figure 12.3 Overnight oximetry recording showing oxygen saturation.

removed to improve airway patency. In young children the insertion of a nasopharyngeal airway with the tip lying behind the tongue but just above the epiglottis can provide an improved upper airway (Figure 12.4). Although it is possible to use a prong beyond infancy, some older children and adults will find the insertion of the prong distressing, and carers may experience keeping the tube in position.

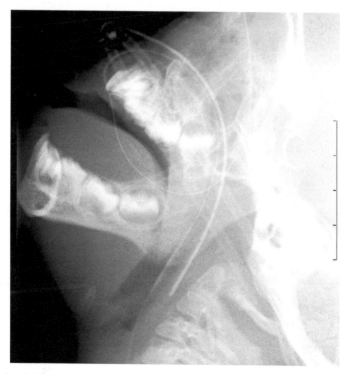

Figure 12.4 Optimum position of a nasopharyngeal airway in a young child.

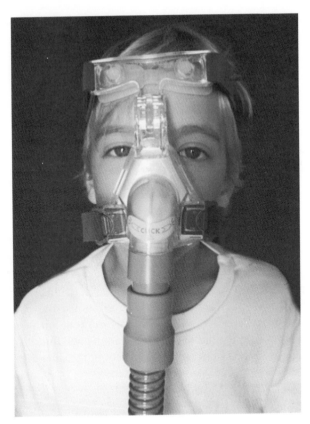

Figure 12.5 Child wearing a CPAP device.

Recently, there has been increasing interest in the use of a nasal or facial mask for the delivery of continuous pressure to maintain patency of the pharynx and supra-glottic area during periods of tone loss in REM sleep. A mask with soft interface of silicone or gel covers the nose or face and is secured by straps linked to a hat-like structure (Figure 12.5). Air is delivered at a predetermined positive pressure during sleep via a simple and portable continuous positive airway pressure (CPAP) device. Cooperation is required, but this mechanism has been successfully used even in individuals with PIMD and can prevent the sequelae of chronic hypoxia.

Oxygen therapy may be used when all other interventions to improve upper airway patency have failed. It has to be recognised that oxygen treatment in itself is not altering the obstruction. It merely elevates the baseline oxygen saturation so that episodes of desaturation are better handled and desaturation is masked to a degree. Delivery of oxygen may remove the central drive to breathe in patients who have been chronically hypoxic and hypercarbic. Monitoring may be required to ensure that an increasing respiratory acidosis with rising carbon dioxide levels is not occurring when oxygen therapy is first introduced. This is not usually problematic in children on low-flow oxygen. High-flow oxygen should not be required.

Chronic changes to lung gas exchange

There are a number of factors associated with PIMD that predispose to chronic parenchymal changes in the lung and interference with the efficient gas exchange of oxygen from the alveolus to the capillaries. These may include recurrent infections, repeated episodes of aspiration or the chronic lung disease of prematurity.

In its mildest form, long-term supplemental oxygen is required. In children with prematurity (and young children who have chronic infective or aspiration changes) there is the potential for new alveolar growth. Sufficient recovery can allow for weaning of the oxygen therapy, provided repeated insults are prevented and somatic growth occurs. Oxygen levels should be titrated to maintain oxygen saturation levels above 93%. More severe or diffuse damage may require the delivery of oxygen under positive airway pressure. This can be delivered via non-invasive or invasive interfaces and is further discussed next.

Long-term ventilation

The remaining two categories of respiratory failure – a central failure to breathe with loss of respiratory drive and a failure of bellows functioning – may both require artificial ventilatory support if the individual is no longer able to maintain effective gas exchange. This may be in the form of a brief rescue from a reversible condition – such as an acute pneumonia or during recovery from spinal surgery. In other circumstances, the changes leading to the ventilatory failure may be irreversible and long-term strategies of respiratory support will need consideration.

Over the last decade, there have been considerable developments in the field of long-term ventilation and the move to providing such support in a domiciliary setting. Improvement in both the interface (how the machine connects to the patient) and the machines to deliver the ventilatory support has resulted in increasing use of positive pressure support for children and adults with PIMD. Significant challenges still remain in both the use of these modalities, especially in the individual with intellectual disabilities and the ethical issues that arise in the introduction of life-saving devices in patients with complex needs.

Non-invasive (mask) interface

A range of masks have been developed to suit the needs of all ages including, more recently, the needs of the younger child. The mask can be either applied to deliver positive pressure via the nose or cover both the mouth and the nose. As discussed earlier, the commonest use for this interface is to deliver a continuous source of positive pressure (CPAP) for upper airway obstruction but bi-level ventilation – delivering a differential pressure level during inspiration and expiration – can also be achieved via a nasal or full-face mask. In effect, one is thus able to support an individual who has limited ability to self-ventilate.

There are significant limitations to the use of mask delivery. Some patients, especially children, will not tolerate the mask and never adjust to its application in spite of patient periods of acclimatisation. For those who require ventilatory support for considerable parts of the day (usually beyond 16 hours a day), it is difficult to achieve. Skin breakdown over pressure points can be troublesome although this problem is less prevalent with the development of gel-based masks and silicone lining systems that do not require a tight seal. Excessive drooling and failure to deal with oral secretions can also be a contraindication to mask use. Recent anecdotal reports suggest that the prolonged use of a mask may result in some distortion of the facial bones and a negative impact on dentition and maxillary growth.

Invasive (tracheostomy) ventilation

Long-term ventilation is most easily delivered by a tracheostomy. The decision to move to a tracheostomy interface for ventilatory support needs to be considered carefully. There are considerable nursing and carer implications. A tracheostomy may provide easy tracheal access for the removal of secretions, prevention of choking episodes and the rapid and easy application of the ventilatory device, but it also presents a risk for accidental obstruction, dislodgement (sometimes with fatal implications) and increases infection risk. Carers and parents need to be fully trained in tracheostomy care.

Home ventilation equipment and additional support

A decision to move to long-term ventilatory support (especially if a tracheostomy is used) will require a needs assessment to determine the best environment for ongoing care of the individual patient. It is recognised that the acute hospital environment (intensive care, high dependency or acute medical ward) is not the best environment for a child and is not in their best interest for long-term support. Any move to long-term ventilatory support should be accompanied by a programme that moves the child either back into their family home or into a suitable long-term placement that can address the child's developmental and emotional growth.

There are recognised common areas that will require the attention of the rehabilitation team in this process from hospital to home. Firstly, the home may need adaptation to accommodate the multiple equipment needs of the child. Fortunately, ventilators are now designed to be small, portable, battery operated and easy to use. Sophisticated settings are very rarely required for home use, and simple machines with basic settings are now commercially available at reasonable cost. Secondly, having a child or adult with multiple needs at home on long-term ventilation (especially if the support is for 24 hours a day via a tracheostomy) requires an additional level of carer input. Many of these individuals will be provided with a package of care that provides additional respite to the parents with a small team of trained carers under the supervision of a nurse.

All patients on long-term ventilation should be reviewed by a centre with expertise in this area to ensure that the evolving needs of the individual and their family are regularly assessed and the inevitable changes that accompany their growth and the underlying condition are accommodated.

Ethical issues

The ability to provide long-term ventilatory support for children and adults with PIMD raises new ethical considerations.

Often one is in a position where you are required to balance three competing pressures: technology (what we can technically and physically achieve); ethics (what we ought to do) and the law (what we are legally obliged to do). The question may be asked: just because we can maintain life, are we required to do so at all costs? At what point do we move from sustaining a life worth living to delaying an inevitable death?

At the heart of all decision regarding the use of long-term ventilation in children with PIMD lies the needs of the child. At all times the child's best interests must be paramount, but these difficult decisions are made harder when the individuals themselves are unable to contribute to the debate. Decisions are made by those who know them best, and as such, these decisions are not necessarily without bias. These issues of consent apply equally to the adult with reduced capacity to provide consent and for whom consenting adults are identified to act in the person's best interests (Department of Constitutional Affairs, 2007). Further reading is provided at the end of the chapter.

Long-term ventilation (especially once a tracheostomy has been fashioned) should improve quality of life (see Chapter 2) and not be simply a means to prolong a life where death is inevitable or life has become intolerable. This can be especially true when life can only be sustained within an intensive care environment. A multidisciplinary approach between all interested parties, with regular reviews, is required for planning strategy, especially when attempting to pre-empt what should occur in a crisis. The concept of ceilings of care is often useful – the teams need to consider how far they will use life-supporting technology for their patient and at what point they will recognise that the best interests of the child (or adult) are no longer being met.

Conclusion

There is no right or wrong thing to do – merely finding the most appropriate approach for a specific individual. There is no 'one size fits all'.

Each person with PIMD requires a tailor-made approach to all the aspects of their respiratory care and lung health.

Further reading

Consent

The Department of Health has published a large number of resources to support consent; these are available on the following web page: http://www.dh.gov.uk/en/policyandguidance/healthandsocialcaretopics/consent/index.htm.

Specific key documents include the following:

DH (2001). *Consent: A Guide for People with Learning Disabilities.* Available at: http://www.dh.gov.uk/dr_consum_dh/idcplg?IdcService=GET_FILE&dID=17040&Rendition=Web (accessed 7 August 2007).

DH (2001). *Seeking Consent: Working with People with Learning Disabilities.* Available at: http://www.dh.gov.uk/dr_consum_dh/idcplg?IdcService=GET_FILE&dID=3330&Rendition=Web (accessed 7 August 2007).

DH (2004). *Consent Form 4 – Form for Adults Who Are Unable to Consent to Investigation or Treatment.* Available at: http://www.dh.gov.uk/dr_consum_dh/idcplg?IdcService=GET_FILE&dID=25735&Rendition=Web (accessed 7 August 2007).

General/respiratory

O'Brien, K., Tate, K., & Zaharia, E. (1991). Mortality in a large southeastern facility for persons with mental retardation. *American Journal on Mental Retardation*, 95(4), 397–403.

Stuart, J.M., Stewart-Brown, L., Harvey, J., & Morgan, K. (1990). Deaths from asthma in the mentally handicapped. *British Medical Journal*, 300(6726), 720–721.

Turner, S., & Moss, S. (1996). The health needs of adults with learning disabilities and the health of the nation strategy. *Journal of Intellectual Disability Research*, 40(5), 438–450.

Yoshikawa, H., Yamazaki, S., & Abe, T. (2005). Acute respiratory distress syndrome in children with severe motor and intellectual disabilities. *Brain and Development*, 27(6), 395–399.

Aspiration

Cass, H., Wallis, C., Ryan, M., Reilly, S., & McHugh, K. (2005). Assessing pulmonary consequences of dysphagia in children with neurological disabilities: when to intervene? *Developmental Medicine and Child Neurology*, 47(5), 347–352.

Frazier, J.B., & Friedman, B. (1996). Swallow function in children with Down syndrome: a retrospective study. *Developmental Medicine and Child Neurology*, 38(8), 695–703.

Platyker, A.C.G. (1998). Gastroesophageal reflux and aspiration syndromes. In Chernick, V., Boat, T.F. (eds), *Kendig's Disorders of the Respiratory Tract in Children* (6th edition). Philadelphia: WB Saunders; 584–600.

Reilly, S., Skuse, D., & Poblete, X. (1996). Prevalence of feeding problems and oral motor dysfunction in children with cerebral palsy: a community survey. *Journal of Pediatrics*, 129(6), 877–882.

Rogers, B., Stratton, P., Msall, M., Andres, M., Champlain, M.K., Koerner, P., & Piazza, J. (1994). Long-term morbidity and management strategies of tracheal aspiration in adults with severe developmental disabilities. *American Journal of Mental Retardation*, 98(4), 490–498.

Non-invasive mask support

Liner, L.H., & Marcus, C.L. (2006). Ventilatory management of sleep-disordered breathing in children. *Current Opinion in Pediatrics*, 18(3), 272–276.

Massa, F., Gonsalez, S., Laverty, A., Wallis, C.E., & Lane, R.J.T. (2002). The use of nasal continuous positive pressure to treat obstructive sleep apnoea. *Archives of Disease in Childhood*, 87(5), 438–443.

Long-term ventilation

Jardine, E., & Wallis, C. (1998). Core guidelines for the discharge home of the child on long-term assisted ventilation in the United Kingdom. UK Working Party on Paediatric Long Term Ventilation. *Thorax*, 53(9), 762–767.

Noyes, J., & Lewis, M. (2005). *From Hospital to Home: Guidance on Discharge Management and Community Support for Children Using Long-Term Ventilation*. Available at: http://www.barnardos.org.uk/from_hospital_to_home.pdf (accessed 7 August 2007).

References

Böhmer, C.J.M., Niezen-de Boer, M.C., Klinkenberg-Knol, E.C., Deville, W.L., Nadorp, J.H., & Meuwissen, S.G.M. (1999). The prevalence of gastro-oesophageal reflux disease in institutionalised intellectually disabled individuals. *American Journal of Gastroenterology*, 94(3), 804–810.

Böhmer, C.J.M., Niezen-de Boer, M.C., Klinkenberg-Knol, E.C., & Meuwissen, S.G.M. (2000). Gastroesophageal reflux disease in intellectually disabled individuals: how often, how serious, how manageable? *American Journal of Gastroenterology*, 95(8), 1868–1872.

Böhmer, C.J.M., Niezen-de Boer, M.C., Klinkenberg-Knol, E.C., Tuynman, H.A.R.E., Voscuil, J.H., Deville, W.L.J.M., & Meuwissen, S.G.M. (1997). Gastro-oesophageal reflux disease in intellectually disabled individuals: leads for diagnosis and the effects of omeprazole therapy. *American Journal of Gastroenterology*, 92(9), 1475–1479.

Department for Constitutional Affairs (2007). *Mental Capacity Act: Code of Practice*. UK: The Stationery Office.

Dreyfuss, P., Vogel, D., & Walsh, N.,(1991). The use of transdermal scopolamine to control drooling: a case report. *American Journal of Physical Medicine and Rehabilitation*, 70(4), 220–222.

Rollins, H. (2006). The psychosocial impact on parents of tube feeding their child. *Paediatric Nursing*, 18(4), 19–22.

Chapter 13

DENTAL CARE AND ORAL HEALTH

Pauline Watt-Smith

Introduction

This chapter aims to identify dental problems which can occur both for the person for their dentist. It will give an overview of the disorders which can result or accompany intellectual disability and aims to provide some understanding of the dental treatment that can be carried out and the different settings in which this treatment may have to be performed. Good oral health in the twenty-first century should be the right of everyone. However, people with an intellectual disability generally have poorer general health than those without a disability and, correspondingly, poorer oral health. Those with a disability are perceived to receive lower-quality oral healthcare than those without an intellectual disability (Davis et al., 2000).

Special care dentistry was never part of the undergraduate curriculum and therefore there was no structured career pathway. In the past, people with intellectual disabilities may have only obtained treatment under general anaesthesia from oral surgeons resulting only in the extraction of teeth. In present times the Community Dental Service has generally provided dental care in dental clinics, but now special care dentistry has been introduced into the undergraduate curriculum in many dental schools, for example, Cardiff Dental Hospital and Dental School. In December 2005, the General Dental Council agreed, in principle, that special care dentistry would be recognised as a speciality. Hopefully, in the future, this will lead to a structured training pathway leading to a consultant-led service.

Learning objectives

At the end of the chapter the reader should:

- understand that prevention of oral disease is much better than treatment;
- appreciate the importance of regular dental attendance to provide optimum treatment rather than crisis management; and
- become familiar with techniques to improve dental care and oral hygiene.

What is oral health?

Oral health is defined as a standard of health of the oral and related tissues which enables an individual to eat, speak and socialise without active disease, discomfort or embarrassment and which contributes to general well-being (Department of Health, 1994).

Shapira et al. (1998) indicated that the poorest standard of oral hygiene is reported in people with intellectual disabilities and functional disabilities. People with disabilities have the right to be able to obtain and maintain the same degree of oral care and oral health as people without disabilities. This will require the dentist to adapt their treatment to individual needs. The dentist needs to be flexible about appointments when possible and needs to act fairly and not make adverse assumptions about the patients or their condition.

The governing body for dental health matters is the General Dental Council (GDC).

The GDC in protecting patients advocates that:

- putting patients' interests first and acting to protect them;
- respecting patients' dignities and choices;
- protecting the confidentiality of patients' information;
- cooperating with other members of the dental team and other healthcare colleagues in the interests of the patients;
- maintaining professional knowledge and competence; and
- being trustworthy.

(GDC, 2005, p. 4)

'Oral health and quality oral health care contributes to holistic health. It should be a right not a privilege' (Clark & Vanek, 1984, p. 213–216).

In oral healthcare and dentistry today, we have the benefit of knowledge with reference to:

- diet;
- importance of fluoride in reducing dental decay;
- importance of daily tooth-brushing regimes;
- importance of interceptive orthodontics to reduce gum disease;
- importance of sugar-free medication;
- school screening in order to monitor the numbers of decayed, missing and filled teeth in children at different ages in their school careers; and
- importance of regular dental check-ups.

Given the right support and opportunity, people with intellectual disabilities are able to utilise all these options. Over the last two decades, there has been a move away from institutionalised care of people with intellectual disabilities and an increase in integration into the community. Correspondingly, there has been a reduction in the number of special schools for people with intellectual disabilities which made it more difficult for dental healthcare professionals to establish the level of need and to plan for preventive dental care. One of the aspects of provision in special schools was the regular inspection of the oral and dental health of the students; these inspections are no longer carried out.

Establishing need and preparing for treatment would be the ideal as opposed to providing emergency dental treatment for the relief of pain. It is every person's right to pain-free dentistry in the twenty-first century, but this is best achieved in a structured way by familiarising the patient with the dentist so that a continuation of dental care is established and fear reduced. For people with a profound intellectual and multiple disability, there is limited choice regarding dental care provision, as the person is totally reliant upon carers for understanding needs, providing oral hygiene or supervising oral hygiene. The reliance on the carer recognising dental decline and then subsequently contacting a dentist, and providing transport to the dental surgery may all be perceived as barriers to oral care.

In this respect, as dentists and other oral healthcare providers, we may need to educate the carers or family in oral care to aid prevention and alert them to person's specific needs. For example, many older family carers may themselves be edentulous and consider multiple extractions the norm without realising that today, as dentists, we are able to offer a full range of treatment tailored to individual needs. Treatment may be offered under local anaesthetic, relative analgesia or sedation, either oral, nasal or intravenous (IV), with general anaesthesia available as a last resort in many cases. However, there are some people with severe or profound intellectual and multiple disabilities for whom general anaesthesia is the only way dental treatment can be provided. Again, this may be planned within the multidisciplinary framework where blood tests and even podiatry procedures may be achieved at the same visit.

During childhood people with profound intellectual and multiple disabilities are generally cared for at home within the family unit, depending on family circumstances and the degree of disability. From birth to age 16 the child will have been assessed by a multidisciplinary team which may comprise physicians, health visitors, speech therapists and dentists, often from the Community Dental Service (CDS). Whilst at school, mainstream or special school, the child will have been screened by the dentist from the CDS at specific ages, three times within their academic career, with their dental need recorded. If the child is not registered with a dentist then the appropriate treatment will be addressed by dentists within the CDS. However, once the child reaches age 16 and leaves school, dental contact is often lost and treatment is often sought on a 'needs' only basis via an access centre rather than continuing care.

Since April 2006 the new National Health Service (NHS) dental contract has resulted in many NHS dentists changing to providing only private treatment at an increased cost to the patient, which further reduces the choice of people with profound intellectual and multiple disabilities in obtaining regular dental care. It can therefore be understood that people with profound intellectual and multiple disabilities are at an increased risk of unnecessary premature loss of teeth, unnecessary gum disease and associated dental pain which will impact on their lives and behaviour. The need for regular dental care can therefore be perceived as an important prerequisite for the patients' general health.

Ethnicity and cultural attitudes to oral health

Another factor that may need addressing is ethnicity and cultural differences within our ever-increasing multicultural society. Different customs and attitudes to oral health exist within different cultures, and as oral healthcare professionals we need to be aware of these. Dietary differences may occur which can impact the patient's oral health. In addition, there may be a language barrier between parent/carer and dentist in providing information on both oral hygiene advice and treatment requirements. Again, a multidisciplinary approach is advisable, including the possibility of providing interpreted written illustrative information on treatment needs. In 1999 the Department of Health issued a paper focusing on epidemiology-based needs assessment, indicating that there would be an expected increase in the number of people with intellectual disabilities from different ethnic groups for treatment (NHS SSI Executive, 1999).

Importance of regular dental care for people with an intellectual disability

Intellectual disabilities can be due to congenital chromosomal aberration, metabolic conditions, intrauterine infections, trauma, cerebral hypoxia at birth or premature birth (see introductory chapter). There are several key syndromes and medical conditions of note in the provision of good oral health, including Down's syndrome, Fallot's tetralogy, Williams' syndrome, Tuberous sclerosis, Prader-Willi syndrome and cerebral palsy.

Down's syndrome

The incidence of Down's syndrome in the UK is 1.5/1000 births. The male to female ratio is 1:1 and 40% of people with Down's syndrome have associated congenital heart defects (British Society for Disability and Oral Health and the Faculty of Dental Surgery, 2001). Dental anomalies include large tongues, congenitally missing or misshapen teeth; for example, conical incisors. People with Down's syndrome tend to have a strong gag reflex and an estimated 20% will have an underactive thyroid.

They may also be immunodeficient and so breastfeeding should be actively encouraged in order to both passively improve the immunodeficient status and improve the jaw and tongue position which will aid oral health in later years. Children with Down's syndrome who have not been breastfed often become habitual mouth breathers with associated tongue protrusion. Habitual mouth breathers often have more gum problems, and people with Down's syndrome are at a higher risk of gum disease due to their already immuno-compromised state. The oral cavity is full of micro-organisms which can be found in large colonies in the gingival crevices surrounding the teeth. In habitual mouth breathers, increased numbers of bacteria are found in the more moist areas of the mouth. With good toothbrushing regimes these bacteria are removed, but if oral care is neglected, or patchy at best, then plaque accumulates on the tooth surfaces as well as around the gum margins resulting in florid inflammation of the gums (gingivitis). If left untreated, this progresses to inflammation of the supporting fibres of the teeth in their sockets, periodontitis, which causes mobility of the teeth and pain. Ultimately, this leads to loss of teeth unless treated and good oral hygiene instigated; people with Down's syndrome are often missing teeth. It is important to maintain the existing dentition as long as possible; denture compliance is problematic, resulting in compromised speech, mastication and poor aesthetics.

People with Down's syndrome may also present with atlanto-axial instability, which for dental treatment in the chair, may pose a problem due to the risk of neck injuries and the potential to cause irreversible spinal injury. A cushion placed under the neck will reduce this risk and make the person more comfortable and at ease.

An estimated 50% of people with Down's syndrome also have hearing problems which can also lead to communication problems. Ineffective communication can lead to distress and disorientation which may in turn lead to presentation of behaviour which makes assessment of dental need difficult. Care will be necessary if treatment is required under general anaesthetic and a full general anaesthetic assessment mandatory. If radiographs are necessary for dental treatment then lateral obliques are the radiograph of choice as intra-oral radiographs can be invasive and difficult for the person to tolerate. This may then distress the person and provide poor radiographic results. A multidisciplinary approach may be necessary to ascertain what action is in the person's best interest particularly with people with severe or profound intellectual disabilities in order to discuss expectations and outcomes.

As mentioned earlier, people with Down's syndrome also have associated cardiac problems which put them at risk of bacterial endocarditis, a potentially life-threatening illness. Previously, depending on the degree of cardiac involvement, antibiotic cover would be required for any dental procedure that was subgingival. This includes deep scaling and root planning to remove hard deposits of calculus. For those who are not allergic to penicillin, a typical antibiotic regime might include 3 g oral amoxicillin 1 hour prior to dental treatment or 1 g amoxicillin via IV. For individuals who are allergic to penicillin 300 mg clindamycin IV given over 10 minutes is more usual. Either regime depends on a degree of compliance from the person and many dental practitioners are reluctant to practise IV procedures therefore making it more difficult for many people with Down's syndrome to obtain the necessary dental care that they require to keep them dentally (and medically) fit. If oral antibiotic therapy is required, the person should arrive 1 hour earlier and be given 3 g amoxicillin under supervision and a nurse sits with the person whilst the antibiotic is ingested. If allergic to amoxicillin then 600 mg clindamycin administered orally is the alternative choice. The latest guidelines on antibiotic cover for dental procedures (Elliott et al., 2005) make it easier to treat these individuals in the dental clinic and is not so invasive for the person as most antibiotic therapy is now advised to be given orally.

Other groups of people with associated intellectual disabilities requiring antibiotic prophylaxis prior to dental treatment are those with Fallot's tetralogy and Williams' syndrome.

Fallot's tetralogy[1]

Fallot's tetralogy comprises four defects:

- Ventricular septal defect
- Pulmonary stenosis
- 'Overriding aorta'
- Compensatory right ventricular hypertrophy

These individuals are at risk of endocarditis, and liaison with their general practitioner and cardiologist is very important prior to dental treatment. They are also at risk of bleeding tendencies due to defective platelet function. They may present with cleft palate or hypodontia (missing teeth) or delayed eruption. They are best treated in a hospital setting where their cardiology problems can best be monitored. General anaesthesia is best avoided, but due to their intellectual disabilities, compliance with treatment in the dental chair can be difficult.

Williams' syndrome[2]

This syndrome comprises cardiovascular abnormalities and intellectual disabilities due to a microdeletion on chromosome 7. People with Williams' syndrome may also suffer from infantile hypercalcaemia which can leave a growth deficiency, osteosclerosis and craniostenosis. They may also suffer from sucking and swallowing problems and benefit from exercises to train the oral muscles perhaps by using an oral screen. Dentally, general anaesthetic is to be avoided.

Tuberous sclerosis[3]

Approximately 25% of people with tuberous sclerosis present with severe intellectual disabilities. This condition presents with café-au-lait spots, skin fibromas and depigmented skin; many of their teeth are pigmented with hypoplastic (thin) enamel. The fibromas may occur in the oral mucosa and other organs including the brain leading to intellectual disabilities, so these individuals are best treated using a multidisciplinary approach and in a hospital setting.

Prader-Willi syndrome[4]

This is a rare syndrome which manifests itself with intellectual difficulties and obesity. Diabetes is a complication so appointments need to be arranged following meals to avoid hypoglycaemia.

---

[1] http://www.dhg.org.uk/information/fallots.aspx
[2] http://www.williams-syndrome.org.uk/
[3] http://www.tuberous-sclerosis.org/
[4] http://www.pwsa.co.uk/

Cerebral palsy[5]

Cerebral palsy is an acquired condition caused by hypoxia or trauma at birth, and it affects one in ten live births and may or may not result in intellectual disabilities. About 50% of people with cerebral palsy have intellectual disabilities, epilepsy, impaired hearing, and vision or speech disability. They have motor impairment, uncontrolled body movements, seizure disorder, sensory dysfunction, and frequently use a wheelchair. Cerebral palsy is the most common congenital physical handicap.

Hemiplegia is common, and people presenting with hemiplegia frequently experience epilepsy; however, they rarely have intellectual disabilities. Conversely, people presenting with quadriplegia with cerebral palsy are often impaired by intellectual disabilities. Their dento-oral features share similar characteristics:

- High-vaulted palates
- Anterior open bite
- Excessive salivation (dribbling or drooling)
- Tooth erosion
- Tooth grinding (bruxism)
- Heightened gag reflex
- Self-injurious behaviour

High-vaulted palate

From a social perspective this affects speech, making it difficult to understand the person and consequently assumptions are made of intellectual impairment when this might not necessarily be the case. Communication difficulties may arise when speech is poorly understood, but many use computerised keyboards so that mutual agreement on treatment planning may be arranged and completed with the person's consent. However, a high-vaulted palate makes it difficult from a dental aspect to construct appliances that fit correctly. Difficulties can occur with eating and swallowing, and close liaison with other healthcare professionals is necessary from birth to encourage feeding and speech for clearer articulation.

Anterior open bite

This condition occurs when, on closure, only the posterior teeth occlude and a large gap occurs between the upper and lower front teeth. It is caused by soft tissue and/or bony abnormality with hyperactivity of the tongue musculature leading to tongue thrust, which in turn causes splaying of the developing teeth and poor oral seal. As a consequence of the poor oral seal, plaque levels increase, particularly at night as there is an associated mouth breathing habit, and gingivitis and caries (decay) may result if left untreated. Aesthetics may be compromised leading to poor self-image and esteem.

---

[5] http://www.scope.org.uk/

Excessive salivation (dribbling or drooling)

Excessive salivation can also result from poor oral seal. It is very seldom due to hypersalivation. It is related to impaired tongue motility and poor neck stability as well as dental abnormalities. It is most frequently associated with drooping head forehead posture reducing the oral seal. Treatment may include physiotherapy, surgery or drug use (Finkelstein & Chrysdale, 1992):

- Physiotherapy may include the use of an oral screen to aid strengthening of the perioral muscles to improve the oral seal. It may also improve swallowing by strengthening the buccinator muscles and upper constrictor muscles of the pharynx.
- Surgery is only planned after close liaison with orthodontists and oral surgeons, and orthognathic surgery may be required to improve the existing jaw relationship to create an optimal oral seal.
- Alternative surgery may involve excision or re-routing of the salivary gland ducts, but this may have a deleterious effect on the teeth, leading to gross decay and difficult restorative problems. If this is decided as the treatment of choice then preventative measures must be put into place as a high priority. This may involve the use of fluoride gels applied in trays to wear at night, fluoride varnishes and fissure sealants. Corsodyl gel may be recommended to be applied at the gum margins as chlorhexidine is bactericidal. Saliva replacing sprays may need to be instigated, as although excessive dribbling or drooling is not to be desired, saliva does play an important role in the mouth in that it is protective of the teeth and gums and is required to aid efficient mastication.
- Pharmacological intervention may be required via the use of hyoscine patches which are placed on the back of the neck. These are more generally used in acquired neurological diseases, for example, multiple sclerosis (MS). People with MS often experience side effects, for example, nausea, leading to poor compliance and rejection.

It can be seen that improvement in the prevention of dribbling or drooling is vitally important to many individuals. It is necessary, however, that radical treatments be avoided in order to balance the onset of other oral side effects and dental complications for the person in the long term. As with all treatment planning nothing should be done in isolation and the long-term benefit to the person should be the major concern. Minimal dental aids may include the use of a mouth prop during treatment, keeping the fingers buccally placed and offering early morning appointments before food is eaten. The effects of dribbling or drooling on the self-esteem of the person cannot be overemphasised as this affects what they eat, where they eat and with whom they will share meals without feeling embarrassment.

Tooth erosion

Erosion of teeth is frequently seen in people with intellectual disabilities. Dental erosion is defined as: *'the irreversible loss of dental hard tissues due to a chemical process of acid dissolution but not involving bacterial plaque acid and not directly associated with mechanical or traumatic factors or with dental caries'* (O'Sullivan & Milosevic, 2007, p. 1).

Many people with intellectual disabilities have a poor diet and consume soft drinks that are acidic in nature or are taking medication that is acidic, for example, vitamin C or iron-containing compounds. Some saliva-replacing substitutes are also acidic (O'Sullivan & Milosevic, 2007).

Intrinsic causes of dental erosion are due to acid reflux, vomiting, and rumination which are seen commonly in people with intellectual disabilities. Dental erosion is commonly seen on the palatal surfaces of central and lateral incisors. These surfaces appear translucent, and if left untreated, both enamel and dentine are eroded and the pulp of the teeth exposed, leading to severe pain.

Dental treatment of erosion can be difficult in people with intellectual disabilities as compliance with the regular restorative techniques needed can be difficult. The management of dental erosion in people with intellectual disabilities again is multidisciplinary and may involve the person's doctor, gastroenterologist, carers to advise them of dietary considerations and dentist to restore the lost enamel or even dentine. If the erosion can be stabilised then dental treatment can be instigated by placing palatal veneers over the lost tooth structure. However, these placements, either in cast metal, porcelain, or a composite filling material, are all technique sensitive and depend on a dry area which can only be achieved by use of a rubber dam to isolate the teeth involved. This may be difficult for individuals with intellectual disabilities to tolerate (Nohl et al., 1997). Again, as with all dental treatment for people with intellectual disabilities, prevention must be a high priority and involve all members of the caring team. Treatment can be provided under sedation and this will be addressed later in this chapter.

Tooth grinding (bruxism)

Tooth grinding is an exhibition of habitual or parafunctional oral behaviour resulting in clenching and grinding of the jaws. In the so-called 'normal' population, tooth grinding can be attributed to habitual or parafunctional behaviour, but is also related to stress. The person may be unaware of grinding their teeth but may experience pain in the temporomandibular joints or persistent headaches during waking. Clinically, there will be evidence of wear on canine teeth, evidenced by a diamond-shaped facet at the incisal edge. Treatment may involve the construction of a hard acrylic splint to be worn at night which protects the teeth and joints from further damage by opening up the vertical dimension of the jaw by 2 mm so that any grinding that occurs is against plastic and not tooth. In people with severe intellectual disabilities, firstly, compliance with construction of and then wearing the splint could be unpredictable. Secondly, daytime bruxing, which is seen mainly in people with very severe intellectual disabilities who have very poor means of communication, has been seen as stimulating neurological activities which may result in light and sound sensations which the person perceives as positive. The noise generated by bruxing is very loud and the damage to the teeth can be extensive.

An alternative form of treatment to the hard plastic splint would be provision of a thickened form of gumshield which is not so technique sensitive to construct and would be easier for carers to fit. There is a danger that the gumshield would not be regularly removed and cleaned and that food debris and plaque would collect under the shield leading to gross decay and pain for the person involved. Sometimes teeth have been extracted to reduce the habitual clenching position, but often the person repositions their jaw so that a new grinding position occurs. It becomes very difficult to successfully treat, as often the person will not open their mouth sufficiently for the carer to remove or insert the gumshield even if it were possible for the dentist to make impressions for the gumshield. This provision of treatment would therefore have to be made on case-selection basis.

Heightened gag reflex

Many people with cerebral palsy and with intellectual disabilities have a heightened gag reflex. This may be due to a tapered palate with labially inclined maxillary teeth due the pressure of the tongue because of abnormal swallowing patterns. Preventative care is very important as often the person has poor arm movement and needs help cleaning the teeth to prevent hyperplastic gum disease and halitosis. Individuals with heightened gag reflex are often mouth breathers so excessive plaque accumulates overnight. Electric toothbrushes may be useful or specially adapted normal brushes. Fluoride toothpaste is very important as fluoride rinses may prove difficult to use.

Aids to provide a successful diagnosis are needed, such as bite-wing radiographs to detect decay between teeth, or peri-apical radiographs when specific information is required about a particular tooth. These techniques may subsequently make the person very uncomfortable. Experience has shown that by placing topical local anaesthetic (e.g. topical lidocaine spray) in the region required for examination reduces the gag reflex so that the procedure is more comfortable for the person. Again, using a mouth prop and keeping the fingers buccally placed may help.

Self-injurious behaviour

Oral self-injury may be seen, especially in children with intellectual disabilities, and it may also be linked to cerebral palsy or other disorders, for example, Lesch-Nyhan syndrome (an inherited disorder seen in males causing delayed motor movement). The degree of damage caused may be severe and permanent (Fenton, 1982).

An obvious cause of pain of dental origin must be investigated and eliminated with treatment implemented within a multidisciplinary framework. Parents and carers must be reassured, symptomatic relief offered, and if there is a good level of compliance, oral aids such as suck-down mouth guards, bite planes and tongue stents constructed. Behavioural management techniques may be instigated and any dental treatment required may have to be done using sedation. In very severe cases of lip biting and associated tongue biting, the only treatment to eliminate pain may

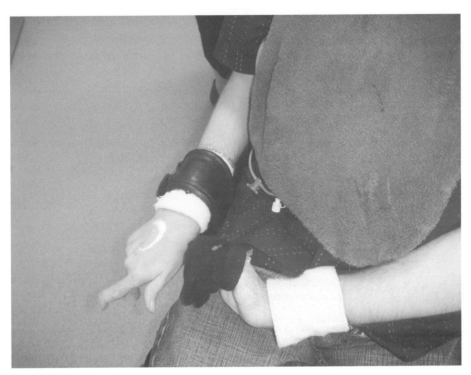

Figure 13.1 Photograph of a person with cerebral palsy showing scarring on hand a result of prolonged self-injury through 'hand biting'.

be to render the person edentulous, but this would have to be agreed within a multidisciplinary framework which would include the person (Figures 13.1–13.3).

There are several other health factors which are of particular concern in relation to achieving good dental health, these include:

Cardiovascular disease

A person with cardiovascular disease is generally on long-term medication. Appointments should be planned to be after the person has received their medication and should be of short duration and kept to time to avoid unnecessary stress. The person should not be treated in the supine position. People with angina may benefit from using their glyceryl trinitrate spray immediately before the dental appointment. Sedation using relative analgesia is acceptable but general anaesthesia is to be avoided in a person who has had a myocardial infarct within the last 3 months.

Hypertension can cause problems for the dentist and the person. Many people become hypertensive in the dental surgery, but severe levels of raised blood pressure, for example, 200/150 should contraindicate treatment that day. Many people with intellectual disabilities are treated under IV sedation, but they are required to attend an assessment appointment first where blood pressure and oxygen saturation

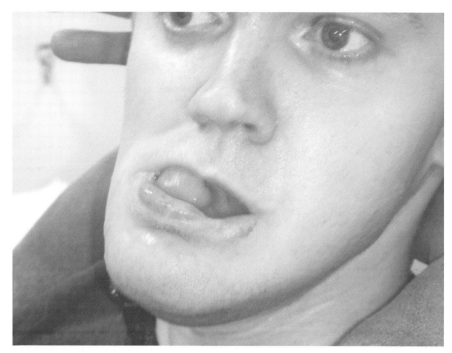

Figure 13.2 Ulceration of tongue and evidence of lip biting of a person with cerebral palsy.

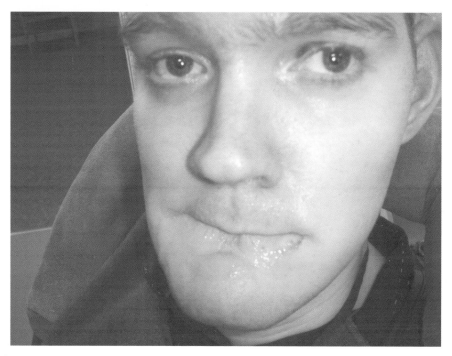

Figure 13.3 Photograph of a man with cerebral palsy following tooth extraction, at his request, eliminating the cause of his oral pain and discomfort.

CHECKLIST FOR DENTAL TREATMENT WITH IV SEDATION

Patient's Name		Date of Assesment	Date of Referral
Date of Birth:		Referred by:	
Telephone Numbers		PDS Access	
		PDS Cont Care	
Home		GDP	
Work		GMP	
Mobile		Other	
Medical History Form Completed		Relevant MH ASA 1 2 3 4	
Consent Form Completed		Urgent YES NO	
IV Information leaflet given		Cardiac problems ☐	
Pre-operative instructions given		COAD ☐	
Emla issued		Liver Problems ☐	
FP17 signed		Bleeding Problems ☐	
Estimate of treatment cost given		Pregnancy ☐	
		Allergies ☐	
Provisional Treatment Plan		Diabetes ☐	
Visit 1		Epilepsy ☐	
		Other ☐	
Visit 2		Medication	
Visit 3		**Blood Pressure Recorded** ☐	
Pre-operation Sedations Required ☐		Weight	
Pre-operative Antibiotic Prophylaxis ☐		**Follow-up Action Required**	
Details		1 ☐	
		2 ☐	
Suitable for single operator/ sedationist Y ☐ N ☐		3 ☐	

Will accept short-notice appointment
    YES   NO
		Lenght of Appointment
		        SHORT LONG	

Signed...   Date...

Figure 13.4 Checklist for dental treatment with IV sedation. (Reproduced with kind permission from Warwickshire PCT.)

levels are measured (see Figure 13.4). Local anaesthetic of lidocaine with 1:80 000 adrenaline is perfectly safe and up to 4 mL can safely be injected. The emergency drug box should always be within easy reach, replenished when necessary and up to date. Oxygen should also be at hand and the cylinders full and be checked on a daily basis.

Cerebrovascular accidents

Every year over 150,000 people in the UK have a stroke (cerebrovascular accident). UK statistics parallel those in the rest of the world (Geddes et al., 1996). Cerebrovascular accidents affect many people over middle age particularly if they have hypertension. Other causes can be thrombosis or as a result of intracerebral/subarachnoid haemorrhage. The result is a neurological defect caused by a sudden interruption of oxygenated blood to the brain. The aftermath can be devastating with hemi- or even quadriplegia and associated speech loss and difficulties in self-care and feeding; some patients require PEG (percutaneous endoscopic gastrostomy) feeding (see Chapter 15). This has an impact on oral health as plaque and calculus build up which requires careful cleaning using high-speed suction and the use of two toothbrushes in order not to bite the operator's fingers. Impaired mobility and diabetes mellitus may also be associated factors.

Multiple sclerosis

Multiple sclerosis (MS) mainly affects younger people with a range of symptoms that affect neurological symptoms in time and site. Approximately 0.15% of the population in the UK have MS. Of these an estimated 20% have benign MS, 20% have relapsing MS, 40% have secondary progressive MS and 15% have the primary progressive form. Symptoms can be of rapid onset or the patient may go into remission for several months. It is, however, particularly distressing leading to paralysis and, eventually, wheelchair necessity. Causes have been attributed to environmental, genetic, familial and geographic. MS is the most common neurological condition affecting about 1 in 1000 young adults (Multiple Sclerosis Society, 2007).

As the disease progresses, people often become disorientated and forgetful and their speech becomes slurred, being able to give a longer appointment without rushing is generally appreciated, providing written instructions, and a written treatment plan is also helpful.

Often there is an associated tremor and treatment may need to be provided under IV sedation. Oral hygiene aids need to be implicated early on with electric toothbrushes proving useful and Corsodyl (chlorhexidine gluconate gel 1%) a useful adjunct to be used at night. The use of custom-made gumshields which can be worn at night with the addition of fluoride gel is extremely helpful in preventing decay, particularly around the gum margins. Once again prevention is not a cure but it is very useful in delaying the onset of severe pain.

People with MS should not be treated fully supine in case of respiratory distress, and they should be given several shorter appointments particularly when they are feeling fatigued with as much treatment carried out as is comfortable for the person. Sometimes using a prop to keep the mouth open helps expedite treatment.

Due to poor swallowing reflex in the later stages of the disease, the patient should not be supine; high suction is required and rubber dam placed if necessary. They are often provided with hyoscine patches as their disease advances to dry excessive saliva, but these have side effects of nausea and are often not well tolerated. Baclofen is often prescribed for painful limb spasms, but this may cause xerostomia and a painful dry mouth. They appreciate being seen by the same dentist for each appointment, as familiarity is important particularly as the disease progresses. Depression is a feature of the disease and so a positive approach from the dental team often helps; exertion, heat, fever, anxiety and infection all exacerbate the disease.

Dementia

Dementia is a progressive, neurodegenerative disease affecting a person's ability to perform normal daily activities and has been described as a variety of syndromes (Ettinger, 2000). One particular dementia of concern is Alzheimer's disease.[6] Over 750 000 people in the general population in the UK have Alzheimer's and 18 000 of these are aged under 65 years (Fiske et al., 2006).

This form of dementia produces a severe reduction in the patient's intellectual capacity and is a progressive disease.

As the disease progresses, the person frequently becomes very frustrated and agitated in new surroundings, including the dental surgery.

They may exhibit complete personality changes making life very difficult for their carer. Drug therapy may include cholinesterase inhibitors and anti-inflammatories, but side effects of these drugs are xerostomia, causing increased plaque deposits and caries (Sreebny & Schwartz, 1997). In edentulous patients denture wearing may become very difficult and painful. As soon as the diagnosis is made, dental treatment plans should be designed to be easily maintainable both by the patient and the carer as the disease progress. Teeth of doubtful prognosis should be extracted early on in the treatment planning stage and the individuals and their carer involved at every stage of the dental treatment. As the disease progresses and the persons become less oriented to the world around them, a compassionate treatment approach is very much appreciated by the persons and their family and health supporter. Familiar routines and seeing the same dentist when possible, close supervision from the general practitioner and family/health supporter all help make the dental visit less stressful for all concerned. Extra time must be allowed for appointments, and in the final analysis, treatment may no longer be available in the surgery and will require to be treated under general anaesthesia after careful assessment.

Autism[7]

Autism is the most severe of the developmental disabilities. In the dental surgery it is very important to familiarise the persons with their new surroundings and this

---

[6] http://www.alzheimers.org.uk/

[7] http://www.nas.org.uk/ and http://www.autismconnect.org/

may take several visits before they will even sit in the dental chair. Again, having the same dental team on hand is very important and 'show, tell, do' is a helpful communication tool (Golding, undated). Children may wish to bring a special toy so that the proposed treatment may be shown on the toy first. A multidisciplinary approach is necessary, and speech and language experts are extremely helpful in preparing the child for their dental visit.

Treatment under local anaesthetic is preferable but alternative treatment protocols may be relevant if the child is completely unapproachable. Direct answers to the child's questions about treatment are important, and only the treatment agreed should be provided so that trust is not lost.

Domiciliary care

For some individuals attending the dental clinic either is not possible or is inadvisable, and it may be beneficial for a domiciliary visit to be made. People who may be eligible for domiciliary dental treatment include individuals who are severely medically compromised, those with Alzheimer's disease living at home, those who have agoraphobia, or are completely house bound; it is important not to presume that because the person has a profound intellectual and multiple disability, they need to be seen at home. However, if attending the dental clinic proves unsuccessful then domiciliary visits can be arranged either by members of the General Dental Service or the CDS.

When considering a domiciliary visit, it is imperative that the area of working is safe for the dentist and dental nurse. Where possible, zone the working area to keep a clean and dirty area. A domiciliary box should always be ready for use and packed with appropriate materials, gloves, local anaesthetic, disposable aprons, notes, forceps and swabs if necessary and also a prescription pad. The Dentalman™ apparatus takes setting up but does have portable suction and an air supply so that drills can be used and fillings done if necessary. Appropriate bags should also be taken to remove clinical waste and a sharps box for needle and anaesthetic disposal. Domiciliary visits take time but are an important part of the dentist's role in caring for special care patients.

From a dental perspective, whatever the cause of intellectual disability there are problems in providing satisfactory dental treatment. These may be summarised as follows:

- Fear
- Lack of time
- Lack of operator skill
- Poor surgery design/access
- Poor communication
- Inability to provide continuing care (both by dentist and carers)
- Devising unrealistic dental treatment plans

Fear

Fear is a large barrier to obtaining, and providing, satisfactory dental treatment for people with intellectual disabilities, and it may not purely relate to the patient. As discussed earlier, people with intellectual disabilities are often deprived of choice. This may relate to choosing which surgery to attend in the first place. Also to be considered is the carer's attitude to dentistry. If the carer has a fear of dentistry then this may be transferred to the patient, and can present problems before the first appointment. Most dentists are familiar with the phrase 'I hate dentists!', so a carer with that outlook will not reassure the person initially. Likewise, the dentist who is afraid of people with disabilities in any form may not want to provide treatment. As healthcare professionals we are committed to doing no harm, but there are many occasions when supervised neglect may occur often out of fear and lack of time to provide the necessary treatment.

To overcome all types of patient/carer fear, it may be necessary to attend the surgery purely to familiarise the person with the dental team and the facility so that they feel more relaxed. It is important for the dentist to be made aware of all aspects of the person's medical condition and if any further physical aids may be required in order to provide treatment safely, for example, hoists, banana boards and turntables. These will have an impact on manual handling requirements. As a result of the medical history, other factors may need to be considered. These may include the following:

- Timing of the appointment
- The need for antibiotic prophylaxis
- Alteration of medication

Timing of appointments

Many people with profound intellectual and multiple disabilities have associated physical disabilities, so preparing for early appointments may be problematic, time of attendance should be considered with each individual concerned.

Similarly, timing is important to consider for people with type 1 diabetes; appointments are best made shortly after mealtimes to reduce the risk of hypoglycaemia.

People may also have difficulty with the concept of time, and waiting patiently in an unfamiliar waiting room may also be problematic. Ideally, appointments should be kept short, effective and to time as much as possible in order to keep the person comfortable.

Need for antibiotic prophylaxis

If antibiotic prophylaxis is required and is the treatment of choice, it must be given at the surgery under the supervision of the dentist. A dental nurse must be available to sit with the person after administration of the antibiotic in case of any untoward reactions.

Alteration of medication

In general, there should be no alteration of a person's existing medication for dental procedures and certainly without consulting their GP or consultant. Occasionally, if someone is taking more than 10 mg prednisolone or another steroid on a daily basis, it may be necessary to double the daily dose if an extraction is planned. Also, if a patient is being administered warfarin then it is necessary to know the current International Normalisation Ratio (INR) before any extraction or deep scaling treatment planned. Generally, the INR is recorded in a book which the carer should have available. An INR of 2.5–3.5 is suitable for treatment in the dental surgery.

Extraction should be as atraumatic as possible and the socket packed with Surgicel™ (oxidised cellulose) and sutured to prevent post-operative bleeding. If the INR has not been registered recently then in many CDS surgeries the Coagulo check is available to give an instant reading, therefore reducing the delay for extraction and alleviating pain more quickly. A post-operative rinse of 1% tranexamic acid, 10 mL three times daily for 3 days, is a useful adjunct to reducing post-operative bleeding in patients on oral coagulants and antiplatelet drugs, for example, clopidogrel which will prolong bleeding so attention should be made to the medical drug history.

Lack of time

People with intellectual disabilities often require more time for their appointments than the general population. This may be due to any of the aforementioned reasons, and for those with physical disabilities they may require more time to transfer to the dental chair in order to be treated more comfortably both for themselves and the operator.

Delay in transport may also affect their treatment, particularly if ambulance transport is involved. In the NHS dental surgery time is money, and there is no remuneration for lengthy appointments for what is often a simple procedure as described by the current NHS dental remuneration scale. Consequently, many people with intellectual disabilities are referred to the CDS for treatment where such financial restraints are not the norm as their services will have been commissioned by the PCT (Primary Care Trust).

Lack of operator skill

Many general dental practitioners are reluctant to treat people with intellectual disabilities because they do not feel comfortable treating someone with whom they may have limited, if any, communication. They may not be familiar with people with intellectual disabilities and the sometime unpredictability of their behaviour and their noise; for example, daytime bruxing may not be easy to accept in an NHS dental surgery (Davies et al., 1988). The undergraduate dental curriculum is being adjusted to include special care dentistry as a specific entity, but many older graduates may have had no training in this area of dentistry and not developed skills to treat their respective group of special needs patients. In the current dental climate, many practitioners are more interested in developing skills in advanced restorative techniques and aesthetic dentistry (such as those seen on television make-over shows) and less in what is often very routine dentistry on difficult patients. This is not a poor reflection on general dental practitioners but is realistic. The General Dental Council in December (2005) approved the addition of Special Care dentistry to the dental specialist register. This will hopefully develop into a consultant-led service with recognised training pathways which will both improve quality of treatment for users and increase numbers of dentists providing special care dentistry within a recognised speciality.

Poor surgery design

Many high-street dental surgeries are located in the first floor premises without lifts making access difficult for people with profound intellectual and multiple disabilities where they use a wheelchair or have limited mobility. The Disability Discrimination Act (1995) made it compulsory to provide lifts and disabled facilities including a loop system for those with hearing impairments as many people with intellectual disabilities have a hearing impairment (see Chapter 11). This has improved facilities for people with intellectual disabilities, but the additional costs can still be an issue borne by the dental practices.

Poor communication

The dental/medical terminology used to explain treatment and procedures can often lead to problems in achieving effective communication between patient/carer and dentist. Where the person has an intellectual difficulty places an additional challenge to establishing effective communication. For successful treatment to be achieved, it is essential that the person or their carer has a full understanding of the treatment on offer, only then can an informed decision be made.

Communication Matters[8] is a resource website which contains resources which can support the communication of oral health instruction especially for those with complex communication needs.

In the past, people with intellectual disabilities were treated mainly by oral surgeons under general anaesthetic and as a result had many teeth extracted to avoid the need for multiple general anaesthetics. Times have changed for the better, and we can now offer our people with profound intellectual and multiple disabilities a whole realm of dental treatments either by local anaesthetic, regional analgesia, oral sedation or IV sedation. The person and their carers are given written information about the treatment that may be involved and a telephone number if queries need answering.

---

[8] http://www.communicationmatters.org.uk/

Information to provide continuing care by dentist and carer

It is generally accepted that carers in care homes and in domiciliary care services change jobs on a fairly regular basis. This makes it difficult to maintain a reasonable and consistent standard of oral health for people therein. Similarly, if there has been a recent change in carer, there may not be anyone familiar to the person, available to accompany them to their treatment. A final result may be an unnecessary extraction which may further reduce the person's self-esteem and increase their fear of dentists. One way that we can positively help is by going in to care homes and in domiciliary care service settings and teach carers how best to brush their charges' teeth and show them the range of different toothbrushing aids now available for use.

One of the important things that as dentists we can do to improve oral health in people with intellectual disabilities and their carers is to educate them on sensible diets. The importance of *five* pieces of fruit and vegetables a day is vitally important to good general health (see Chapter 15). The problem is that many people with profound intellectual disabilities are reliant on others to provide their food and drink; it is important that choices are made which do not compromise dental health. For those who take liquid medications, it is important to ask for sugar-free versions of the medication where these are available.

The introduction of fluoride into drinking water (1 ppm) has greatly reduced dental decay, and the associated use of fluoride toothpaste also has helped reduce decay. For those people who are PEG fed or have swallowing difficulties (see Chapter 14), non-foaming toothpastes are available which makes brushing their teeth easier.

Dental treatment for people with intellectual disabilities

As mentioned earlier, the first visit to the dental surgery for someone with intellectual disabilities may simply be to see the clinic and meet the dental team in order to familiarise themselves with the different surroundings.

Initially, an oral assessment is necessary, and where there are severe or profound intellectual disabilities, this will involve a multidisciplinary approach possibly involving psychiatrists, physicians, dietitians, speech and language therapists, physiotherapists, family and carers. This approach should result in a maintainable treatment plan which is acceptable to patient, family and carers and reduce the need for crisis management.

Ideally, treatment is best carried out under local anaesthetic in the dental chair. For those people who use a wheelchair and are able to transfer to the dental chair there are several aids which can be used including banana boards, turntables and hoists. When planning to transfer a person using a hoist, it is advisable to ask them to arrive with their sling already in place which reduces discomfort for them outside of their familiar surroundings and preserves their dignity. The use of a cushion to add extra neck support is also helpful (Figures 13.5–13.6).

Some people who use very large powered wheelchairs are too heavy to be transferred to the dental chair and this does make dentistry challenging for the operator.

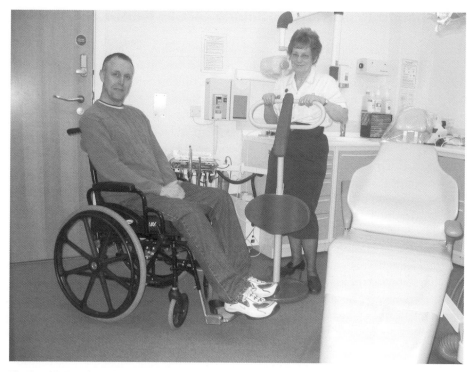

Figure 13.5 Photograph showing the rotating turntable ready for use by patient.

There are specially designed ramps which can be fitted in the surgery to allow the person to be treated in their wheelchair without causing the operator to work in a possibly contorted position in order to obtain access to the mouth; these are, however, very costly.

There are also headrest adaptations which can be attached to the handles of wheelchairs which allow the person to be treated in their chair if treatment is only going to be of short duration.

Some people with intellectual disabilities have a computer screen on the table of their wheelchair, and this can be used as a positive communication aid when ascertaining treatment needs.

If dental treatment is impossible under local anaesthetic then it is possible to provide treatment using either:

- relative analgesia;
- oral sedation;
- intravenous sedation (midazolam only in primary care);
- multiple route midazolam (DSTG, 2000);
- oral and IV sedation; and
- intranasal (Figure 13.5) and IV sedation.

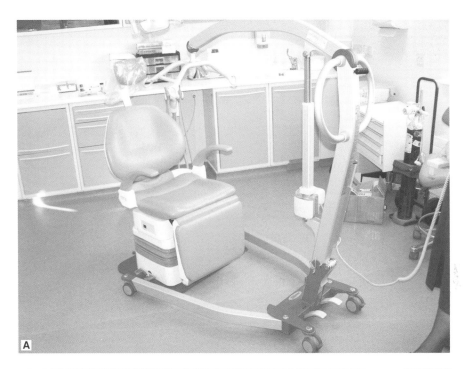

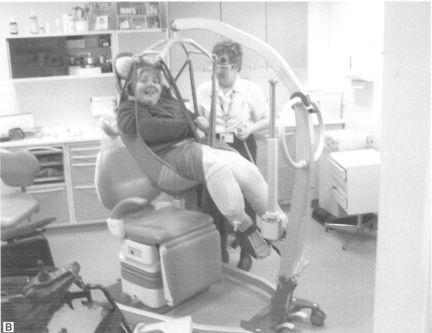

Figure 13.6 (a–c) Series of photographs showing the use of a hoist to transfer a person from their wheelchair safely to the dental chair for ease of treatment.

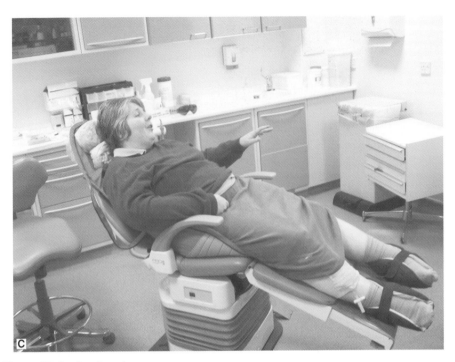

Figure 13.6 Continued

The person may also be premedicated using oral diazepam +/− IV midazolam.

The individuals undergoing treatment who require sedation particularly are classified for fitness and risk, as described by the American Society for Anaesthesiologists, and anyone whose sum of their medical condition adds up to ASA111 should not be sedated outside a specialist facility.

The American Society of Anaesthesiologists (ASA) physical status classification system (ASA, undated):

ASAI A patient without systemic disease, a normal healthy patient

ASAII A patient with mild systemic disease that does not affect their lifestyle

ASAIII A patient with moderate systemic disease that limits activity but is not incapacitating

ASAIV A patient with incapacitating systemic disease that is a constant threat to life

ASAV A moribund patient not expected to survive 24 hours, with or without medical intervention

ASAVI A clinically brain dead patient awaiting organ retrieval surgery

Any of these methods of sedation are acceptable for people in the dental surgery assessed at ASAI or ASAII as long as there are two nurses present, one to monitor the person and one to assist the operator. The nurse monitoring should have a certificate in conscious sedation for dental nursing. Sedation logbooks must be kept

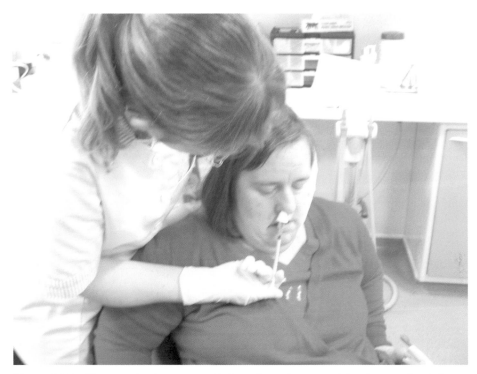

Figure 13.7 Photograph of a person with Down's syndrome receiving intranasal sedation.

up to date and all staff fully trained both in the procedure and in how to deal with emergencies. The emergency drug box should always be easily accessible and oxygen cylinders full.

A pre-operative assessment appointment is necessary before sedation appointments. The person must be accompanied to the appointment, full instructions of the procedure are given and written instructions are also provided (Figure 13.7).

As a final resort general anaesthesia may be the only means of providing dental treatment when the person is totally non-compliant but preservation of teeth is our main priority. A full range of routine dental treatments can be carried out in a theatre setting under the supervision of a consultant anaesthetist, and this may have to be provided annually or every other year for some patients (Figure 13.8).

Consent

Consent must be obtained before an investigation or treatment can be commenced. In the case of someone with severe or profound intellectual disabilities, who is deemed unable to give informed consent, then a decision needs to be reached in their 'best interest'. To support this decision-making process, the Department of Health developed *consent form 4* (Department of Health, 2004) which the family member or advocate will sign together with the health professional proposing the treatment. The dentist who signs this form will have to justify why they are planning

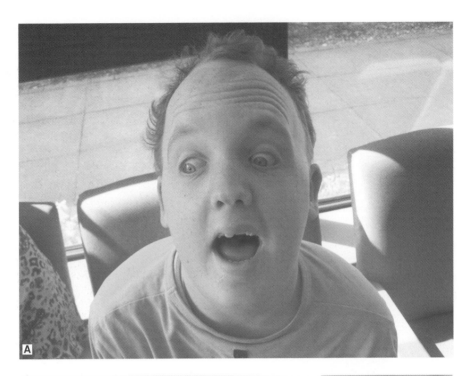

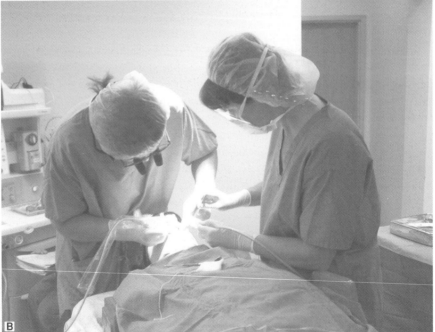

Figure 13.8 Series of photographs showing dental treatment under general anaesthetic for a patient with severe intellectual and multiple disabilities.

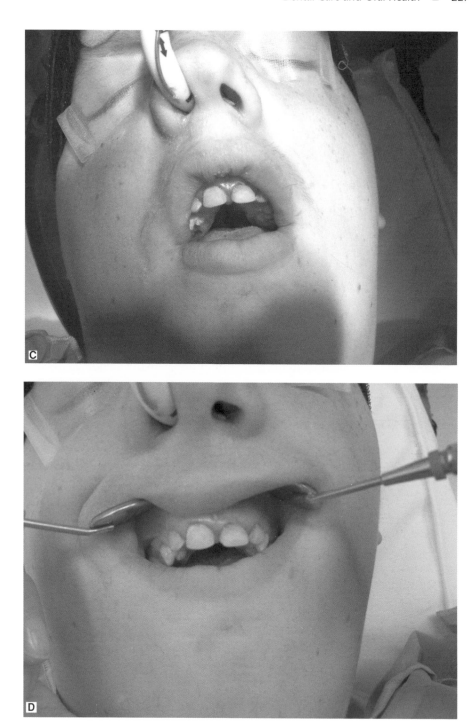

Figure 13.8 Continued

to provide the treatment suggested and this is generally to relieve the patient of pain (Shuman & Bebeau, 1994).

If treatment is unable to be carried out under sedation then general anaesthesia must be planned. All general anaesthetics carry a risk and patients are best assessed by the anaesthetist and consent obtained. An anaesthetist best assesses people with profound intellectual and multiple disabilities whose combined medical history classifies them as ASAIII, and their treatment is carried out in a district general hospital even if it is under sedation. It is advisable to provide written post-operative treatment instructions and hand these to a named carer and document all details of the procedures performed.

All dental treatment modalities that are available to able-bodied people are to be offered to those with intellectual disabilities. However, the result of dental treatment must always be 'to do no harm' and consequently treatment plans must be devised that are easily maintainable by the patient and or carer. If dentures are to be provided, it is easy to get the technician to insert the patient's name in the dentures, and this reduces the number of lost dentures particularly on hospital wards or in institutions. The materials that we have at our disposal now for restoring teeth have also improved in their ease of placement, and some contain fluoride which can leach out and remineralise the margins of the cavity.

Dentistry itself has changed radically over the last 30 years. The emphasis now is on prevention and minimal tooth preparation rather than extending cavities to prevent further decay.

Providing domiciliary dental care

To increase the success of a consultation with a person with profound intellectual and multiple disabilities, it may be valuable to carry out an initial oral hygiene assessment at their home. Carrying out the initial assessment in their own familiar surroundings gives the operator and the person time to become better acquainted before seeing them for the first visit in the unfamiliar dental surgery. An oral health assessment form is useful to record the outcome of the assessment (Figure 13.9).

Working with carers and building a good rapport with them aids treating the patient more successfully and improves the prognosis for oral health maintenance.

People with profound intellectual and multiple disabilities may have difficulty holding their mouth open voluntarily and as a result may clamp their mouths tightly, making access difficult. The use of a Bedi wedge™ (Figures 13.10 and 13.11) which can be worn on the dentists' finger as they examine and clean their patients' teeth is helpful and can be washed and given to the carer to help with oral hygiene for that particular person.

The use of two toothbrushes is another means of providing oral hygiene measures when the person is not able to hold their mouth open with routine toothbrushing (Figure 13.12).

The Collis Curve toothbrush™ is another useful aid to clean both sides of the teeth at once (Figure 13.13); this makes it much easier for carers, to help with maintaining better oral hygiene for their clients.

ORAL HEALTH ASSESSMENT

This brief dental examination has been carried out away from the dental surgery and without the benefit of radiography

NAME: D.O.B.

Consent given for assessment   yes ☐ no ☐ **best interest** ☐

Pain in mouth   yes ☐ no ☐
Teeth ☐   Gums ☐   Soft tissues ☐

Soft Tissue Problems/Pathology   yes ☐ no ☐

Missing Teeth   yes ☐ no ☐

Filled Teeth   yes ☐ no ☐

Untreated decay   yes ☐ no ☐

Fractured teeth/fillings   yes ☐ no ☐

Gingival Singd   yes ☐ no ☐

Edentureless   yes ☐ no ☐

Denture problems   yes ☐ no ☐

Treatment urgency

Maintenance ☐   Non-urgent appointment ☐   Urgent appointment ☐

Signed...   **Date**..................................

Checklist before appointment

Updated Medical History Form   ☐ **Current Drugs List** ☐ **Other**................ ☐

Appointment sent/received   ☐

Date of Appointment..

Figure 13.9 Example of the oral health assessment form that is used during patient's oral health screening in residential homes or hospitals. (Reproduced with kind permission from Warwickshire PCT.)

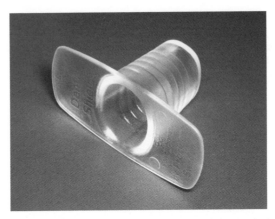

Figure 13.10 The Bedi wedge can be placed on the dentist's finger during examination and cleaning. (Reproduced with permission from Dr R. Bedi.)

When sedation is used then a McKesson mouth prop™ can be placed between the person's teeth and a full range of treatment can be carried out without fearing that the person will close their mouth and injure either themselves or the operator (Figure 13.14).

Dental materials have improved greatly in the recent years, and many small cavities can be treated using newer materials which do not even involve any drilling.

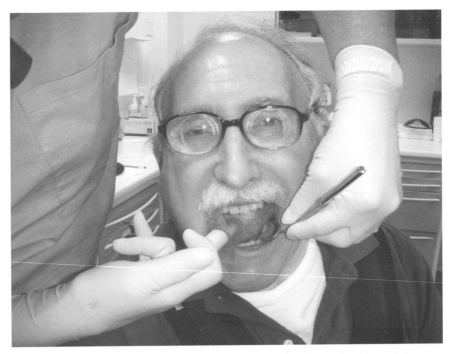

Figure 13.11 Photograph illustrating the use of Bedi wedge in a patient's mouth for examination and cleaning.

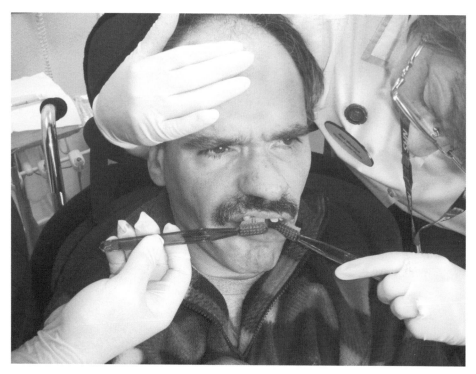

Figure 13.12 Photograph showing the use of two toothbrushes to provide oral hygiene measures in a patient with profound intellectual difficulties.

Even for large cavities, we now have materials that bond to tooth substance so that once the cavity is decay free, the tooth can be restored more easily. Some of the materials used leach out fluoride and help remineralise lost tooth substance.

Most specialist dentists can provide a range of leaflets containing information on products to use for dry mouths, denture care, and oral healthcare for patients.

The Collis Curve toothbrush

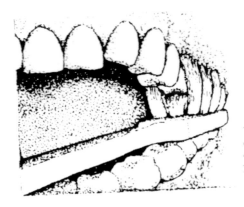

The curved design of the bristles allows you to clean all three sides of your teeth at the same while eliminating the danger of poking the bristles into your gums.

Figure 13.13 The Collis Curve toothbrush. (Reproduced with permission from Dr C. Collis.)

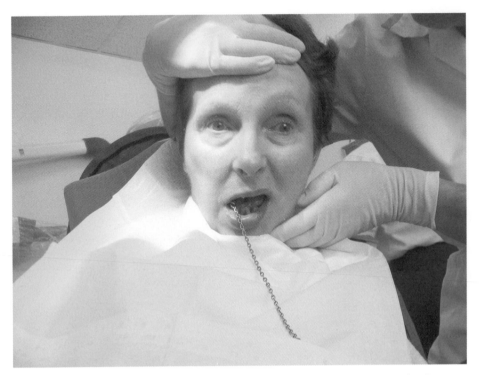

Figure 13.14 Photograph showing the use of the McKesson mouth prop to maintain constant opening of the patient's mouth for routine dental treatment.

Conclusions

The dental treatment needs of people with profound intellectual and multiple disabilities are no different from those of the rest of the population. Prevention and dietary education are always the best options, and this is where there are differences as people with severe or profound intellectual and multiple disabilities have to rely on others to provide their dental care. As caring healthcare professionals, it is our responsibility to provide as much information regarding oral care as possible and take the responsibility of offering regular recall appointments to monitor oral health. In an increasingly ageing population to retain natural teeth is much better and easier to manage than dentures, and this is particularly applicable to people with severe or profound intellectual and multiple disabilities.

Important points to remember:

- that all people have a right to good oral care;
- this care may need to be tailored to their specific needs but should not be inferior to that provided to the general public;
- that prevention is better than cure;
- that diet and smoking cessation are very important to good oral health; and

- that unrealistic dental treatment plans cannot be executed. Providing dental treatment that is simple and easily maintainable by person and their carer is in their best interests.

Further reading

British Dental Health Foundation (2005). *Dental Care for People with Special Needs*. Available at: http://www.dentalhealth.org.uk/faqs/leafletdetail.php?LeafletID=37 (accessed 7 November 2007).

Clifford, T.J., Warsi, M.J., Burnett, C.A., & Lamey, P.J. (1998). Burning mouth in Parkinson's disease sufferers. *Gerodontology*, 15(2), 73–78.

Department of Health (2005). *Choosing Better Oral Health: An Oral Health Plan for England*. Available at: http://www.dh.gov.uk/en/Publicationsandstatistics/Publications/PublicationsPolicyAndGuidance/DH_4123251 (accessed 7 August 2007).

Disability Discrimination Act (2005). Available at: http://www.opsi.gov.uk/acts/acts2005/20050013.htm (accessed 7 August 2007).

Disability Rights Commission (2005). *Disability Equality Duty*. Available at: http://www.drc.org.uk/employers_and_service_provider/disability_equality_duty.aspx (accessed 7 August 2007).

National Institute of Dental and Craniofacial Research (NIDCR) (2007). *Dental Care Every Day: A Caregiver's Guide*. Available at: http://www.nidcr.nih.gov/HealthInformation/DiseasesAndConditions/DevelopmentalDisabilitiesAndOralHealth/DentalCareEveryDay.htm (accessed 7 November 2007).

Useful websites

BDA Smile – the BDA patient information website, it provides independent dental advice for children, teenagers, adults and the over 50s – http://www.bdasmile.org/

British Dental Association (BDA) – the professional association for dentists in the UK – http://www.bda.org/

British Dental Health Foundation – a UK-based independent charity working to bring about improved standards of oral health care – http://www.dentalhealth.org.uk/

British Society of Dental Hygiene and Therapy (BSDHT) – the professional association to represent the dental hygienists and therapists (formerly the British Dental Hygienists' Association, BDHA) – http://www.bdha.org.uk/

British Society of Disability in Oral Health (BSDH) – A UK based society which works with other organisations to raise awareness of the barriers to oral health of people with disabilities http://www.bsdh.org.uk/

Human Rights Act (1998). Available at: http://www.opsi.gov.uk/ACTS/acts1998/19980042.htm.

National Institute of Dental and Craniofacial Research (NIDCR) (2006). *Oral Conditions in Children with Special Needs: A Guide for Health Care Providers*. Available at: http://www.nidcr.nih.gov/HealthInformation/DiseasesAndConditions/ChildrensOralHealth/SpecialNeeds.htm. This page presents a series of images depicting stages of oral development, oral trauma, oral infections and gingival overgrowth.

National Institute of Dental and Craniofacial Research (NIDCR) (2007). *Special Care Resources*. The page provides links to a series of excellent resources. http://www.nidcr.nih.gov/HealthInformation/SpecialCareResources/

References

American Society of Anesthesiologists (ASA) (undated). *ASA Physical Status Classification System*. Available at: http://www.asahq.org/clinical/physicalstatus.htm (accessed 31 October 2007).

British Society for Disability and Oral Health and the Faculty of Dental Surgery (2001). *Clinical Guidelines and Integrated Care Pathways for the Oral Health Care of People with Learning Disabilities*. Available at: http://www.rcseng.ac.uk/fds/clinical_guidelines/documents/icppld.pdf (accessed 1 July 2008).

Clark, C.A., & Vanek, E.P. (1984). Meeting the health care needs of people with limited access to care. *Journal of Dental Education*, 48(4), 213–216.

Davies, K.W., Holloway, P.J., & Worthington, H.V. (1988). Dental treatment for mentally handicapped adults in general practice: parents and dentists' views. *Community Dental Health*, 5, 381–387.

Davis, R., Bedi, R., & Scully, C. (2000). ABC Oral Health Care for patients with special needs. *BMJ*, 321(7259), 19–26.

Dental Sedation Teachers Group (DSTG) (2000). *Standards in Conscious Sedation for Dentistry*. Available at: http://www.dstg.co.uk/teaching/standards-oct-02/ (accessed 31 October 2007).

Department of Health (1994). *An Oral Health Strategy for England*. London: Department of Health.

Department of Health (2004). *Consent Form 4 – form For Adults Who Are Unable to Consent to Investigation or Treatment*. Available at: http://www.dh.gov.uk/dr_consum_dh/idcplg?IdcService=GET_FILE&dID=25735&Rendition=Web (accessed 7 August 2007).

Disability Discrimination Act (1995). Available at: http://www.opsi.gov.uk/acts/acts1995/1995050.htm (accessed 7 August 2007).

Elliott, T.S, Foweraker, J., Fulford, M., Gould, F.K., Perry, J.D., Roberts, G.J., Sandoe, J.A.T., & Watkin, R.W. (2005). *Guidelines for the Prevention of Endocarditis: Draft for Consultation*. Birmingham: British Society for Antimicrobial Chemotherapy (BSAC).

Ettinger, R.L. (2000). Dental management of patients with Alzheimer's disease and other dementias. *Gerodontology*, 17(1), 8–16.

Fenton, S.J. (1982). Management of oral self mutilation in neurologically impaired children. *Special Care in Dentistry*, 2(2), 70–73.

Finkelstein, D.M., & Crysdale, W.S. (1992). Evaluating and management of the drooling patient. *Journal of Otolaryngology*, 21(6), 414–417.

Fiske, J., Frenkel, H., Griffiths, J., & Jones, V. (2006). Guidelines for the development of local standards of oral health care for people with dementia. *Gerodontology*, 23(Suppl 1), 5–32.

Geddes, J.M., Fear, J., Tennant, A., Pickering, A., Hillman, M., & Chamberlain, M.A. (1996). Prevalence of self reported stroke in a population in northern England. *Journal of Epidemiology Community Health*, 50(2), 140–143.

General Dental Council (2005). *Standards for Dental Professionals*. Available at: http://www.gdc-uk.org/NR/rdonlyres/6F3D848E-F31A-4A8C-AEFA-C4D78D06B618/20453/Standardsfordentalprofessionals.pdf (accessed 7 August 2007).

Golding, M. (undated). *Dental Care and Autism*. Available at: http://www.nas.org.uk/content/1/c4/86/15/dentalcareandautismfinal2.pdf (accessed 31 October 2007).

Multiple Sclerosis Society (2007). *About MS*. Available at: http://www.mssociety.org.uk/about_ms/index.html (accessed 7 August 2007).

NHS SSI Executive (1999). *Epidemiologically Based Needs Assessment*. London: Department of Health.

Nohl, F.S., King, P.A., Harley, K.A., & Ibbetson, R.J. (1997). Retrospective survey of resin-retained cast metal Palatal Veneers for the treatment of Anterior tooth wear. *Quintessence International*, 28(1), 7–14.

O'Sullivan, E. & Milosevic, A. (2007). *Clinical Guideline on Dental Erosion: Diagnosis, Prevention and Management of Dental Erosion*. Available at: http://www.rcseng.ac.uk/fds/clinical_guidelines/documents/erosion_guideline.pdf (accessed 1 July 2008).

Shapira, J., Efrat Berkley, D., & Mann, J. (1998). Dental health profile of a population with mental retardation in Israel. *Special Care Dentistry*, 16(4), 149–155.

Shuman, S.K., & Bebeau, M.J. (1994). Ethical and legal issues in special patient care. *Dental Clinics of North America*, 38(3), 553–575.

Sreebny, L.M., & Schwartz, S.S. (1997). A reference guide to drugs and dry mouth 2nd edition. *Gerodontology*, 14(1), 33–47.

Chapter 14

DYSPHAGIA AND PEOPLE WITH PROFOUND INTELLECTUAL AND MULTIPLE DISABILITIES

Hannah Crawford

Introduction

When working with people with profound intellectual and multiple disabilities (PIMD), nurses need to be aware of the signs and symptoms of many health conditions, in order support these individuals appropriately, and to request intervention from other agencies. In February 2004, the NHS National Patient Safety Agency (NPSA) published a report describing patient safety issues for people with intellectual disabilities (National Patient Safety Agency, 2004). The report detailed five priority risk areas, one of which was swallowing difficulties or 'dysphagia'. Dysphagia can be defined as:

> ...eating and drinking disorders which may occur in the oral, pharyngeal and oesophageal stages of deglutition. Subsumed in this definition are problems positioning food in the mouth and in oral movements, including sucking, mastication and the process of swallowing. Eating and drinking is a highly complex, multi-system skill involving anatomic stability, neuromuscular control and co-ordination, sensory perception, gastrointestinal function, cardio-respiratory support and integration from the autonomic nervous system (RSCLT, 2006, p. 320).

Research has highlighted health risks associated with dysphagia (Cook & Kahrilas, 1999). For people with PIMD, health risks associated with dysphagia include chest infections, chronic lung disease, asphyxia, obstructive sleep apnoea and hypoxemia in oral feeding (Eyman et al., 1990; Rogers et al., 1994; Beange et al., 1995; Hollins et al., 1998; Aziz & Cambell-Taylor, 1999). More recent documents (Department of Health, 1998; Department of Health, 2001b) emphasise that illnesses in adults with intellectual disabilities are often underreported or misdiagnosed. The NPSA report raised the profile of dysphagia within the PIMD population and highlighted the need to think about solutions to improve safety and service provision for this population.

For people with PIMD dysphagia is often an associated difficulty. Speech and language therapists, when surveyed, report that people who have cerebral palsy and/or PIMD make up the highest proportion of their dysphagia caseloads (Watson, 2004; Crawford, 2006).

Learning objectives

At the end of the chapter the reader should:

- understand what is meant by 'normal' eating and drinking;
- recognise the signs and symptoms of dysphagia;
- develop their knowledge of associated conditions;
- develop their knowledge in relation to assessment and management of dysphagia within a multidisciplinary framework; and
- develop an appreciation of the implications for nursing practice.

The normal swallow

To understand the normal swallow it is important to consider the anatomy and physiology of the pharynx. The image overleaf presents a Saggital section of the pharynx, depicting the location of the key physiological components that facilitate normal swallowing (Figure 14.1). The normal swallow tends to be categorised into stages. However these stages are interrelated, they can overlap, and one can be happening alongside another. They are generally classified as the oral preparatory stage, the oral stage, the pharyngeal stage and the oesophageal stage.

The oral preparatory stage is when food and drink is being prepared in the mouth before transfer backwards to swallow. This stage includes chewing, tasting, mixing food and/or drinks with saliva, and is a voluntary stage. This stage is variable in length depending on factors such as hunger or thirst, texture and consistency of the food or drink, the amount of teeth someone has and their oral hygiene, the strength and range of movement of the structures in the mouth, the amount of saliva produced and how long the person wants to keep the food or drink in their mouth.

The oral stage describes the stage where the food or drink is gathered into a 'ball' or bolus and transferred to the back of the mouth ready to be swallowed. At this stage it is important to achieve oral closure in order to create pressure in the mouth, to enable to bolus to be squeezed backwards. This closure is usually created by closing the lips, but in some cases may be created by pressing the tip of the tongue against the back of the top teeth. Alongside oral closure, there will be closure of the jaw and there will muscular tension in the cheeks. The tongue then forms into a shape that creates a central groove in which the bolus is squeezed along. This is done by gradually squeezing the tongue along the palate in what is often described as a 'stripping' motion. As the bolus is moving along the palate, the soft palate will make contact with the pharyngeal wall, in order to close the entrance into the nasal passage, therefore preventing the bolus passing this way.

This is where the pharyngeal stage begins, at which stage the swallow 'proper' is triggered. As the bolus moves over the back of the tongue, it moves into a pocket formed by the base of the tongue and the epiglottis, called the valleculae. In addition

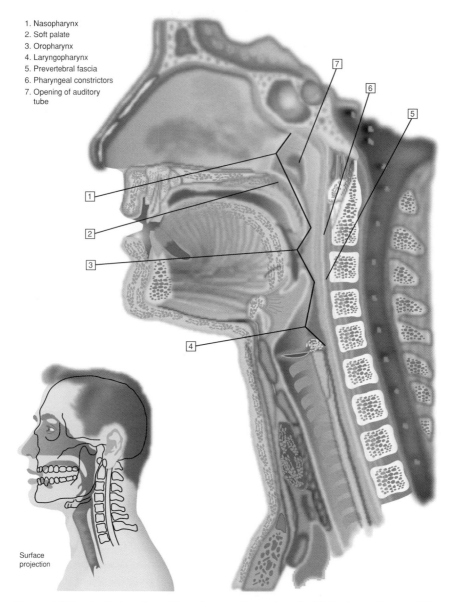

1. Nasopharynx
2. Soft palate
3. Oropharynx
4. Laryngopharynx
5. Prevertebral fascia
6. Pharyngeal constrictors
7. Opening of auditory tube

Surface projection

Figure 14.1 Sagittal section of the pharynx. (Reproduced with kind permission of Elsevier Inc.)

the pharyngeal constrictor muscles help to squeeze the bolus through along with gravity, alongside the action of the tongue base squeezing against the pharyngeal walls.

There are differences between individuals as to where exactly the swallow is triggered. The trigger of the swallow reflex or the efficiency of the swallow is not related to the gag reflex (Bleach, 1993), as has previously been suggested. Although some people can delay the trigger of their swallow reflex, once the bolus moves into the pharynx it becomes an involuntarily controlled mechanism. At this stage the larynx is very important in the swallow movement. As the bolus moves into the valleculae, the epiglottis drops down and covers the airway, or trachea. The larynx is pulled upwards and forwards by the movement of the hyoid bone. This movement can be felt, and often observed, as the 'Adam's apple' or larynx rising up and down at the point of swallow. At this point, the vocal cords within the larynx are also closed. This ensures that within an efficient swallow there are two stages of closure and therefore protection of the airway – the closure by the epiglottis and the closure of the vocal cords. This upward and forward movement of the larynx and the force of the bolus opens the upper oesophageal sphincter, the muscle ring at the top of the oesophagus, allowing the bolus to pass through the pharynx into the oesophagus, and consequently the oesophageal stage of the swallow begins (Figure 14.1).

When eating large mouthfuls, the bolus may be transferred in a 'piecemeal' fashion. The individual will prepare a small part of the mouthful into a bolus, while storing the remainder in the cheeks. Once this piece has been transferred backwards and swallowed, the process will start again until the whole mouthful has been cleared.

The oesophageal stage is described as beginning at the upper oesophageal sphincter and ends when the bolus passes through the lower oesophageal sphincter as into the stomach. The duration of this stage varies between 8 and 20 seconds (Logemann, 1998). The bolus is transferred down the oesophagus by the peristaltic action of the oesophageal muscles and is assisted by gravity. This stage is under involuntary control.

Dysphagia

In the general population, dysphagia can be caused by many conditions (Cook & Kahrilas, 1999). These include stroke, Parkinson's disease, amyotrophic lateral sclerosis, dementia, encephalitis, trauma, the side effects of medication, radiation, myasthenia gravis and tumours (Marks & Rainbow, 2001).

There are variations in estimates as to the proportion of people with intellectual disabilities who have dysphagia, from 36% (Hickman, 1997) to 73% (Rogers et al., 1994). Studies have indicated that dysphagia is particularly prevalent in people with profound and multiple intellectual disabilities. Chadwick et al. found that 62.5% of their study cohort had severe to profound disabilities, with 92.5% of their cohort having limited mobility (Chadwick et al., 2002). For people with profound and multiple intellectual disability, some of the main causes of dysphagia, in addition to those listed earlier, include cerebral palsy, Rett syndrome and the effects of medication (Sokoloff & Pavlakovic, 1997; Schechter, 1998).

Dysphagia can occur in the mouth, in the laryngeal/pharyngeal area, or in the oesophagus, or in some or all of these stages (RSCLT, 2006). The signs, symptoms and results of dysphagia can include coughing on food or drink, choking, difficulty triggering a swallow to complete absence of a swallow, chest infections, weight loss, dehydration, malnutrition, aversion to food, difficulties chewing, rushing food or long mealtimes, difficulty taking medication and changes in behaviour at mealtimes. A checklist of signs and symptoms of concern is included (Appendix 14.1). Logemann

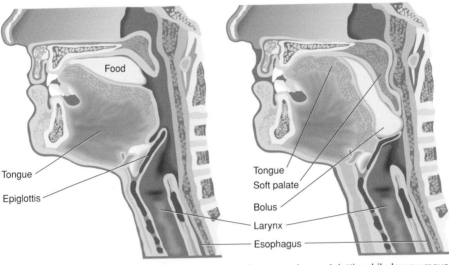

Bolus (food) pushed backward towards palate by tongue

Bolus reaches epiglottis while larynx moves upward and forward. Soft palate closes off nasopharynx.

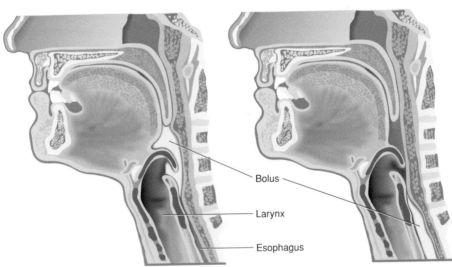

Pharyngeal constrictors contract and knead bolus into the esophagus. Epiglottis prevents bolus from entering the larynx. Trickle of food shown here entering esophagus, but is prevented from going farther by closure of ventricular folds.

Peristaltic contraction of esophagus moves bolus towards stomach and epiglottis begins to return to resting position.

Figure 14.2   Stages of swallowing. (Reproduced with kind permission of Elsevier Inc.)

Table 14.1 Oral stage of swallowing.

Observed problem	Possible causes
Food loss from the mouth	Tongue thrust reflex Weak lip closure Reduced tongue control
Food pocketing in the cheeks	Reduced tone in cheeks Reduced tongue control Weak tongue movements
Difficulty forming food into a bolus	Reduced tongue control Weak and/or reduced tongue movements
Difficulty chewing	Reduced side-to-side tongue movement Reduced jaw movements
Difficulty moving food backwards in mouth	Reduced tongue control
Food sitting in the mouth	Weak and/or reduced tongue movements
Food sticking in roof of mouth	High-arched palate Reduced strength and range of movement of tongue resulting in inability to squeeze tongue to the roof of the mouth
Food coming down the nose	Reduced movement of the soft palate

Adapted from Logemann (1998).

(1998) identified the common presentations of dysphagia, and their anatomical causes, some of these are listed in the Tables 14.1–14.3.

In people with cerebral palsy, and particularly those who have profound and multiple intellectual disabilities, dysphagia is highly prevalent. Figures vary, but suggest approximately 60% of people with cerebral palsy have dysphagia (Rogers et al., 1994; Hickman, 1997). In a study of speech and language therapists' dysphagia caseload, 75% reported this client group to be represented on their caseload (Crawford, 2006). The presentation of dysphagia may be at the oral, pharyngeal or oesophageal stages, or may involve all of these stages.

In people with Rett syndrome, dysphagia was found to be a significant difficulty (Morton et al., 1997; Sugerman Issacs et al., 2003). The difficulties observed include significant oral stage problems, swallowing air which leads to a bloated stomach, discomfort and the bringing up of wind and some pharyngeal stage problems.

Assessment of dysphagia

Assessment of dysphagia is usually undertaken by a speech and language therapist, although many other professionals assess elements of the mealtime, as is demonstrated later. Assessment techniques include taking a detailed case history from the people who know the individual well. This will take into account the description of the presenting difficulties, a summary of the current meals and drinks taken and how this happens, any recent changes that have affected eating and drinking, and any reports of respiratory difficulties. It will take into account oral status and hygiene,

Table 14.2 Pharyngeal stage of swallowing.

Observed problem	Possible causes
Struggling to swallow	Weak and/or reduced movement of the base of the tongue
Coughing/choking before the swallow	Weak, reduced or uncoordinated movements of the base of the tongue, larynx and pharynx leading to difficulties controlling food/drink. This leads to airway penetration and/or aspiration before the swallow In its most extreme form, this may result in a completely absent swallow
Coughing/choking during the swallow	Difficulty achieving airway closure either due to reduced elevation of the larynx, or difficulties with the movement of the valleculae. This leads to airway penetration and/or aspiration during the swallow
Coughing/choking after the swallow	Reduced, weak and/or uncoordinated movements of the tongue base, larynx and pharynx leading to residue building up in the 'pockets' in the pharynx. This then enters the airway and can be either coughed out or aspirated Poor opening of upper oesophageal sphincter resulting in food/drink not passing into oesophagus and leading to airway penetration or aspiration of the residue

It is essential to note that food and/or drink can be silently aspirated. This means that before, during or after the swallow, material can enter the lungs. Silent aspiration takes place when the individual does not cough or choke or show any other outward signs that this is happening. Aspiration would be defined as material entering the lungs with some outward sign, such as coughing, choking, respiratory disturbance or an increase in secretions. Aspiration and silent aspiration over time may result in chest infections or aspiration pneumonia

Adapted from Logemann (1998).

Table 14.3 Oesophageal stage of swallowing.

Observed problem	Possible causes
Undigested or partly digested food coming back up. May appear like vomiting, retching or regurgitating	Oesophageal stricture
	Achalasia Reduced peristalsis
Discomfort after meals	Reflux
Poor appetite	Hiatus hernia *Helicobacter pylori* Upper or lower oesophageal sphincter dysfunction

Adapted from Logemann (1998).

medication, hearing and visual status and cognitive skills. The SLT will investigate any associated difficulties that could impact on eating and drinking. Direct assessment will normally be undertaken within the individual's familiar environments. Assessment aims to gather information about the individual's physiological and neurological functioning with respect to eating and drinking. It will include a detailed examination of the oral and facial structures and observe the effect of position at mealtimes. Following this the individual will usually be observed at several mealtimes in order to determine how he or she usually eats and drinks and what the presenting difficulties are. Assessment also aims to determine whether factors such as the environment, feeding methods, particular support staff, methods of communication at mealtimes, types of food/drink and fatigue effect the individual's skills and abilities. Management strategies are often trialled at the end of the assessment period.

In some cases it may be necessary to recommend instrumental assessment in order to provide further information about skills and difficulties. In regular use by speech and language therapists and radiology departments is the videofluoroscopy swallow study X-ray, sometimes referred to as the modified barium swallow. It is good at identifying aspiration (Mathers-Schmidt & Kurlinski, 2003) and normal swallows, but is not as good at identifying how functionally useful the swallow is. Studies conclude that videofluoroscopy remains the gold standard. There are other methods that can be used as an adjunct to the clinical assessment, but there is still debate in the literature as to their reliability (Langmore et al., 1991; Mathers-Schmidt & Kurlinski, 2003; Tohara et al., 2003).

These methods include the following:

- *Fibre endoscopic evaluation of swallowing*: This is where an endoscope is passed through the nasal passage and the swallowing process is observed via a camera on the end of the scope. This is a sensitive tool for some areas of assessment (Mathers-Schmidt & Kurlinski, 2003), but it is more physically invasive than videofluoroscopy swallow study and therefore may not be available as an assessment technique for use with many individuals with PIMD.
- *Pulse oximetry*: This is where a small oxygen saturation reader is placed on an extremity, for example, the client's finger. Oxygen saturation levels are observed during the meal, and conclusions drawn regarding respiratory compromise, if the saturation levels drop. Findings for the reliability for this method of assessment are inconclusive as yet (Sherman et al., 1999; Smith, 2002; Tohara et al., 2003).
- *Cervical auscultation*: This is where a stethoscope is placed on the neck so as to be able to listen to the client's breathing and events during the swallow. Conclusions are drawn from the sounds that are heard. Many speech and language therapists use this tool as an adjunct to their clinical assessment, but findings are not yet consistent as to its reliability (Tohara et al., 2003).

Management of dysphagia

In general, people with dysphagia are managed by providing direct advice to improve their skills, and advice about techniques to carry out when swallowing. For

people with profound and multiple intellectual disabilities, difficulties with comprehension and/or retention of information may mean that it is more appropriate to
use what are called 'compensatory techniques' (Logemann, 1998). Compensatory
techniques are techniques that families/carers can employ to support people with
dysphagia. These can include the following:

- Changes in postures to facilitate a safe swallow
- Physical support methods at mealtimes
- Changes in food textures
- Thickening fluids
- Changes in feeding regime, for example, small meals at regular intervals
- Adapting the environment
- Adapting utensils

In very severe cases of dysphagia, the provision of non-oral nutrition and/or hydration can be considered.

When managing people with dysphagia, and profound and multiple intellectual
disabilities, management decisions should always be made with reference to what
the client would want for themselves. Decisions should be made in order to maximise
safety, facilitate best possible functioning and maintain and develop skills. Management should always be directed by quality-of-life considerations (Schechter, 1998;
RSCLT, 2006). In some cases, it may not be possible to ensure all these criteria are
met. For example, a management route that includes thickening normal liquids to
attempt to reduce aspiration may be considered the safest route for an individual.
However, it may be felt by all involved that this route is not the most appropriate option for an individual, given what he would want for himself and what is
perceived to be his best quality of life. As a multidisciplinary team working with a
client, it is necessary to discuss this issue and arrive at an acceptable management
option that balances risks and benefits of the chosen route.

Ethics and best interests

In cases where it is not possible to determine what an individual would want and
they are not able to consent to assessment and treatment themselves, agreement
must be reached on a course of action that is felt to be in the best interests of
the individual. No one else can consent on behalf of another person, regardless
of whether the individual lacks capacity to make a decision for themselves, and
regardless of any relationship with the individual, for example, partner, parent and
child (Department of Health, 2001a). There may be disagreement among the people
involved as to the best intervention route. In these cases it is essential to attempt to
overcome differences through discussion. Any agreed route of intervention should
be made bearing in the mind the client's best interests (Brown, 2002), and should be
an ethical route of intervention. The intervention should aim to consider the four
principles of medical ethics (Beauchamp & Childress, 2004):

Autonomy: Where possible, the individual should be encouraged to make their own informed choices, acting as an individual.

Beneficence: The benefits and risks of the intervention should be considered, and intervention should be decided on with reference to the benefits for the patient.

Non-maleficence: The intervention should avoid harm, or the harm should be minimal, and the benefit should far outweigh the harm.

Justice: The intervention should be balanced in terms of risks, benefits and cost, and all individual clients should be treated in a similar and fair fashion.

It may be necessary, where an intervention is agreed that involves a significant level of risk for an individual, to complete a risk assessment and management plan. This should always be a multidisciplinary process. The assessment should document all the benefits and risks of the intervention, and should clearly detail the review schedule, what constitutes an increase in risk, and the recommended action should risk increase. An example of a risk assessment and monitoring form is included (Appendix 14.2), with a completed form as an example. Other similar resources are available on the NPSA website.[1]

Multidisciplinary intervention

Assessment and management of dysphagia should always be multidisciplinary. Many professionals have key roles within dysphagia intervention. In order to make sound and ethical risk management decisions that are person centred, there needs to be a multidisciplinary discussion. Discussion should be between the person, if possible, the family, the carers, the support staff and the multidisciplinary team.

Roles within assessment and management of dysphagia tend to be as shown in Table 14.4.

Working in partnership with carers

When working with people with profound and multiple intellectual disabilities, their difficulties with comprehension often result in a need for everyone involved with them to work together to ensure a mutual understanding of their eating and drinking recommendations. The responsibility for day-to-day care falls on their family and/or direct care staff. The literature has indicated that while aspiration pneumonia is associated with dysphagia (Langmore et al., 1998; Marik, 2001), its impact and severity is often influenced by a number of factors, including the reliance on other people for feeding. For people with profound and multiple intellectual disabilities, it is likely that they will be reliant on others for mealtime support (Hickman, 1997). Aziz & Campbell-Taylor (Aziz & Cambell-Taylor, 1999) suggest that the

---

[1] http://www.npsa.nhs.uk/

Table 14.4 Roles of multidisciplinary team members within assessment and management of dysphagia.

Person	Role
Client	Must remain central in assessment and all management decisions
Family	Their knowledge of their relative must inform all assessment and management. Family may refer their relative for assessment, and are important in the implementation and monitoring of recommendations and their relative's health and well-being
Support staff, e.g. befrienders and home helps	Their knowledge of the client may help inform assessment and management decisions. They also may be important in implementing recommendations and may have useful information that may help when monitoring the client's condition and response to recommendations
Speech and language therapist	They are the lead professional in the assessment and management of dysphagia. They will take information from all involved to build a case history, will carry out assessment and give advice on appropriate management of dysphagia. They will monitor and review clients. In many cases they coordinate multidisciplinary dysphagia intervention, and will often liaise with professionals in primary care, e.g. medics. They will direct the GP in the prescription of thickening agents, if required
Physiotherapist	They will assess and offer recommendations for the best positioning for individuals at mealtimes. As part of this role they may liaise with wheelchair/seating services or providers. They are also responsible for the assessment and monitoring of chest status and the provision of chest care guidelines
Occupational therapist	They will assess an individual and give advice or recommendations for appropriate utensils at mealtimes. This is often done in liaison with the speech and language therapist if the utensil is to ameliorate dysphagic conditions, e.g. the use of the spout of a cup to control liquid flow. They may also assess the individual's ability to take part in the task of eating or drinking, and give advice as to skill development and any appropriate support that is required. They may liaise with wheelchair/seating services
Dietitian	They will assess nutritional and hydrational status and advise accordingly. They will direct the GP in the prescription of supplements if required. They will give advice as to balanced menus, in particular when individuals are on modified diets. In individuals who are non-orally fed, or have a combination of oral and non-oral intake, they will work to ensure an appropriate intake, appropriate feeds and how these should be paced throughout the day
Nurse	They can be responsible for identifying individuals who are displaying dysphagic symptoms and referring to the appropriate professional. They will be responsible for monitoring an individual's health status, and are regularly in contact with service providers. Community nurses can work alongside the rest of the multidisciplinary team to monitor the implementation of recommendations. As care coordinators they will lead regular reviews and will facilitate risk assessment and management

(continued)

Table 14.4 (Continued) Roles of multidisciplinary team members within assessment and management of dysphagia.

Person	Role
Social worker	They may be responsible for identifying individuals who are displaying dysphagic symptoms and referring to the appropriate professional. They may be responsible for identifying appropriate service providers and are regularly in contact with them. Social workers can work alongside the rest of the multidisciplinary team to monitor the implementation of recommendations. As care coordinators they will lead regular reviews and will facilitate risk assessment and management
Psychologist	They will assess and provide intervention for people who have eating and drinking difficulties that are associated with emotional or psychological difficulties. They may also provide support for families for whom the assessment process, its findings, recommendations and implications may be difficult
Day care staff	They may be responsible for identifying individuals who are displaying dysphagic symptoms and referring to the appropriate professional. They will also be responsible for implementing recommendations, for monitoring their success, for monitoring the health status of their client and for feeding back information to the relevant professional
Respite staff	They may be responsible for identifying individuals who are displaying dysphagic symptoms and referring to the appropriate professional. They will also be responsible for implementing recommendations, for monitor their success, and for monitoring the health status of their client and for feeding back information to the relevant professional
General practitioners	They will be responsible for identifying individuals who are displaying dysphagic symptoms and for referring onto the relevant professionals. They are responsible for prescribing supplements and thickening agents, and for considering the impact of different medications on the individual. They are central in the management and monitoring of the individual's health, and should be part, or informed of, any multidisciplinary risk management decisions. All professionals involved in the assessment and management of dysphagic individuals should inform the GP of assessment findings, management decisions and concerns about the individual's health
Other medics	These may include psychiatrists, gastroenterologists, physicians, surgeons, radiologists, respiratory medics and ENT surgeons, who all have specialist roles within dysphagia assessment and management
Advocate	They are independent individuals who work to develop a relationship with the client, and where required represent the client's views, interests, rights and wishes

task of supporting individuals at mealtimes is often given to inexperienced and junior members of staff. Research has indicated that staff tend to underestimate their clients' difficulties (Cumella et al., 2000; Kerr et al., 2003) which would have implications for the identification and management of dysphagia.

Studies focusing on carers' knowledge of and ability to follow dysphagia recommendations show that compliance ranges between 76 and 82%, with variations in levels dependent on carer, type of recommendation and venue (Chadwick et al., 2002, 2003, 2006, 2007).

These studies also show that carers' ability to follow recommendations is not necessarily associated with whether they know what the exact recommendations are for an individual, but indicate that a general understanding of dysphagia and the significant health risks that are associated are linked with a higher level of compliance (Chadwick et al., 2002). In addition, carers find some types of recommendations easier to follow than others. An example of an accessible guideline sheet is included (Appendix 14.3).

Associated considerations

Respiration

For people with profound and multiple intellectual disabilities, chest infections are the leading causes of death (Cooper et al., 2004; NHS Scotland, 2004). Chest infections can be due to a variety of reasons, which may include dysphagia, because aspiration can lead to chest infections, aspiration pneumonia and death. Other contributing factors can be asthma, poor positioning, skeletal changes, immobility and ageing. A poor chest status may be indicative of dysphagia and may on its own be a reason for referral for an assessment of eating and drinking. Additionally, although individuals may not have dysphagia, they may have respiratory difficulties which make it difficult for them to coordinate their breathing with their swallowing and may lead to dysphagic symptoms.

Asphyxia

Asphyxia is a common reason for referral for an eating and drinking assessment. Asphyxiation is when something blocks the airway and intervention is required to remove the blockage. This can occur on food or non-food material. It could be assumed that an individual who aspirated more regularly than other people is at greater risk of asphyxiation, if ingesting solid substances that are not adapted. For people with an intellectual disability, the mortality rate due to asphyxia has been noted as significant (Carter & Jancar, 1984), with one study recorded it as 1.87% (Hollins et al., 1998). A recent study has suggested that fast eating, cramming food and early loss of food into the pharynx before swallowing may result in a higher risk of asphyxiation for individuals with intellectual disabilities (Samuels & Chadwick, 2006).

Oral health

Oral health is of particular importance when considering dysphagia in people with profound and multiple intellectual disabilities. Studies have shown (Langmore et al., 1998; Marik, 2001) that one of the key indicators for the development of aspiration pneumonia in dysphagic patients is oral hygiene. If individuals are aspirating dangerous pathogens harboured in dirty teeth, the negative impact of this on the lungs is intensified. It is of particular importance, therefore, to ensure that people with dysphagia have clean teeth, healthy gums and regular dental check-ups. This remains true for people who receive their nutrition and hydration non-orally, for example, through an NG (nasogastric) tube or a PEG (percutaneous endoscopic gastrostomy) tube, although advice should be sought from dental staff to ensure the use of safe brushing techniques and safe cleaning agents to use.

People with intellectual disabilities are at a greater risk for poor oral health, unmet oral health needs, and attend the dentist less frequently than the general population (Arnold et al., 2000; Fiske et al., 2000; Royal College of Surgeons of England, 2001; Royal College of Surgeons of England's joint Advisory Committee for Special Care Dentistry, 2003). For people with PIMD and dysphagia, the methods of management of dysphagia can have a significant impact on oral health. These include:

- the high risk of dental infection and decay, due to lengthy mealtimes and therefore oral retention of food;
- exposure to 'free sugars' released when food is modified (e.g. mashed);
- sugar-dense food supplements, medications containing sugar and gastroesophageal reflux and vomiting corroding the teeth (Bernal, 2005; Gabre et al., 2005);
- a high level of oral bacteria due to mouth breathing, infections as noted earlier, and side effects of medication (Bernal, 2005); and
- difficulties with oral care due to the dependence on others, and to impaired oral reflexes (Bernal, 2005).

Gastroesophageal considerations

People with PIMD have a higher incidence of gastroesophgeal problems than the general population, and those with more complex physical and intellectual disabilities have more problems than people with less complex disabilities (Galli-Carminati et al., 2006).

These include the effects of medication on functioning, *Helicobacter pylori*, ulcer, hiatus hernia, oesophagitis, gastritis, heartburn, dyspepsia, achalasia and oesophageal stricture. These can have implications on an individual's ability or motivation to swallow. They may result in a difficulty in swallowing because food is getting stuck in the oesophagus and may result in pain in the chest and/or back area. They may produce complicating symptoms, such as regurgitation of food, which can come as far as the mouth, or may be aspirated, causing an individual to cough as it compromises the airway. The literature indicates that gastroesophageal reflux disease and *H. pylori* are of particular concern for people with intellectual disabilities.

Gastroesophgeal reflux disease (GERD) is common in people with intellectual disabilities (Cooper et al., 2004), with up to 50% of people with intellectual disabilities exhibiting signs of the condition on testing (Bohmer et al., 2000). Symptoms of GERD commonly include heartburn, regurgitation, persistent vomiting, vomiting blood, food refusal, recurrent pneumonia, dental erosion and behaviour difficulties at mealtimes. Other less common symptoms include asthma, chronic cough, laryngitis and chest pain (Vaezi, 2005). GERD may be more difficult to identify and manage in people with PIMD because of their difficulty in reporting symptoms. Management can be complicated by:

- poor positioning making reflux more likely;
- reduced oesophageal peristalsis and delayed gastric emptying, which may be as a result of compromised motor functioning or as a result of medication;
- constipation causing backflow;
- dysphagia;
- tube feeding; and
- reduced salivary flow resulting in an increase in acid in the oesophagus.

Long-term reflux can lead to the development of Barrett's oesophagus, and in severe cases adenocarcinoma, so identification of GERD is crucial.

H. pylori is a common bacterium that grows in the intestine and lives in the gastrointestinal tract. Many people carry the bacteria, and it is more common where people live in very close contact with each other and where hygiene and sanitation may be compromised. It is particularly common in people with intellectual disabilities (Scheepers at al, 2000) and is more common in people who live or have lived in institutions. It is a bacterial infection of the stomach, which causes symptoms such as indigestion, bloating and fullness, mild nausea which may be relieved by vomiting, belching and regurgitation and feeling very hungry 1 to 3 hours after eating (National Library of Medicine, undated). Clinically, individuals often cough and bring up thick, but clear phlegm, despite presenting with a clear chest. It is suggested that the higher levels of stomach cancer that exist in people with intellectual disabilities may be the result of a higher level of *H. pylori* (Duff et al., 2001).

Dementia

There is debate in the literature as to prevalence of dementia in people with intellectual disabilities. Researchers discriminate between people who have Down's syndrome and people who do not, when reporting prevalence figures.

People with intellectual disabilities, without Down's syndrome

Researchers do not agree as to the prevalence rates with figures of between 6.1% for a 60+ age group (Janicki & Dalton, 2000) and 70% for an 85- to 94-year age group (Cooper, 1997). Zigman et al. (2004) in their study quote lower rates of dementia in the non-Down's syndrome population than those found by other researchers, and report that they were slightly lower than those found in the general population.

Comparison of studies and subsequent conclusions are difficult because the studies use different methodologies, different assessment criteria and tools, and stratify age groups differently.

That said it is important to consider that in many cases of dementia, dysphagia is a factor for patients at some stage of the disease process. Clinically, there has been a belief that dysphagia is a symptom that appears only terminally, but more recent research indicates that this may not be the case (Priefer & Robbins, 1997; Ikeda et al., 2002; Marik & Kaplan, 2003).

People with Down's syndrome

Researchers agree that there is a clear link between Down's syndrome and the development of Alzheimer's disease, with reported prevalence rates varying from approximately 3–10% in the 40–49 age range, 13–47% in the 50–59 age range, 30–50% in the 60+ age range (Holland et al., 2000; Tyrrell et al., 2001).

In most studies dysphagia is not directly identified, although eating and drinking competence is sometimes assessed in terms of activities of daily living. It is also not clear from some studies what details were included in broad categories such as activities of daily living, or 'self-care skills', or 'other' (Holland et al., 2000) which potentially may include eating and drinking. In some studies this is assessed as how capable individuals are in preparing meals. Dysphagia may not have been identified because in most studies the tools used do not probe for it. However, dysphagia is suggested by observations made in some studies. Cosgrave et al. (2000) report one participant who has a gastrostomy in situ, and a small amount of study participants who they have 'end stage' data on, are all fully dependent on feeding tubes, indicating significant difficulties. They also discuss the opinion that the end stage of dementia has been lengthened by preventative treatments for aspiration pneumonia, suggesting that dysphagia may indeed be a significant consideration for some time, with many patients. Aspiration pneumonia is widely acknowledged to be a complication of chronic/severe dysphagia (Langmore et al., 1998).

It is clear that when caring for people with dementia, dysphagia should be considered from diagnosis onwards, due to its potentially life-threatening complications. Management decisions in dysphagia and dementia should always take into account presenting symptoms, discomfort, distress and quality of life. They should be made within a multidisciplinary framework, and taking into account the individual's own views, where possible, any advance directives, and the views of significant others. There should be no predetermined treatment route for individuals with dementia and dysphagia or treatment routes that are not accessible because someone has a diagnosis of dementia. All options should be considered from texture modification, positioning changes, appropriate support at mealtimes, and in the more severe cases, non-oral feeding support.

Other reported features of, or associated with dementia include changes in personality, memory loss, spatial disorientation, epilepsy, urinary incontinence, decline in general mental functioning, decline in daily living skills, loss of person's hygiene skills, decline in language skills and the ability to feed oneself. There is some variation in patterning of these difficulties across the mild/moderate/severe spectrum, but authors claim that the pattern of dementia may not be different to that of the general population (Holland et al., 1998; Cosgrave et al., 2000; Holland et al., 2000; Tyrrell et al., 2001; McCarron et al., 2005).

Implications for nurses

Nurses working with people with PIMD have a central role in their care, whether they are community, residential or inpatient based. It is essential that nurses understand the process of normal swallowing and are able to identify signs and symptoms of concern. Nurses may be responsible for supporting individuals at mealtimes and on an ongoing basis, so they need to be aware of the complex needs of people with dysphagia and theory behind recommendations that are made. Nurses also need to be aware of the conditions associated with dysphagia, which may predispose their clients to more severe dysphagia. This will allow nursing staff to identify individuals who are risk of having dysphagia, or who are displaying signs and symptoms of dysphagia, to refer to the appropriate agency when necessary. It will allow them to support individuals sensitively and skilfully at mealtimes, monitor their skills, feed back appropriate information to relevant professionals and play a key part in any multidisciplinary discussion.

Conclusion

Dysphagia is a significant health issue for people with profound and multiple intellectual disabilities. Chest infections, one of the primary consequences of dysphagia, are the leading cause of death for people with intellectual disabilities. Dysphagia is a collection of symptoms, which on occasion, may require careful identification and differential diagnosis. As such it is essential that 'front-line' staff, such as nurses, are knowledgeable about dysphagia, its signs, symptoms and consequences. This will ensure the provision of optimum intervention for people with profound and multiple disabilities in a timely and appropriate manner.

Appendix 14.1 Signs and symptoms potentially indicating dysphagia.

Urgent difficulties	Non-urgent difficulties
Current pneumonia	Food refusal
History of pneumonia	Oral stage problems, e.g. food loss from the mouth
Current chest infection	Behavioural difficulties at mealtimes
History of chest infections	Fast eating
History of serious choking (e.g. hospital/ paramedics)	Occasional coughing when eating/drinking
Coughing at every meal/every drink	Gradual weight loss
Sudden weight loss	Long mealtimes
BMI < 15	Difficulty feeding self
Sudden change in eating/drinking skills	
Respiratory distress when eating/drinking	Urinary tract infections

Appendix 14.2 Example of a risk assessment form.

	Name and signature	Role/profession
Activity that may be causing risk		
Benefits of undertaking activity		
Risks associated with undertaking activity		
Action plan to minimise risk		
	Name and signature	Role/profession
Individuals agreeing and involved with action plan		
Risk review schedule		

Example of a risk monitoring form.

Date of review	Individuals present	Risk level
		Stable/changing action:
		Stable/changing action:
		Stable/changing action:

Examples of completed forms

		Role/profession
Activity that may be causing risk	Eating and drinking	
Benefits of undertaking activity	Maintaining QOL Maintaining positive interactions	
Risks associated with undertaking activity	Development of a chest infection Choking incident Weight loss Reduced QOL	
Action plan to minimise risk	Dietary modifications Positioning and support recs Close MDT monitoring	
	Name and signature	Role/profession
Individuals agreeing and involved with action plan		Parents, SLT, physio, OT, day centre staff Discussion with general practitioner (GP) re plan
Risk review schedule	6 weekly	

Date of review	Individuals present	Risk level
03/05	SLT, day centre staff, parents	Stable/changing Action: continue to monitor
05/05	SLT, physio, OT	Stable/changing `chesty' presentation Action: discuss concerns with GP
07/05	SLT, physio, day centre staff, parents, care coordinator	Stable/changing pneumonia and serious choking incident Action: refer for physician opinion on PEG

Appendix 14.3 Eating and drinking guidelines.

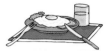

NAME:

The following guidelines should be followed when....................is eating and/or drinking

- Ensure....is sitting upright
- ....should receive a soft moist diet
- ....should have regular small sips of normal liquid
- ....should have his teeth cleaned 3 times a day

We understand, and agree to follow these recommendations. We agree to contact the Speech & Language Therapist on....................if we have any concerns about........................or if staffing personnel change.

Signature   Print name   Date

Glossary

Apnoea: A general term meaning the cessation of breathing (Marcovitch, 2006).

Asphyxia: Asphyxia means literally absence of pulse, but the name is given to the whole series of symptoms which follow stoppage of breathing ... obstruction of the air passages may occur as the result of (the entry of) a foreign body (Marcovitch, 2006).

Aspiration: The taking of foreign matter into the lungs with the respiratory current (Merriam-Webster, 2005a).

Aspiration pneumonia: A disease of the lungs that is characterised especially by inflammation and consolidation of lung tissue followed by resolution, is accompanied by fever, chills, cough and difficulty in breathing and is caused chiefly by infection. In this case the infection is caused by the material aspirated (National Library of Medicine, 2007).

Bolus: A soft mass of chewed food (Merriam-Webster, 2005b).

Client: A generic term used to refer to people who are the recipients of dysphagia services. It is not intended as a label for the people who use the services.

Dysphagia: A difficulty, discomfort or pain when swallowing (Marcovitch, 2006).

Hypoxemia: Deficient oxygenation of the blood (Merriam-Webster, 2005c).

Oesophagus: The oesophagus, or gullet, is the muscular tube linking the throat to the stomach, down which passes swallowed food and drink (Marcovitch, 2006).

Pharynx: Another name for the throat ... (strictly it is the) cavity into which the nose and mouth open above, from which the larynx and gullet open below, and in which the channel for the air and that for the food cross one another (Marcovitch, 2006).

Acknowledgements

Thanks to Paula Leslie and Tracy Lazenby for advice on content and editing, and to Janet Telford for all her support.

Further reading

Crawford, H. (2006). ALD and dysphagia: the need for evidence-based care. *RCSLT Bulletin*, January (645), 14–15.

National Patient Safety Agency (undated). *Dysphagia*. Available at: http://www.npsa.nhs.uk/health/resources/dysphagia (accessed 27 September 2007).

References

Arnold, C., Brookes, V., Griffiths, J., Maddock, S., & Theophilou, S. (2000). *Guidelines for Oral Health Care of People with Physical Disability*. Report of BSDH Working Group. Revised Jan 2000. Available at: http://www.bsdh.org.uk/guidelines/physical.pdf (accessed 23 August 2007).

Aziz, S.J., & Cambell-Taylor, I. (1999). Neglect and abuse associated with undernutrition in long-term care in North America: causes and solutions. *Journal of Elder Abuse and Neglect*, 10(1/2), 91–117.

Beange, H., McElduff, A., & Baker, W. (1995). Medical disorders of adults with mental retardation: a population study. *American Journal on Mental Retardation*, 99(6), 595–604.

Beauchamp, T.L., & Childress, J.F. (2004). *Principles of Biomedical Ethics* (5th edition). Oxford: Oxford University Press.

Bernal, C. (2005). Maintenance of oral health in people with learning disability. *Nursing Times*, 101(6), 40–42.

Bleach, N.R. (1993). The gag reflex and aspiration: a retrospective analysis of 120 patients assessed by videofluroscopy. *Clinical Otolaryngology*, 18(4), 303–307.

Bohmer, C.J.M., Klinkenberg-Knol, E.C., Niezen-de-Boer, M.C., & Meuwissen, S.G.M. (2000). Gastroesophgeal reflux disease in intellectually disabled individuals: how often, how serious, how manageable? *The American Journal of Gastroenterology*, 95(8), 1868–1872.

Brown, L. (2002). Best interest – best practice. *RCSLT Bulletin*, November, 6.

Carter, G., & Jancar, J. (1984). Sudden deaths in the mentally handicapped. *Psychological Medicine*, 14(3), 691–695.

Chadwick, D.D., Jolliffe, J., & Goldbart, J. (2002). Carer knowledge of dysphagia management strategies. *International Journal of Language and Communication Disorders*, 72(3), 345–357.

Chadwick, D.D., Jolliffe, J., & Goldbart, J. (2003). Adherence to eating and drinking guidelines for adults with intellectual disabilities and dysphagia. *American Journal on Mental Retardation*, 108(3), 202–211.

Chadwick, D.D., Jolliffe, J., Goldbart, J., & Burton, M.H. (2006). Barriers to compliance among caregivers of adults with learning disabilities and dysphagia. *Journal of Applied Research in Intellectual Disabilities*, 19(2), 153–162.

Cook, I.J., & Kahrilas, P.J. (1999). AGA technical review on management of oropharyngeal dysphagia. *Gastroenterology*, 116(2), 455–478.

Cooper, S.A. (1997). High prevalence of dementia among people with learning disabilities not attributable to Down's syndrome. *Psychological Medicine*, 27(3), 609–616.

Cooper, S.A., Melville, C., & Morrison, J. (2004). People with intellectual disabilities: their health needs differ and need to be recognised and met. *BMJ*, 329(7463), 414–415.

Cosgrave, M.P., Tyrrell, J., McCarron, M., Gill, M., & Lawlor, B.A. (2000). A five year follow-up study of dementia in persons with Down's syndrome: early symptoms and patterns of deterioration. *Irish Journal Psychiatric Medicine*, 17(1), 5–11.

Crawford, H. (2006). ALD and dysphagia: the need for evidence-based care. *RCSLT Bulletin*. January.

Crawford, H., Leslie, P., & Drinnan, M. (2007). *Compliance with Dysphagia Recommendations by Carers of Adults with Intellectual Impairment*. Available at: http://www.springerlink.com/content/b13127xj338t3467/ (accessed 28 September 2007).

Cumella, S., Ransford, N., Lyons, J., & Burnham, H. (2000). Needs for oral care among people with intellectual disability not in contact with community dental services. *Journal of Intellectual Disability Research*, 44(1), 45–52.

Department of Health (1998). *Signposts for Success in Commissioning and Providing Health Services for People with Learning Disabilities*. London: Department of Health.

Department of Health (2001a). *Reference Guide to Consent for Examination or Treatment*. London: Department of Health.

Department of Health (2001b). *Valuing People: A New Strategy for the 21st Century*. London: Department of Health.

Duff, M., Scheepers, M., Cooper, M., Hoghton, M., & Baddely, P. (2001). *Helicobacter pylori*: has the killer escaped from the institution? A possible cause of increase stomach cancer in a population with intellectual disability. *Journal of Intellectual Disability Research*, 45(3), 219–225.

Eyman, R., Grossman, H., Chaney, R., & Call, T. (1990). The life expectancy of profoundly handicapped people with mental retardation. *The New England Journal of Medicine*, 323(9), 584–589.

Fiske, J., Griffiths, J., Jamieson, R., & Manger, D. (2000). *Guidelines for Oral Health Care for Long-Stay Patients and Residents Report of BSDH Working Group*. Available at: http://www.bsdh.org.uk/guidelines/longstay.pdf (accessed 23 August 2007).

Gabre, P., Norman, C., & Birkhead, D. (2005). Oral sugar clearance in individuals with oral motor dysfunctions. *Caries Research*, 39(5), 356–362.

Galli-Carminati, G., Chauvet, I., & Deriaz, N. (2006). Prevalence of gastrointestinal disorders in adult clients with pervasive developmental disorders. *Journal of Intellectual Disability Research*, 50(10), 711–718.

Hickman, J. (1997). ALD and dysphagia: issues and practice. *Speech and Language Therapy in Practice*, Autumn, 8–11.

Holland, A.J., Hon, J., Huppert, F., Stevens, F., & Watson, P. (1998). Population-based study of the prevalence and presentation of dementia in adults with Down's syndrome. *British Journal of Psychiatry*, 172, 493–498.

Holland, A.J., Hon, J., Huppert, F.A., & Stevens, F. (2000). Incidence and course of dementia in people with Down's syndrome: findings from a population-based study. *Journal of Intellectual Disability*, 44(2), 138–146.

Hollins, S., Attard, M.T., von Fraunhofer, N., McGuigan, S., & Sedgwick, P. (1998). Mortality in people with learning disability: risks, causes, and death certification findings in London. *Developmental Medicine and Child Neurology*, 40(1), 50–56.

Ikeda, M., Brown, J., Holland, A.J., Fukuhara, R., & Hodges, J.R. (2002). Changes in appetite, food preference, and eating habits in frontotemporal dementia and Alzheimer's disease. *Journal of Neurology, Neurosurgery and Psychiatry*, 73, 371–376.

Janicki, M.P., & Dalton, A.J. (2000). Prevalence of dementia and impact on intellectual disability services. *Mental Retardation*, 38(3), 276–288.

Kerr, A.M., McCulloch, D., Oliver, K., McLean, B., Coleman, E., Law, T., Beaton, P., Wallace, S., Newell, E., Eccles, T., & Prescott, R.J. (2003). Medical needs of people with intellectual disability require regular reassessment, and the provision of client- and carer-held reports. *Journal of Intellectual Disability Research*, 47(2), 134–145.

Langmore, S.E., Schatz, K., & Olson, N. (1991). Endoscopic and videofluroscopic evaluations of swallowing and aspiration. *Annals of Otology Rhinology and Laryngologyl*, 100, 678–681.

Langmore, S.E., Terpenning, M.S., Schork, A., Chen, Y., Murray, J.T., Lopatin, D., & Loesche, W.J. (1998). Predictors of aspiration pneumonia: how important is dysphagia? *Dysphagia*, 13(2), 69–81.

Logemann, J.E. (1998). *Evaluation and Treatment of Swallowing Disorders*. Austin, TX: Pro-ed Publishing.

Marcovitch, H. (2006). *Black's Medical Dictionary* (41st edition). London: A & C Black (Publishers) Limited.

Marik, P., & Kaplan, D. (2003). Aspiration pneumonia and dysphagia in the elderly. *Chest*, 124(1), 328–336.

Marik, P.E. (2001). Aspiration pneumonitis and aspiration pneumonia. *New England Journal of Medicine*, 344(9), 665–671.

Marks, L., & Rainbow, D. (2001). *Working with Dysphagia*. Brackley: Speechmark Publishing.

Mathers-Schmidt, B.A., & Kurlinski, M. (2003). Dysphagia evaluation practices: inconsistencies in clinical assessment and instrumental examination decision-making. *Dysphagia*, 18(2), 114–125.

McCarron, M., Gill, M., McCallion, P., & Begley, C. (2005). Health co-morbidities in ageing persons with Down's syndrome and Alzheimer's disease. *Journal of Intellectual Disability Research*, 49(7), 560–566.

Merriam-Webster (2005a). *MedlinePlus Medical Dictionary. Aspiration*. Available at: http://www2.merriam-webster.com/cgi-bin/mwmednlm?book = Medical&va = aspiration (accessed 1 October 2007).

Merriam-Webster (2005b). *MedlinePlus Medical Dictionary. Bolus*. Available at: http://www2.merriam-webster.com/cgi-bin/mwmednlm?book = Medical&va = Bolus (accessed 1 October 2007).

Merriam-Webster (2005c). *MedlinePlus Medical Dictionary. Hypoxemia*. Available at: http://www2.merriam-webster.com/cgi-bin/mwmednlm?book = Medical&va = hypoxemia (accessed 1 October 2007).

Morton, R.E., Bonas, R., Minford, J., Kerr, A., & Ellis, R.E. (1997). Feeding ability in Rett syndrome. *Developmental Medicine and Child Neurology*, 39, 331–335.

National Library of Medicine (2007). *MedlinePlus A.D.A.M Medical Encyclopaedia. Aspiration Pneumonia*. Available at: http://www.nlm.nih.gov/medlineplus/ency/article/000121.htm (accessed 1 October 2007).

National Patient Safety Agency (2004). *Understanding the Patient Safety Issues for People with Learning Disabilities*. London: Department of Health.

NHS Scotland (2004). *Health Needs Assessment Report: People with Learning Disabilities in Scotland*. Glasgow: NHS Scotland.

Priefer, B., & Robbins, J. (1997). Eating changes in mild-stage Alzheimer's disease: a pilot study. *Dysphagia*, 12(4), 212–221.

Rogers, B., Stratton, P., Msall M., Andres, M., Champlain, M., Koerner, P., & Piazza, J. (1994). Long term morbidity and management of strategies of aspiration in adults with severe developmental disabilities. *American Journal on Mental Retardation*, 98, 490–498.

Royal College of Surgeons of England (2001). *Clinical Guidelines and Integrated Care Pathways for the Oral Health Care of People with Learning Disabilities*. Available at: http://www.rcseng.ac.uk/fds/docs/icppld.pdf (accessed 23 August 2007).

Royal College of Surgeons of England's joint Advisory Committee for Special Care Dentistry (2003). *A Case of Need: Proposal for a Speciality in Special Care Dentistry*. Available at: http://www.bsdh.org.uk/misc/ACase4Need.pdf (accessed 23 August 2007).

RSCLT (2006). *Communicating Quality 3: RCSLT's Guidance on Best Practice in Service Organisation and Provision*. London: Scotprint.

Samuels, R., & Chadwick, D.D. (2006). Predictors of asphyxiation risk in adults with intellectual disabilities and dysphagia. *Journal of Intellectual Disability Research*, 50(5), 362–370.

Schechter, G. (1998). Systemic causes of dysphagia. *Otolaryngologic Clinics of North America*, 31(3), 525–535.

Scheepers, M., Duff, M., Baddeley, P., Cooper, M., Hoghton, M., & Harrison, J. (2000). *Helicobacter pylori* and the learning disabled. *British Journal of General Practice*, 50(459), 813–814.

Sherman, B., Nisenboum, J.M., Jesberger, B.L., Morrow, C.A., & Jesberger, J. (1999). Assessment of dysphagia with the use of pulse oximetry. *Dysphagia*, 14(3), 152–156.

Smith, S. (2002). Seeing is believing. *RCSLT Bulletin*, April, 5–7.

Sokoloff, L.G., & Pavlakovic, R. (1997). Neuroleptic-induced dysphagia. *Dysphagia*, 12(4), 177–179.

Sugerman-Issacs, J., Murdock, M., Lane, J., & Percy, A. (2003). Eating difficulties in girls with Rett syndrome compared with other developmental disabilities. *Journal of the American Dietetic Association*, 103(2), 224–230.

Tohara, H., Saitoh, E., Mays, K., Kuhlemeier, K.V., & Palmer, J.B. (2003). Three tests for predicting aspiration without videofluorography. *Dysphagia*, 18(2), 126–134.

Tyrrell, J., Cosgrave, M., McCarron, M., McPherson, J., Calvert, J., Kelly, A., McLaughlin, M., Gill, M., & Lawlor, B. (2001). Dementia in people with down's syndrome. *International Journal of Geriatric Medicine*, 16(12), 1168–1174.

Vaezi, M. (2005). Atypical manifestations of gastroesophageal reflux disease. *Medscape General Medicine*. Available at: http://www.medscape.com/viewarticle/506303 (accessed 23 August 2007).

Watson, F. (2004). Learning disabilities and dysphagia: the patient safety agenda. *RCSLT Bulletin*, December.

Zigman, W.B., Schupf, N., Devenny, D.A., Miezejeski, C., Ryan, R., Urv, T.K., Schubert, R., & Silverman, W. (2004). Incidence and prevalence of dementia in elderly adults with mental retardation without down's syndrome. *American Journal on Mental Retardation*, 109(2), 126–141.

Chapter 15

NUTRITION, HYDRATION AND WEIGHT

Siân Burton, Susan Cox and Sue M. Sandham

Introduction

Good nutrition is recognised as an important factor in maximising and maintaining health. In people who have a profound intellectual and multiple disability (PIMD), there is a higher prevalence of polarised weight distribution compared with the general population, as well as nutrition-related health problems such as coronary heart disease, type 2 diabetes, chronic constipation and dental caries (Bryan et al., 2000; Parsons, 2002; Bradley, 2005; Melville et al., 2005). As yet there is no nationally recognised nutrition risk screening in PIMDs, but it is generally accepted that improving recognition of these problems before they become a case for crisis management would be beneficial (Bryan et al., 1996).

In children there is evidence suggesting that early intervention is of benefit (Campbell & Kelsey, 1994; Sullivan & Rosenbloom, 1996). For example, regular nutrition assessments by the nurse, dietitian, speech and language therapist (SALT) should reduce the occurrence of the following which cause morbidity and mortality:

- Malnutrition
- Aspiration pneumonia
- Recurrent chest and urinary infections
- Dehydration
- Chronic constipation

Learning outcomes

The reader will be able to:

- identify the key nutritional concerns in people who have PIMDs;
- understand the need for good multi-professional working in addressing these nutritional concerns;
- appreciate the contribution of good food to quality of life, morbidity and mortality;
- identify the methods of administering artificial nutrition support; and

- be aware of the specific nutritional consequences of the main syndromes associated with an intellectual disability.

Nutrition risk assessment

Effective screening for the risk of malnutrition detects both over- and undernutrition. Indeed nutritional screening is not a new concept, with the first screening tool developed in 1979 by Mullen and colleagues (Mullen et al., 1979). At present there is just one screening tool specifically developed for adults with an intellectual disability which assesses nutritional adequacy as well as under- and overnutrition (Bryan et al., 1996).

However, a key issue to appreciate is that nutritional screening is not intended to be 100% accurate, does not replace clinical judgement but informs it, and serves to raise awareness of a person's nutritional status (Wright, 2002; Bartholomew et al., 2003; Williams, 2005).

The National Institute for Clinical Excellence Guideline 32 recommends that nutritional screening is undertaken at least annually for all adults in community care homes (National Institute for Clinical Excellence, 2006). Although supported/assisted accommodation as such are not directly mentioned, it is worth considering undertaking such risk assessments for individuals with PIMDs (Dimascio et al., 2004).

⋆ *Training by a dietitian is needed before using a nutrition risk assessment tool.*

For individuals who are nutritionally at risk, a full assessment of nutritional status is required and undertaken by the specialist dietitian working with individuals with PIMDs (Thomas & Akobeng, 2000). This involves critical scrutiny of the following:

- Medical history, including biochemical and haematological status
- Family history
- Nutrition history
- Medication history
- Weight history
- Behavioural history related to food and fluids
- Dental and oral function
- Physical mobility
- Sensory function

Figure 15.1 illustrates the contribution of members of the multi-professional team (MPT) in enabling the person to achieve and maintain optimal nutritional status.

Malnutrition is defined as *the provision of food, which satisfies an individual's requirements for essential nutrients including fluid in order to achieve and maintain optimum health*. Malnutrition is a general term for the medical condition caused by an improper or insufficient food intake.

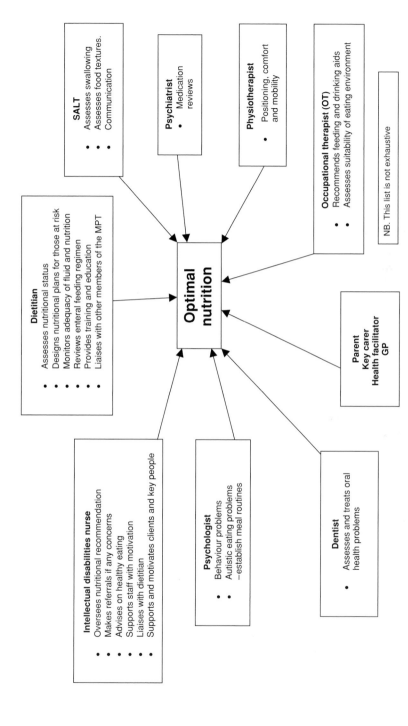

Figure 15.1 Summary of contributions of multi-professional team members.

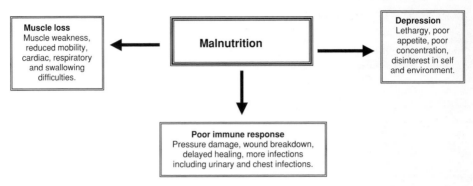

Figure 15.2   Clinical consequences of malnutrition.

In this chapter we will be using the word 'malnutrition' to describe 'undernutrition'. Thus, an individual will experience malnutrition if the appropriate amount, kind or quality of nutrients comprising a healthy diet is not consumed for an extended period of time.

Malnutrition can mean both under and overnutrition though it is more commonly used to refer to the presence of undernutrition.

Malnutrition is often not identified simply because weight checks are not being undertaken on a routine basis (Thomas & Bishop, 2007).

★ *Ensure the people you support have regular weight checks.*

The clinical consequences of malnutrition are summarised in Figure 15.2; if left untreated, malnutrition will ultimately result in death.

How do we identity malnutrition and obesity?

For the general population the body mass index (BMI) is the usual method of assessing if an adult is within the ideal parameter of the weight for height standards. In people with an intellectual disability, BMI has not been found to be a totally appropriate or accurate measurement (Bryan et al., 1996; Samson-Fang & Stevenson, 2000). Nonetheless, BMI can be used as a guide, in conjunction with a diet and weight history, to assess nutritional status. This assessment should be carried out by a registered dietitian.

The formula to calculate BMI is:

weight (kg)/height (m)^2 and can be interpreted as shown in Table 15.1.

As previously mentioned, it is not unusual for the majority of adults with PIMDs to be under (or over) these ideal BMI figures. Due to the severe muscle wasting in cerebral palsy and other conditions, the normal ideal for that person can be a BMI of 15.

Table 15.1 Interpretation of BMI.

BMI	Interpretation
>40 kg/m^2	Morbid obesity
>30 kg/m^2	Obesity
25–29 kg/m^2	Overweight
19–24.9 kg/m^2	Ideal for general population
<18.5 kg/m^2	Underweight

Source: British Dietetic Association (2006).

Height

An accurate height measurement with a stadiometer can be difficult to obtain when a standing height is not feasible. Supine length can be a good alternative provided that the person is straight, though a rough height using a tape measure over a curved spine may be considered better than no measure at all (Carter et al., 2006).

Segmented methods of obtaining height such as demispan and knee height can be especially useful as most people with PIMDs are unable to stand. For children with spinal curvature, segmented measures such as the upper arm (also known as the tibial length), knee height and lower leg can be used to assess height. Studies using these alternative height measurements have found good correlation with a standing height or supine length (Spender et al., 1989; Stevenson, 1995; Sullivan & Rosenbloom, 1996, Stewart et al., 2006).

There are other documented methods of assessing and monitoring nutritional status in both adults and children such as the use of anthropometric measurements which assess body composition, i.e. fat and muscle (Sampson-Fang & Stevenson, 2000; Todorovic & Micklewright, 2004; Stewart et al., 2006). These measurements are summarised in Table 15.2.

However it is generally recognised that there is no absolute method in PIMDs due to atypical body shape. A practitioner trained and experienced in such methodology is essential to obtain accurate measurements though in routine practice such measurements can be difficult and impractical to undertake as clothing and spinal jackets need to be removed (Stewart et al., 2006).

Table 15.2 Anthropometric measurements.

Description	Use
Mid-arm circumference – MAC	Indicator of whole body fat stores. Repeated measurements indicative of change in nutritional status. Sensitive to short-term changes
Triceps skin-fold thickness – TSF	As above
Mid-arm muscle circumference – MAMC	Measure of lean tissue derived from MAC and TSF measurements
Subscapular skin-fold thickness – SST	Indicator of whole body fat stores. Repeated measures indicative of change in nutritional status – better reflection of long-term changes

Weight

Ramp or hoist scales are useful for wheelchair users, but no matter which type of scales is used they must be calibrated and serviced annually (Stewart et al., 2006). Monthly weighing is advisable, increasing in frequency if any trend is identified. In children weight measurement can be carried out by using balance scales and/or an electronic balance. This measurement together with the length or height can be plotted along the Child Growth Foundation centile charts.

Nutritional status

One of the best indicators of a shift in nutritional status in adults is to see if there has been a 5–10% weight change over the last 6 months. This often suggests the need for a referral to a dietitian to investigate the dietary habits of that person and identify any problems quickly.

★ *Loose/tight fitting clothes and jewellery are an indicator of altering weight status.*

Many children with PIMDs have weights below the bottom centile (0.4th centile). Specific centile charts have been developed for children with cerebral palsy and could be used to guide clinical practice. However, the original research study by Krick et al. (1996) had a small sample size and caution is recommended in their use (Stewart et al., 2006).

Observation of children at mealtimes can be very informative, enabling the nurse to check posture and the eating environment. Also, a child's inability to cope with textures commensurate with age can be indicative of poor feeding competence and possible nutritional inadequacy. Such children's nutritional status should be checked at least every 3–6 months by the dietitian in order to start dietetic intervention or monitor that already in place (Stallings & Zemel, 1996).

Medication and effects on nutritional status

People who are most at risk from drug–nutrient interactions include those who are:

- malnourished;
- dehydrated;
- on long-term medication;
- children; and
- elderly.

Nearly all medication has the potential to cause side effects, some of which can be minimal while others can be more noticeable. The drugs most commonly used in intellectual disabilities and their impact on nutritional status are shown in Appendix 15.1.

Nutritional requirements

A healthy diet provides sufficient energy and nutrients (including fluid) to maintain normal physiological functions and allows for growth and replacement of body tissues. People with PIMDs have the same basic dietary requirements as everybody else: carbohydrates and fat for energy, protein for growth, tissue replacement and to maintain a good autoimmune system. Fluid and fibre are also essential to maintain good gut motility. Additionally, vitamins and minerals are necessary in small amounts for enzyme function and growth, with calcium and vitamin D being especially important for the growth and maintenance of bone health.

Under- and overnutrition are the common nutritional problems in intellectual disabilities (Department of Health, 2001). There is often huge variation between an individual's needs and that specified in reference tables which are used to estimate average nutritional requirements. Such recommendations for the general population are not usually applicable for people with PIMDs due to the presence of atypical body size and shape, activity levels and effects of medication. For these reasons alone, the dietitian should assess nutritional status at least once a year for adults but more frequently for children and indeed in any person after illness or surgery (Wake, 2003). All care staff should have received training on the fundamentals of nutrition care. They also need to engage in specific training in relation to the needs of their individual clients (Department of Health, 2001; Dickson, 2002).

Key points

- Give a wide variety of foods of the appropriate texture to ensure provision of a full range of nutrients including fluid.
- Weight change is the best indicator of too many or too few calories or energy.
- Allow sufficient time for each individual to enjoy their meals.

★ *People with PIMDs often require at least three times as long to eat and drink.*

It is important that where parents are caring for a relative with PIMDs at home, they should be highly involved in the nutritional planning and their son or daughter's preferences, and wishes should be keenly adhered to wherever possible. The individual's preferences are paramount and both professionals and carers need to acquire the skills to assist people with PIMDs to make choices, leading to the enhancement of personal self-worth and independence (Johansson, 2001). The use of photographs, information in accessible formats and objects of reference can be invaluable in this regard (Jackson & Jackson, 1999).

Children with PIMDs need intensive nutritional monitoring by a paediatric dietitian (Stewart et al., 2006). For children with cerebral palsy of whom up to 30% have severe feeding difficulties, the dietitian is a key member of the MPT (Hartley & Thomas, 2003).

Menu planning

Enjoyment of mealtimes and encouragement of the pleasures of eating should be the focus at all times. Incorporating an individual's choice and their favourite meals into dietary planning can significantly enrich a person's quality of life.

People with PIMDs should have the same foods as the general population whenever possible. Often food will need to be softened and moistened, pureed and enriched. Even a pizza can be enjoyed if made using a savoury sponge or scone base.

Forward planning is recommended as this allows for the incorporation of the widest range of foods and nutrients into the diet. Meal plans with a minimum of a 2-week cycle can be based on a day's typical structure as shown in Figure 15.3; guidelines for healthy eating are shown in Appendix 15.2.

Three small main meals and three snack meals should be given each day. This will give a more even distribution of nutrients and energy. Large meals are best avoided in people with PIMDs as they can contribute to a range of gastrointestinal problems (Morton et al., 1999).

Where possible include red meat at least three times a week for iron and zinc content. It is advisable not to give tea, coffee or caffeine-based drinks with or within an hour of the lunch and evening meal as these drinks reduce absorption of iron (Nelson & Poulter, 2004). A good source of vitamin C at each meal such as fruit juice, citrus or berry fruits, green vegetables can improve iron absorption. Oily fish such as sardines, salmon and pilchards provide essential fats including long-chain omega-3 fatty acids and should be on the menu at least once a week.

★ *Encourage self-feeding wherever possible as this promotes independence.*

Other key issues

- Offer finger foods where possible.
- Most people with PIMDs need assistance with eating, and the food usually needs to be well chopped and soft.
- Those with very poor oral motor skills or dysphagia are likely to need a gastrostomy.

Hydration

The human body is approximately 75% water (Thomas & Bishop, 2007). People can survive without food for weeks but last for only a few days without fluid. Water intake includes that which is consumed in food and beverages as well as small volumes of water from food oxidation and tissue breakdown (Grandjean, 2004).

Most of us need to drink between 1.5 and 2.0 L of fluid daily and we need more in hot weather, when taking exercise or when suffering from diarrhoea. Some of this fluid intake should be fresh drinking water as too much strong tea, coffee and cola drinks (which contain caffeine) may be dehydrating especially in people who are

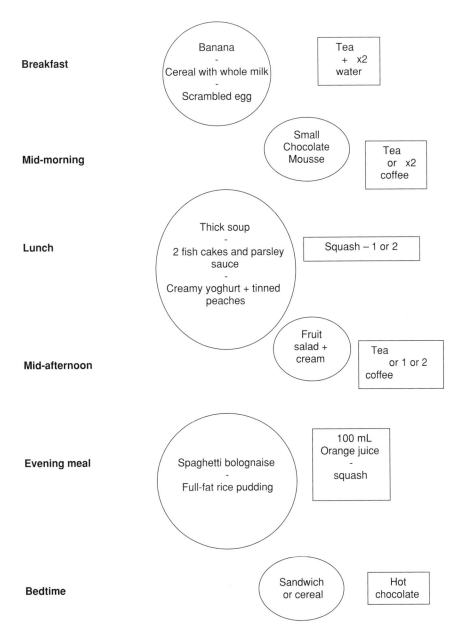

Breakfast

Banana
-
Cereal with whole milk
-
Scrambled egg

Tea + x2 water

Mid-morning

Small Chocolate Mousse

Tea or x2 coffee

Lunch

Thick soup
-
2 fish cakes and parsley sauce
-
Creamy yoghurt + tinned peaches

Squash – 1 or 2

Mid-afternoon

Fruit salad + cream

Tea or 1 or 2 coffee

Evening meal

Spaghetti bolognaise
-
Full-fat rice pudding

100 mL Orange juice
-
squash

Bedtime

Sandwich or cereal

Hot chocolate

Figure 15.3 A day's typical meal structure.

not used to high intakes of caffeine (Royal College of Nursing & National Patient Safety Agency, 2007).

To maintain hydration most adults need 8–10 glasses or mugs of fluid daily. For people with swallowing problems, fluid is surprisingly difficult to manage. In these circumstances a referral to a SALT or dietitian will be necessary to ascertain if a proprietary thickening agent is appropriate.

Dehydration

This occurs when the fluid intake is less than the body requires. As a general rule, 1 L more needs to be taken than is excreted in the urine to avoid dehydration. Extra fluid must always be taken in hot weather, and dry continence pads are an indication of dehydration. Symptoms due to dehydration include:

- headache;
- dark urine;
- frequent urinary tract infections;
- mild confusion;
- fatigue; and
- oliguria/anuria.

⋆ *If a child or adult has not passed any urine for 24 hours, contact the general practitioner. This can suggest severe dehydration.*

Constipation

Constipation is a very common problem for children and adults with PIMDs. There is no clear definition of constipation but it is generally accepted that it means either hardness of stools or delayed/slow peristalsis through the gastrointestinal tract (Claydon, 1996). According to Sullivan & Rosenbloom (1996), chronic constipation in PIMDs can lead to:

- impaired appetite;
- increased convulsions (epileptic seizures);
- incontinence due to pressure on the bladder;
- diarrhoea (though this can be overflow due to constipation and partial obstruction);
- vomiting; and
- challenging behaviour.

Actual defecation depends on various muscle functions that operate by voluntary and involuntary control. Diet alone can rarely prevent constipation in people with PIMDs due to the high prevalence of reduced gut motility. However, good dietary and lifestyle practices can be hugely beneficial. These include plenty of fluid, insoluble fibre found in whole grain cereals, soluble fibre in fruit and vegetables and keeping as active as possible. However, laxatives may be necessary and their use considered prior to the person being subjected to enemas and suppositories. The treatment and management of continence is further explored in Chapter 16.

⋆ *Pure bran is not recommended as it can reduce the motility of the gut.*

Food and fluid textures must be adapted to individual needs, and it is important that if the SALT has undertaken a swallowing assessment (see Chapter 14), the recommended eating and drinking plan is enforced. The dietitian's role is to ensure that any food and fluid intake or nutrition support satisfies the individual's nutritional

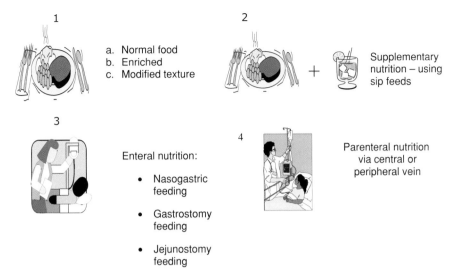

1

a. Normal food
b. Enriched
c. Modified texture

2

+ Supplementary
nutrition – using
sip feeds

3

Enteral nutrition:

- Nasogastric feeding

- Gastrostomy feeding

- Jejunostomy feeding

4

Parenteral nutrition
via central or
peripheral vein

Figure 15.4   Nutrition support.

needs irrespective of texture or route of administration as in enteral tube feeding (ETF).

Nutrition support

There are four methods of providing nutrition support which can be used exclusively or in combination depending on the person's clinical condition. These are summarised in Figure 15.4.

Method 1

Normal food.   Eating a good variety of foods is the first step in nutrition support. Some people may be overwhelmed with the traditional three meals a day approach. Consider using a larger plate so the normal food portion appears small or offering smaller meals more often. Individuals with cerebral palsy for instance manage three smaller main meals a day plus three in-between snacks. Make sure that attention is paid to the appearance as we often 'eat with our eyes' and if it looks good enough to eat then it will more than likely be eaten. Have a positive approach to offering food; your likes or dislikes will affect the person's attitude towards food. For people with sensory impairments, take the time to describe the food being offered, encouraging choice as far as possible.

★ *Take the time to support each individual to make good food choices.*

Enriched.   Some people are unable, for a variety of reasons, to take sufficient normal food to meet their nutritional needs. Factors such as illness can reduce appetite whilst poor oral health can lead to taste changes, discomfort when chewing and

Table 15.3 Enriching food and drink with everyday ingredients.

Food item	Protein	Energy	Can be used in
Skimmed milk powder	√	√	Milk shakes, milk drinks, on cereals, white sauces like custard or parsley sauce, milk puddings
Cream	X	√	Sauces, soups, mashed potato, stews and casseroles. Desserts or fruit smoothies
Crème fraîche	X	√	As above
Grated cheese	√	√	Mashed potato, sprinkled on soups, cheese sauce
Butter/margarine	X	√	Mashed potato, dotted on vegetables, spread liberally on bread or toast
Full cream milk in place of low-fat milk	X	√	Beverages, milk shakes, on cereals and in cooking
Glucose	X	√	As a substitute for ordinary sugar. It is less sweet so can use twice as much **Do not use for people with diabetes or impaired glucose tolerance**
Liquidised meat and poultry	√	√	Soups, gravies, sauces as well as stews and casseroles
Pulses including baked beans	√	√	Soups, stews, casseroles and gravy
Smooth peanut butter	√	√	As above
Full-fat yoghurt	√	√	Stews, casseroles, fruit smoothies
Full-fat mayonnaise, salad crème	X	√	Sandwich/jacket potato fillings

swallowing. An individual's nutritional requirements may increase as a result of disease, for example, cystic fibrosis or during episodes of mania/hyperactivity. Medications also affect the overall nutritional intake. Food and fluids may need to be enriched in order to maintain nutritional status.

★ *Skimmed milk powder is a good source of protein and calcium, can be added to drinks and sauces without increasing satiety.*

The protein and energy content of ordinary meals on the menu can be improved in quick and easy ways. The same choices can be offered from the menu but with the addition of readily available ingredients. See Table 15.3.

★ *Liquidised fruit drinks are a good way to increase vitamin and mineral intake. Add a carrot as well for extra vitamin A.*

Modified texture. To meet the body's needs for nutrients, the person must be able to chew and safely swallow enough food and fluids in order to satisfy individual metabolic demands. If the person has difficulties with swallowing, some of the indications include:

- choking;
- coughing during or just after eating/drinking;
- regurgitation;
- frequent chest infections; and
- 'bubbly chest'.

If any of the mentioned indications are present then seek advice from the speech and language therapist. A modified texture diet may be advised. The dietitian may also be involved to undertake a full nutrition assessment. Should the person need to follow a modified texture/consistency diet with or without thickened fluids then the advice given may be based on the agreed national descriptors produced by the British Dietetic Association and the Royal College of Speech and Language Therapists (British Dietetic Association, 2003). These are summarised in Tables 15.4 and 15.5.

★ Pureed food requires fortification to increase calorie and or protein content of the diet.

High-risk foods

- Food with a stringy fibrous texture such as pineapple, runner beans, celery and lettuce.
- Vegetable and fruit skins, beans such as broad beans, baked and soya, black-eyed peas, garden peas, tomatoes and grapes.
- Mixed consistency foods such as cereals which do not blend with milk, for example, muesli. Minced beef with thin gravy, soup with lumps.
- Crunchy foods such as toast, flaky pastry, dry biscuits and crisps.
- Crumbly items such as bread crusts, pie crusts, crumble and dry biscuits.
- Hard foods such as boiled sweets, chewy sweets and toffees, nuts and seeds.
- Husks such as sweetcorn and granary bread.

Thickeners

Some foods become too runny when they are pureed and may require the addition of thickeners to achieve a uniform consistency and appropriate texture. Natural food thickeners may be used, for example, cornflour, arrowroot, instant mashed potato, or alternatively a commercial thickening product can be obtained on prescription.

★ Follow manufacturer's instructions carefully as some thickeners continue to thicken after mixing.

Commercial thickeners as recommended by the SALT or dietitian can be used to alter the consistency of beverages as well. See Table 15.5.

Table 15.4 National descriptors for food textures.

Texture	Key points
Texture A – liquidised	Food needs to be liquidised/pureed to a smooth, pouring consistency. It should be of a uniform consistency, similar to cream of tomato soup or thin custard The mixture should be sieved to ensure any remaining lumps, skin, bones or bits of food are removed **Avoid high-risk foods**
Texture B – puree	Food is pureed to a smooth consistency which drops rather than pours from the spoon. It should be a similar consistency to soft whipped cream or thick custard It is advisable to sieve all foods to ensure any remaining lumps, skin, bones or bits of food are removed A thickener may be required to maintain the stability **Avoid high-risk foods**
Texture C – soft smooth/puree	Food is smooth, soft and thick enough to eat off a fork or spoon. It should be a similar consistency to smooth, creamed mashed potato or a mousse will hold its own shape on a plate The puree food can be moulded, layered or piped. Requires no chewing. It is advisable to sieve foods to ensure there are no lumps **Avoid high-risk foods**
Texture D – moist/mashable	Food should be soft and moist with some variation in texture. It should be of similar consistency to stewed apple and thick custard or flaked fish in sauce Meat will require pureeing in order to make it soft enough. Requires little or no chewing and be soft enough to be easily mashed with a fork **Avoid high-risk foods**
Texture E – soft diet	Food should be soft and moist enough to be broken into small pieces with a fork. Requires some chewing The addition of a thick gravy/sauce for savoury foods or custard/double cream may be required to moisten the food Dishes can have mixed consistencies, i.e. solids and sauces/gravies, e.g. casseroles **Avoid high-risk foods**

Reproduced from *Nutrition and Modified Diets*, 20–28, copyright 2006, with permission of the Department of Nutrition and Dietetics (East Division) ABM NHS Trust.

Method 2: supplementary feeding

Oral dietary supplements are usually provided in the form of milk or fruit-based energy and nutrient-dense drinks (Green, 2000). They are often called 'sip-feeds' and can be available on prescription. However, the provision of such supplements needs to be carefully considered as there is evidence to indicate that they are being used inappropriately and without any evaluation of their effectiveness (Kayser-Jones et al., 1998; McCombie, 1999; National Institute for Clinical Excellence, 2006). Bartholomew et al. (2003) have developed a hierarchy of nutrition support

Table 15.5 Consistency of beverages.

Texture	Key points
Stage 1	To be drunk through a straw
	Can be drunk from a cup if advised/preferred
	Leaves a thin coat on the back of a spoon
Stage 2	To be taken from a cup
	Leaves a thick coat on back of a spoon
Stage 3	To be taken with a spoon

Source: British Dietetic Association (2003).

to assist in the decision-making process as there are many reasons for a poor intake including a carer's lack of cooking skills. The hierarchy of nutrition support for the community is shown in Table 15.6.

★ *Prescribed sip feeds are not meal replacements (unless directed by the dietitian) and are for named individual use only.*

Method 3: enteral tube feeding

When the person is unable orally to take enough nutrition (including fluids) to satisfy their own metabolic requirements then administering nutrition via a feeding tube is indicated. This may be due to loss of appetite, malabsorption, intermittent or permanent memory loss, dysphagia or chewing difficulties where the consumption of ordinary food and fluids is either inadequate and/or results in aspiration which compromises the safety of that person (National Patient Safety Agency, 2004).

Such ETF is possible as long as the person has a functioning gastrointestinal tract, as with other procedures; consent is required as identified within Chapter 1.

Routes of administration

Feeding tubes can be inserted along different parts of the gastrointestinal tract depending on the person's clinical condition and the length of time that such feeding will be required. Nasogastric feeding is considered a short-term measure with gastrostomy used in the longer term.

Table 15.6 The hierarchy of nutrition support for the community.

Alteration of meal size, texture and frequency of meals
Alteration of cooking practices
Supplementation of foods using normal household ingredients
Use of home-made sip feeds
Supplementation with prescribed products under the supervision of the dietitian

Reproduced from *British Journal of Nursing*, Introduction of a Community Nutrition Risk Assessment Tool, 12(b), 351–358, copyright 2003 with permission of BJN.

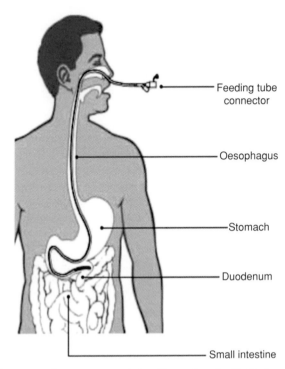

Feeding tube
connector

Oesophagus

Stomach

Duodenum

Small intestine

Figure 15.5 Placement of a naso-enteric tube. (Reproduced with kind permission from Abbott Nutrition, 2001.)

Orogastric: This is used in infants whereby the tube is passed through the mouth and into the stomach before each feed and then removed to reduce the risk of aspiration.

Naso-enteric: A tube inserted through the nose into the stomach (nasogastric) or into the duodenum (nasoduodenal) or into the jejunum (nasojejunal placement).

Figure 15.5 shows the position of a feeding tube after insertion through the nasal cavity into the gastrointestinal tract. The actual position will vary depending on the tube used and may end up resting in the stomach, duodenum or the jejunum.

Enterostomy: This describes an opening into the stomach or jejunum through which the tube is passed. The technique for creating a gastrostomy under local anaesthetic is called percutaneous endoscopic gastrostomy (PEG). Likewise a je-junostomy under local anaesthetic is called a percutaneous endoscopic jejunostomy (PEJ).

★ *Most people with PIMDs who are enterally tube fed will have a gastrostomy tube in situ.*

Figure 15.6 shows the position of the PEG after insertion through the skin and stomach wall into the stomach, a procedure which takes place under local or general anaesthetic.

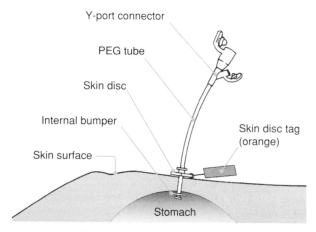

Y-port connector

PEG tube

Skin disc

Internal bumper

Skin disc tag
(orange)

Skin surface

Stomach

Figure 15.6 Position of the PEG tube. (Reproduced with kind permission from Abbott Nutrition, 2001.)

Feeding tubes

These are available in a variety of diameters and lengths, and the one used will depend on the route of administration, the individual's age and more importantly in people with PIMDs, body size and any anatomical variances such as scoliosis.

Other feeding equipment

A range of feeding equipment known as plastics or ancillaries is required which includes:

- administration or 'giving' sets;
- right-angled feeding sets;
- syringes;
- feeding pumps; and
- oral/enteral syringes

Unlike the enteral tube feed, the ancillaries are not available on prescription.

In preparing the person for home enteral tube feeding, the dietitian will provide a written explanation of the feeding regimen as well as the person's requirements for ancillaries and their span of use. However for the continued safety of each person on ETF whether in home or hospital, it is vital that the correct equipment and in particular syringes are used for the administration of bolus feeds and/or medicines (National Patient Safety Agency, 2007). Delivery of feed and ancillaries again is subject to variation though is often via a contracted ETF company home-delivery service.

★ *Liquid preparations of medications should be used wherever possible to reduce the risk of particles blocking the enteral feeding tube.*

Feeding regimens

Enteral feeds are prescribed formulations in sterile containers. They contain the recommended nutrients in a set volume and vary in their composition. For example, a feed can be classed as being one of the following, though many variations are available:

- Standard feed – 1 kcal/mL
- Complete feed – 1 or 1.2 kcal/mL with full complement of vitamins, minerals and fibre in 1 or 1.2 L of feed
- High-energy feed – 1.5 kcal/mL
- Concentrated – 2 kcal/mL
- High-fibre feed – 1 to 1.5 kcal/mL
- Elemental feed – rarely used

★ *Only sterile feed preparations are put down the ETF tubes. No liquidised food items.*

The preparation chosen by the dietitian will be matched to the individual's (adult or paediatric) nutritional needs. The feeding regimen will be planned by the dietitian and will include the following:

- The individual's nutritional goals
- Type of feed to be used
- Total volume per 24 hours
- Rate of administration in mL/hour
- Mode of administration, i.e. continuous pump-assisted feeding or bolus feeding with or without pump
- Volume of pre-feed and post-feed flushes
- Volume of premedication and postmedication flushes
- Additional water to ensure fluid requirements are met
- Type of water to use
- Addition of any supplements such as a fat emulsion to increase the energy content of the chosen feed

★ *Freshly drawn tap water or cooled boiled water may be used in ETF except in jejunostomy feeding when only sterile water should be used.*

Recent recommendations advise monitoring every 3–6 months for individuals who are stable (Todorovic & Micklewright, 2004; National Institute for Clinical Excellence, 2006). However, local variations will apply and close liaison between the intellectual disabilities nurse and the dietitian is essential for the continued well-being of the person with PIMDs.

Administration of medications in ETF

If the individual is still able to swallow safely then oral medications should still continue to be taken this way. When drugs need to be administered via a feeding tube, the following steps will help to ensure safe practice. For adults a 50-mL oral/enteral syringe is usually recommended as smaller syringes can collapse or split a feeding tube due to too much pressure being exerted (British Association for Parenteral and Enteral Nutrition and the British Pharmaceutical Nutrition Group, 2004). In order to minimise the risk of tube occlusion, it is recommended that a pulsating flushing technique is used (White & Bradnam, 2007):

- If the person is on continuous feeding, switch off the feed.
- Flush tube with *at least* 30-mL water.[a]
- Prepare medicines as instructed – see Table 15.7.
- Administer one medication at a time.
- Flush tube after each administration of a drug with *at least* 10-mL water.[a]
- Flush tube with at least 30-mL water[a] after last drug given.
- Check to see if there needs to be a break before restarting the feed.
- Restart the feed.

Table 15.7   Preparing medicines for administration via enteral feeding tube.

Drug presentation	Required preparation	Rationale
Soluble tablet	Dissolve in 10–15 mL water[a] Administer down the tube	Prevent tube blockage
Liquid	Shake well and for viscous liquids dilute with an equal volume of water[a] Administer immediately and do not allow to stand	Prevent tube blockage
Tablet	Crush[b,c] uncoated and sugar-coated preparations well using a pestle and mortar or equivalent Mix with 10–15 mL water[a] then administer down the tube Rinse container and draw up water into the syringe and flush down the tube[a]	Prevent tube blockage Ensure whole dose given
Capsule	Open capsule,[b,c] tip contents into medicine pot Mix with 10–15 mL water[a] then administer down the tube Rinse container and draw up water into the syringe and flush down the tube[a]	Prevent tube blockage Ensure whole dose given

[a]Cool boiled or sterile as per local instructions.
[b]Or as per local instructions.
[c]Crushing tablets and opening capsules usually falls outside a drug's product licence. In such cases the prescriber and the practitioner accept liability for any adverse effects experienced by the client as a result of such administration.

★ *Correct tube flushing techniques with adequate volumes of water result in minimal tube occlusions.*

Method 4: parenteral feeding

Is a method of administration whereby nutrition is delivered via a central or peripheral vein, used when the person's gastrointestinal tract is non-functioning. It is a highly specialised mode of feeding and used rarely for a person with PIMDs.

In practice, even though PEJ feeding is starting to be used more especially in people who are at high risk of aspiration pneumonia, the most common mode of ETF to be encountered by the intellectual disabilities nurse will be via a PEG – especially in the case of people with gastro-oesophageal reflux disorder (GORD) which is a significant problem for children and adults with PIMDs (Morton et al., 1999; Glasgow University Affiliation Programme, 2002). GORD causes great discomfort and affects nutritional status by altering the person's eating habits. The presence of GORD and direct aspiration (DA) of food due to oral and pharyngeal motor problems indicates the likelihood of the need for a PEG.

People with epilepsy and challenging behaviour (CB) may have a PEG inserted to be used during times when food and/or fluid is refused. In epilepsy, for example, some people remain 'flat' for days and not able to take nutrition orally. Challenging behaviour can be exhibited in any person with PIMDs if the situation is conducive (Field & Lohr, 1990). The nutritional implications of CB can be due to adipsia, breath holding, pica, incontinence, repetitive movements and teeth grinding (Didden et al., 1997). When behaviour escalates, staff may be unable to persuade the person to eat or drink and medication may make oral intake impossible. PEG feeding may then be used on a *prn* or *pro nata* basis in order that nutrition and hydration are maintained during periods of crisis.

There are many other conditions/syndromes impacting on the nutritional status of people with PIMDs where the adequacy of an individual's diet is such that supplementation or artificial tube feeding may be required. These are summarised in Table 15.8.

The main exception to this will be the person with Prader-Willi syndrome (PWS) which is characterised by a compulsion to eat and drink at all times. The individual is driven to episodic binging and continuously seeking out sources of food to try and reach satiety, which unfortunately very rarely occurs.

As discussed by Gravestock (2000), binge eating as well as other behaviours symptomatic of eating disorders (EDs) including pica, extreme food faddiness or refusal and rumination/regurgitation have not received much attention or study in people with an intellectual disability, apart from PWS, and have been all too readily subsumed as part and parcel of any underlying genetic syndrome or CB. However, professionals and carers need to have access to training to increase awareness of ED and how to refer to specialised services for the continued well-being of the people they support. Up to 19% of adults have diagnosable ED in the community with up to 35% having obesity and up to 43% being significantly underweight. Even

Table 15.8 Nutritional consequences of syndromes associated with an intellectual disability.

Key syndrome	Symptoms affecting nutritional status	Nutritional consequences	Issues	Action
Autistic spectrum disorder A lifelong disability affecting social and communication skills, often accompanying some degree of intellectual disability The 'triad of impairments': 1. Poor social interaction 2. Poor social communication 3. Poor imagination	Need very structured environment Obsessive desire for order and familiarity Rigid thinking Inflexible Cannot cope with change Easily distracted from eating, changed visual perceptions Poor social skills	Eating will be affected by changes in routine Very fussy with food choices, obsessions with one colour or flavour Eating in different environments, such as at home, at school or college will affect their willingness to eat Won't try unfamiliar foods Some individuals may be sensitive to additives such as caffeine, food colourings and preservatives (Vojdani et al., 2003) Problems with self-feeding, want to eat all day rather than just at mealtimes	Limited variety of foods. Confused by choice Position of food on the plate has to be the same Will gorge on foods they do like Challenging behaviour may be caused by some food colourings and preservatives though evidence is anecdotal Various 'special dietary modifications' have been recommended for the treatment of autism (Richardson, 2004). These may be beneficial in some cases although the evidence is limited	Detailed nutritional assessment by specialist dietitian especially with individuals who eat less than 20 different foods (Isherwood & Thomas, 2002) Individual eating plans with regular monitoring and review Identification of nutritional deficiencies A multi-professional approach to feeding issues, especially in children, is essential with involvement from general practitioner, psychology, SALT, occupational therapist, home carers, school staff and the extended family to ensure adequate nutrition
Cerebral palsy Disability resulting from damage to the brain before, during or shortly after birth. Outwardly manifested by muscular un-coordination and speech disturbances. People with cerebral palsy may or may not have an intellectual disability	Children with spastic and dyskinetic cerebral palsy have problems with muscular control. This affects sucking, swallowing, chewing and also bowel action	As babies they are hard to feed and have faltering growth. This is often a lifelong trait. Consequently they have issues with nutrition and development (Sullivan & Rosenbloom, 1996)	Texture modification, food supplementation and ultimately enteral feeding may be required to maintain health and quality of life	Dietetic intervention and regular monitoring are needed. Close liaison and coordination between health professionals to support the whole family is essential

(continued)

Table 15.8 (Continued) Nutritional consequences of syndromes associated with an intellectual disability.

Key syndrome	Symptoms affecting nutritional status	Nutritional consequences	Issues	Action
Down syndrome A congenital condition caused by the presence of an extra chromosome. Characterised by a moderate to severe intellectual disability, distinct facial and physical characteristics plus a range of health problems	People with Down syndrome are seen to age more quickly, which affects their appetite and enjoyment of food (Holland & Benton, 2004) Diabetes and coeliac disease are more common in the Down syndrome population (Book et al., 2001; Selby, 2001)	Babies are difficult to feed, floppy and frail (Marder, 1996)	Feeding difficulties when young Good nutrition essential for healthy immune systems Weight control and long-chain omega-3 fatty acids valuable for healthy cardiac systems (Siscovick et al., 2000) Adequate fibre intake aids gut motility and reduces incidence of constipation (Cohen, 1999) Diet forms an essential part of treatment in diabetes and is the complete treatment in coeliac disease. Correct dietetic support, appropriate information, training of carers and regular monitoring by dietitian are essential Sudden onset of ageing can affect nutritional intake and has a dramatic effect on weight (Yang et al., 2003)	Paediatric dietitians assess, advise and monitor feeding in babies and children with Down syndrome if there are problems Specialist dietitians can assess, educate and motivate carers and individuals they support to ensure that a healthy well-balanced diet is followed Any extra nutritional needs can be identified and advice is given to ensure appropriate intakes are maintained

Epilepsy Characterised by disturbances in brain function causing repeated brain seizures manifesting as episodic loss of consciousness, abnormal motor phenomena, psychic or sensory disturbances. Many people with intellectual disabilities also experience some form of epilepsy	30–50% people with intellectual disabilities have some form of epilepsy (Department of Health, 2001).	Tonic-clonic seizures where convulsions and loss of consciousness can affect food intake, resulting in poor nutritional status	Loss of consciousness can mean that meals may be missed. Either repeated or intense seizures can cause significant weight loss In children with epilepsy who are resistant to medication, there is some evidence to indicate that a ketogenic diet may be helpful (Freeman et al., 1998)	Epileptic seizures must be considered as the cause of unexplained weight loss. In some cases supplemental feeding and possibly enteral feeding may be necessary Ketogenic diets (high fat, low carbohydrate) are complex and difficult to establish and maintain. Experienced paediatric dietetic, medical and biochemical monitoring is essential

Dietetic advice is essential when diabetes or coeliac disease is diagnosed. The specialist dietitian in intellectual disabilities has the skills essential to provide adequate and ongoing advice and support to all personnel involved with support for the individual

(*continued*)

Table 15.8 (Continued) Nutritional consequences of syndromes associated with an intellectual disability.

Key syndrome	Symptoms affecting nutritional status	Nutritional consequences	Issues	Action
Prader-Willi syndrome This is a complex genetic disorder, characterised by poor muscle tone, immature physical and sexual development. People with PWS become emotionally unstable, have excessive appetites and some degree of intellectual disability	A disruption in the function of the hypothalamus results in the inability to recognise satiety. Consequently, people with PWS are at risk of morbid obesity Babies born with PWS are often frail and have problems suckling	Excessive weight gain begins between the ages of 1 and 6 years when parents see that their children are now eating well and find it difficult to accept guidelines on food restriction (Prader-Willi Association of Australia, 2005) Behavioural problems, such as tantrums and obsessive-compulsive disorder, will also affect the way parents cope with their child who has PWS. People with PWS have an obsessive compulsion to eat and can resort to pica if food is unavailable (Einfeld et al., 1999) Because of poor muscle tone they lead inactive lives. Their requirements for energy are often less than their non-PWS peers Hormone replacement therapy often required for delayed or incomplete puberty can also affect weight gain	Global developmental delay affects mobility in children. If appropriate advice and support is provided to parents of young children and strict guidelines set in place at an early age, people with PWS need not become obese. Access to health promotion information at an early age is essential A number of obese young PWS are diagnosed with maturity onset diabetes of the young and often require insulin Increased risk of osteoporosis, dental caries and abdominal disorders, such as appendicitis, can be missed because of their high pain tolerance (Gellatley, 1996)	In PWS the MPT is essential to provide lifelong support

Rett syndrome This is a childhood neurodevelopmental disorder characterised by an apparently normal child developing symptoms between 7 and 18 months of age such as loss of purposeful use of hands, hand flapping, poor muscle tone, gastric abnormalities, seizures and a degree of intellectual disability (Nomura and Segawa, 2005) Occurs almost exclusively in girls (Renieria et al., 2003)	Problems with the mechanics of eating. Breathing issues, e.g. hyperventilation and breath holding Biting, chewing, swallowing and self-feeding are all affected by very poor muscle tone	Babies are born poor sucklers and have faltering growth Majority of surviving babies are female Nutritional intake is an issue from birth	Poor food intakes and poor muscle tone mean that texture modification of food and thickened drinks may be needed. They will often need to be fed which is time-consuming Constipation is also very common	Dietary adequacy is paramount and regular assessments needed during childhood to support growth SALT intervention to identify appropriate texture will be needed Dietary interventions to consider appropriate fibre and micronutrient intakes are important into adulthood
Tourette syndrome A neurological disease of unknown origin characterised by chronic muscular tics, vocal tics and is socially stigmatising. Often combined with obsessive-compulsive behaviour and attention deficiency disorder	See 'Autistic spectrum disorder'	Nutritional intakes are likely to be poor Many individuals will have feeding issues	Psychological aspects affecting food intake Physical problems affecting eating and feeding.	The MPT will provide essential support to families and individuals
Fragile X syndrome An inhibited mental development, moderate to severe intellectual disability. Autistic-like behaviour with physical and behavioural features and delayed speech	See 'Autistic spectrum disorder'	Nutritional intake may be poor		The MPT will provide essential support to families and individuals

(continued)

Table 15.8 (Continued) Nutritional consequences of syndromes associated with an intellectual disability.

Key syndrome	Symptoms affecting nutritional status	Nutritional consequences	Issues	Action
Non-treated phenylketonuria (PKU) PKU is a rare inherited condition in which there is a build-up of the essential amino acid phenylalanine in the blood stream due to an enzyme deficiency. High levels of phenylalanine in the blood can affect brain development. Since 1969 all babies born in the UK are given the Guthrie test at between 6 and 14 days after birth	People who have not had dietetic treatment for PKU suffer brain damage and severe intellectual disabilities They often have CB, food aversions and low body weight	Challenging behaviours affect food intake	It is possible to reintroduce a low-phenylalanine diet which can improve nutritional status and cognitive abilities in some individuals (MacDonald, 2006)	The specialist dietitian's knowledge and experience is essential to establish the low-phenylalanine diet. Consistent monitoring and thorough training of staff and carers is essential (National Society of Phenylketonuria, 2004)
Klinefelter syndrome Males have an extra X chromosome (Smyth & Bremner, 1998)	Reduced muscle power and stamina and intellectual disabilities	More prone to depression, thyroid disease, diabetes, osteoporosis, asthma and heart disease (Horowitz et al., 1992)	These individuals are often difficult to feed, get tired easily and need carers to be patient and persevere with feeding	Nutritional status needs constant monitoring

though the prevalence amongst people with PIMDs is unknown, we need to accept the possibility that EDs do exist and take the appropriate action.

Conclusion

Nutritional status in children and adults with PIMDs is an essential component of care, and both over- and undernutrition are the most common nutritional pathologies (Stallings & Zemel, 1996). Eating and drinking are fundamental essentials to life. We all need to consume a range of nutrients such as protein, carbohydrate, fat, vitamins, minerals, fibre and fluid to supply the body with the vital resources required for anatomical, physiological and psychological functioning. People with profound and multiple intellectual disabilities are no different with respect to their requirements for nutrition excellence though require more support from a range of professional and non-professional staff to enable them achieve and maintain correct nutritional balance.

The challenge that lies before us is to be cognisant of the value of maximising each person's nutritional status and to be aware of the vital role we play in this process. All members of the MPT need to be sensitive to any changes in eating and drinking habits at an early stage so that the relevant health professionals can be involved and effective nutrition strategies implemented.

As a key member of the MPT, the nurse trained in intellectual disabilities is ideally situated to take forward such strategies to identify any nutritional problems, due to their close involvement with the people they support. This could be by observation at mealtimes or just listening to the person. In her address to the World Health Organization, Johansson, representing Inclusion International (Sweden), vocalised her belief that all people can and want to communicate and that it is up to professionals and carers to help people with profound intellectual disabilities to do so (Johansson, 2001).

Any concerns regarding eating behaviour should be documented and a referral made to the dietitian as soon as possible. Good communication and close partnership working with the dietitian can help to stem any insidious decline in nutritional status.

Remember that people who are dependent on others for their nutrition are at greater risk of unintentional nutritional inadequacies as a result of many factors (Thomas & Bishop, 2007). These include:

- lack of variety leading to taste fatigue;
- being fed too quickly;
- inappropriate textures being offered;
- inflexible mealtimes;
- being overfaced with large meals;
- insufficient time given to eat and drink;
- too frequent use of ready meals due to inexperience of carers;
- lack of attention to personal likes and dislikes; and
- insufficient monitoring of food and fluid intake including ETF.

In conclusion, all members of the MPT have a responsibility to ensure that each individual's nutritional status is preserved irrespective of any difficulties encountered in eating or the need for alternative feeding practices such as PEG. Poor nutrition must not be an accepted consequence for the person with profound and multiple intellectual disabilities.

Appendices

Appendix 15.1   Medications commonly used in intellectual disabilities and their effect on nutritional status.

Type of drug	Examples of drug	Nutritional-related side effects
Antipsychotics	Chlorpromazine HCl Clozaril Haloperidol Risperidone	Drowsiness, apathy, confusion, depression Gastrointestinal disturbances, dry mouth, weight gain
Anticonvulsants/ antiepileptics	Carbamazepine[a] Lamotrigine Topiramate Phenytoin[a]	Nausea, vomiting, constipation, diarrhoea, abdominal pain, oedema, appetite changes, confusion, weight gain, dry mouth, weight loss
Antidepressants – tricyclics	Amitriptyline Imipramine	Loss of appetite, constipation, weight gain, dry mouth
Antidepressants – monoamine-oxidase inhibitors	Phenelzine Isocarboxazid Tranylcypromine	As above plus strict adherence to special diet as certain foods need to be avoided
Antidepressants – selective serotonin re-uptake inhibitors	Citalopram Paroxetine Fluoxetine	Taste disturbance, increased salivation, rhinitis Fluoxetine – changes in blood sugars
Anxiolytics	Diazepam Lorazepam	Salivation changes, constipation, diarrhoea, vomiting
Hypnotics	Chloral hydrate Nitrazepam Temazepam	Drowsiness, confusion, gastric irritation
Antimuscarinics	Atropine sulphate Dicycloverine HCl Hyoscine	Constipation, dry mouth, nausea, vomiting
Mood stabilisers	Lithium carbonate Lithium citrate	Weight gain, excessive thirst, oedema
Laxatives – bulk forming	Ispaghula husk Methyl cellulose	Flatulence, abdominal distension, gastrointestinal obstruction or impaction
Laxatives – stimulant	Bisacodyl Senna	Diarrhoea, hypokalaemia
Laxatives – osmotic	Movicol Lactulose	Long-term use can interfere with the absorption of fat-soluble vitamins. Flatulence, abdominal discomfort

Source: Joint Formulary Committee (2007).
[a]Interacts with tube feeding. Feed to be stopped 2 hours before and after each dose.

Appendix 15.2   Guidelines for healthy eating.

Food	Amount	Notes
Bread, breakfast cereal, potato, pasta, rice	At least one portion at each meal	Offer a variety of wholemeal and white bread. Pasta, rice and instant potato are useful store cupboard items.
Vegetables, salad, fruit	At least one portion a day	Aim for 5 portions of fruit & vegetables each day. Tinned and frozen fruit & vegetables can be used for convenience.
Meat, fish, egg, beans	Two to three portions a day	Try to have oily fish, e.g. pilchards, mackerel, sardines at least once a week. Choose lean meats and cut off any visible fat
Milk, cheese and dairy foods	Two portions a day	Semi-skimmed milk is generally recommended. Powdered or long-life milk is useful, store cupboard items
Butter, margarine, spread	Limit amount	Both contain similar amounts of fat – do not use too much. Or use a low-fat spread.
Food containing sugar	Limit amount	
Fluids	Eight cups or glasses per day	Water, unsweetened juice or squash, milk, tea, coffee

Reproduced with kind permission from the Community Dietitians, Bristol South & West NHS Primary Care Trust, copyright 2006.

Further reading

Bamford Review of Mental Health and Learning Disability (Northern Ireland) (2005). Available at: http://www.rmhldni.gov.uk/ (accessed 1 July 2008).

Barasi, M. (2007). *Nutrition at a Glance*. London: Wiley-Blackwell.

Crawley, H. (2007). *Eating Well for Children and Adults with Learning Disabilities*. Abbots Langley: Caroline Walker Trust.

General Medical Council. *Withholding and Withdrawing Life-Prolonging Treatments: Good Practice in Decision-Making*. Available at: http://www.gmc-uk.org/guidance/library/witholding_and_withdrawing/witholding_lifeprolonging_guidance.asp (accessed 30 September 2007).

Bro Morgannwg Inclusive Communication Initiative (2006). *Health Challenge Wales – Accessible Information on Healthy Living*. Available at: http://new.wales.gov.uk/subsite/healthchallenge/resource/accessible-info/?lang=en (accessed 30 September 2007).

Hirano, I., & Richter, J.E. (2007). Practice parameters committee of the American College of Gastroenterology. ACG practice guidelines: esophageal reflux testing. *American Journal of Gastroenterology*, 102(3), 668–685.

Learning Disabilities Advisory Group (2001). *Fulfilling the Promises*. Cardiff: LDAG.

Royal College of Nursing (2006). *Meeting the Health Needs of People with Learning Disabilities: Guidance for Nursing Staff*. London: RCN Publication.

Scottish Executive (2000). *The Same as You*. Available at: http://www.scotland.gov.uk/ldsr/docs/tsay-00.asp (accessed 3 October 2007).

Welsh Assembly Government (2007). *Statement on Policy and Practice for Adults with a Learning Disability.* Cardiff: WAG.

Useful websites

Bristol Learning Difficulties Website – http://www.bristollearningdifficulties.nhs.uk/
British Association for Parenteral and Enteral Nutrition – http://www.bapen.org.uk/
British Dietetic Association – http://www.bda.uk.com/
Children – http://www.pinnt.com/halfpinnt_main.htm
Clear – consultancy group working to provide advice and training regarding making information accessible – http://www.clearforall.co.uk/
National Association for Epilepsy – http://www.epilepsynse.org.uk/
Parenteral and Enteral Nutrition Group – http://www.peng.org.uk/
Patients on Intravenous and Nasogastric Nutrition Therapy Adults – http://www.pinnt.com/
Rett Syndrome Association – website of the national association – http://www.rettsyndrome.org.uk/
SCOPE – disability organisation for cerebral palsy in England and Wales – http://www.scope.org.uk/
The Caroline Walker Trust – website providing dietetic information particularly targeted towards vulnerable groups and people who need special help – http://www.cwt.org.uk/index.html

References

Bartholomew, C.M., Burton, S., & Davidson, L.M. (2003). Introduction of a community nutrition risk assessment tool. *British Journal of Nursing*, 12(6), 351–358.

Book, L., Hart, A., Black, J., Feolo, M., Zone, J.J., & Neuhausen, S.L. (2001). Prevalence and clinical character of coeliac disease in Down's syndrome. *American Journal of Medical Genetics*, 98(1), 70–74.

Bradley, S. (2005). Tackling obesity in people with learning disability. *Learning Disability Practice*, 8(7), 10–14.

British Association for Parenteral and Enteral Nutrition and The British Pharmaceutical Nutrition Group (2004). *Administering Drugs Via Enteral Feeding Tubes: A Practical Guide.* Available at: http://www.bapen.org.uk/pdfs/drugs%26enteral/practical-guide-poster.pdf (accessed 3 August 2006).

British Dietetic Association (2003). *National Descriptors for Texture Modification in Adults.* Birmingham: British Dietetic Association and the Royal College of Speech and Language Therapists.

British Dietetic Association (2006). *BMI Calculator.* Available at: http://www.bdaweightwise.com/lose/lose_bmi.aspx (accessed 9 August 2006).

Bryan, F., Allan, T., & Russell, L. (2000). The move from long-stay learning disability hospital to community homes; a comparison of clients nutritional status. *Journal of Human Nutrition and Dietetics*, 13(4), 265–270.

Bryan, F., Jones, J.M., & Russell, L. (1996). Reliability and validity of a nutrition screening tool to be used with clients with learning difficulties. *Journal of Human Nutrition and Dietetics*, 11(1), 41–50.

Campbell, M.K., & Kelsey, K.S. (1994). The PEACH survey: a nutrition screening tool for use in early intervention. *Journal of the American Dietetic Association*, 94 (10), 1156–1158.

Carter, C., Allott, K., Almond, S., Hall, K., Stewart, L., & Shaw, V. (2006). *Enteral Feeding in Children with Cerebral Palsy*. Wiltshire: Nutricia Clinical Care.

Claydon, G. (1996). Constipation in disabled children. In Sullivan, P.B., & Rosenbloom, X. (eds), *Feeding the Disabled Child*. London: MacKeith Press; 106–116.

Cohen, W.I. (1999). Health care guidelines for individuals with Down syndrome. *Down Syndrome Quarterly*, 4(3), 1–16.

Department of Health (2001). *Valuing People – A New Strategy for Learning Disability for the 21st Century*. London: HMSO.

Dickson, K. (2002). Moving on, an important relationship between levels of staff training and diets among people with learning disabilities. *Learning Disability Practice*, 5 (2), 11–13.

Didden, R., Duker, P., & Korzilius, H. (1997). Meta-analytic study on treatment effects for problem behaviours with individuals who have mental retardation. *American Journal of Mental Retardation*, 101(4), 387–399.

DiMascio, F., Hamilton, K., & Smith, L. (2004). *The Nutritional Care of Adults with a Learning Disability in Care Settings – A Professional Consensus Statement*. Birmingham: British Dietetic Association.

Einfeld, S.L., Smith, A., Durvasala, S., Florio, T., & Tonge B.J. (1999). Behaviour and emotional disturbances in Prader-Willi syndrome. *American Journal of Medical Genetics*, 82(2), 123–127.

Field, M.J., & Lohr, K.N. (eds) (1990). *Clinical Practice Guidelines: Directions for a New Program*. Washington, DC: National Academy Press.

Freeman, J.M., Vining, E.P.G., Pillas, D.J., & Pyzik, P.L. (1998). The efficacy of the ketogenic diet. *Pediatrics*, 102(6), 1358–1363.

Gellatley, M. (1996). *How to Provide a Healthy Diet for People with Prader-Willi*. London: Prader-Willi Association.

Glasgow University Affiliation Programme (2002). *The Contribution of Practice Nurses to Support the Health Needs of People with Learning Disabilities*. Glasgow: University of Glasgow.

Grandjean, A. (2004). *Water Requirements, Impinging Factors and Recommended Intakes*. World Health Organisation. Available at: http://www.who.int/water_sanitation_health/dwq/nutwaterrequir.pdf (accessed 18 August 2006).

Gravestock, S. (2000). Eating disorders in adults with intellectual disability. *Journal of Intellectual Disability Research*, 44(6), 625–637.

Green, S. (2000). Oral dietary supplements. *JCN Online*, 14 (3), 1–5. Available at: http://www.jcn.co.uk (accessed 5 July 2006).

Hartley, H., & Thomas, J.E. (2003). Current practice in the management of children with cerebral palsy: a national survey of paediatric dietitians. *Journal of Human Nutrition and Dietetics*, 16(4), 219–224.

Holland, T., & Benton, M. (2004). *Ageing and Its Consequences for People with Down's Syndrome*. Middlesex: Down's Syndrome Association Publication.

Horowitz, M., Wishart, J.M., O'Loughlin, P.D., Morris, H.A., & Norden, B.E.(1992). Osteoporosis and Klinefelter's syndrome. *Clinical Endocrinology (Oxford)*, 36(1), 113–118.

Isherwood, E., & Thomas, K. (2002). *Dietary Management of Autistic Spectrum Disorder*. Birmingham: British Dietetic Association.

Jackson, E., & Jackson, N. (1999). *The Use of Photography in the Care of People with a Learning Disability*. London: Jessica Kingsley Publishers.

Johansson, E. (2001). *Rethinking Care: From the Perspective of Disabled People. Appendix 4: Presentations*. Available at: http://whqlibdoc.who.int/hq/2001/a78624_appendix4.pdf (accessed 12 August 2006).

Joint Formulary Committee. (2007). *British National Formulary* (54th edition). London: British Medical Association and Royal Pharmaceutical Society of Great Britain.

Kayser-Jones, J., Schell, E.S., Porter, C., Barbaccia, J.C., Steinbach, C., Bird, W.F., Redford, M., & Pengilly, K. (1998). A prospective study of the use of liquid oral dietary supplements in nursing homes. *Journal of the Geriatric Society*, 46(11), 1378–1386.

Krick, J., Murphy-Miller, P., Zeger, S., & Weight, E. (1996). *Pattern of Growth in Children with Cerebral Palsy*, 96(7), 680–685.

MacDonald, A. (2006). Phenylketonuria: practical dietary management. *Journal of Family Healthcare*, 16(3), 83–88.

Marder, L. (1996). *Gastro-intestinal Problems in Children with Down's Syndrome-Newsletter*. London: Down's Syndrome Association Publication.

McCombie, L. (1999). Sip feeding prescribing in primary care: an audit of current practice in greater Glasgow Health Board, Glasgow, U.K. *Journal of Human Nutrition and Dietetics*, 12(3), 201–212.

Melville, C.A., Cooper, S.A., McGrother, C.W., Thorp, C.F., & Collacott, R. (2005). Obesity in adults with Down syndrome. *Journal of Intellectual Disability Research*, 49(2), 125–133.

Morton, R.E., Wheatley, R., & Minford, J. (1999). Respiratory tract infections due to direct and reflux aspiration in children with severe neurodisability. *British Journal of Nursing*, 41(5), 329–334.

Mullen, R.L., Buzby, G.P., Matthews, D.C., Smale, B.F., & Rosata, E.F. (1979). Reduction of operative morbidity and mortality by preoperative nutritional assessment. *Surgical Forum*, 30(5), 80–82.

National Institute for Health and Clinical Excellence (2006). *Nutrition Support in Adults – Clinical Guideline 32*. London: National Institute for Health and Clinical Excellence.

National Patient Safety Agency (2004). *Understanding the Patient Safety Issues for People with Learning Disabilities*. London: NPSA.

National Patient Safety Agency (2007). *Promoting Safer Measurement and Administration of Liquid Medicines via Oral and Other Enteral Routes*. London: NPSA.

National Society of Phenylketonuria (2004). *Management of Phenylketonuria, Consensus Document for the Treatment and Management of Children, Adolescents and Adults with Phenylketonuria*. London: NSPKU.

Nelson, M.J., & Poulter, J. (2004). Impact of tea drinking on iron status in the U.K. *Journal of Human Nutrition and Dietetics*, 17(1), 43–52.

Nomura, Y., & Segawa, M. (2005). Natural history of Rett syndrome. *Journal of Child Neurology*, 20(9), 764–768.

Parsons, T. (2002). Weight management for health. *Learning Disability Practice*, 5(8), 28–37.

Prader-Willi Association of Australia (2005). *Management Strategies*. Available at: http://www.pws.org.au/general.html#judy (accessed 4 August 2006).

Renieria, A., Meloni, I., Longo, I., Ariani, F., Mari, F., Pescucci, C., & Cambi, F. (2003). Rett syndrome: then complex nature of a monogenic disease. *Journal of Molecular Medicine*, 81(6), 346–354.

Richardson, A.J. (2004). Clinical trials of fatty acid treatment in ADHD, dyslexia, dyspraxia and the autistic spectrum. *Prostaglandins, Leukotriennes and Essential Fatty Acids*, 70(4), 383–390.

Royal College of Nursing & National Patient Safety Agency (2007). *Water for Health: Hydration Best Practice Toolkit for Hospitals and Healthcare*. Available at: http://www2.rcn.

org.uk/__data/assets/pdf_file/0003/70374/Hydration_Toolkit_-_Entire_and_In_Order.pdf (accessed 30 September 2007).

Samson-Fang, L.J., & Stevenson, R.D. (2000). Identification of malnutrition in children with cerebral palsy: poor performance of weight-for-height centiles. *Developmental Medicine and Child Neurology*, 42(3), 162–168.

Selby, P. (2001). *Diabetes and Down's Syndrome*. Middlesex: Down's Syndrome Association Publication.

Siscovick, D.S., Raghunathan, T.E., King, I., Weinmann, S., Bovbjerg, V.E., Kushi, L., Cobb, L.A., Copass, M.K., Psaty, B.M., Lemaitre, R., Retzlaff, B., & Knopp, R.H. (2000). Dietary intake of long chain n-3 polyunsaturated fatty acids and the risk of primary cardiac disease. *American Journal of Clinical Nutrition*, 71(1), 2085–2125.

Smyth, C.M., & Bremner, W.J. (1998). Klinefelter syndrome. *Archives of Internal Medicine*, 158(12), 1309–1314.

Spender, Q.W., Cronk, C.E., Charney, E.B., & Stallings, V.A. (1989). Assessment of linear growth in children with cerebral palsy; use of alternative measures to height and length. *Developmental Medicine and Child Neurology*, 31(2), 206–214.

Stallings, V., & Zemel, B.S. (1996). Nutritional assessment of the disabled child. In Sullivan, P.B., & Rosenbloom, L. (eds), *Feeding the Disabled Child*. London: MacKeith Press, 62–76.

Stevenson, R.D. (1995). Use of segmented measures to estimate stature in children with cerebral palsy. *Archives of Pediatric and Adolescent Medicine*, 149(6), 658–662.

Stewart, L., McKaig, N., Dunlop, C., Daly, H., & Almond, S. (2006). *Dietetic Assessment and Monitoring of Children with Special Needs and Faltering Growth: A Professional Consensus Statement by The British Dietetic Association Specialist Paediatric Group*. Birmingham: The British Dietetic Association.

Sullivan, P.B., & Rosenbloom, L. (1996). An overview of the feeding difficulties experienced by disabled children. In Sullivan, P.B., & Rosenbloom, L. (eds), *Feeding the Disabled Child*. London: MacKeith Press; 1–10.

Thomas, A.G., & Akobeng, A.K. (2000). Technical aspects of feeding the disabled child. *Current Opinion in Clinical Nutrition and Metabolic Care*, 3(3), 221–225.

Thomas, B., & Bishop, J. (eds) (2007). *Manual of Dietetic Practice* (4th edition). London: Blackwell Sciences.

Todorovic, V., & Micklewright, A. (eds) (2004). *A Pocket Guide to Clinical Nutrition* (3rd edition). Birmingham: PEN Group Publications.

Vojdani, A., Pangborn, J.B., Vojdani, E., & Cooper, E.L. (2003). Infections, toxic chemicals & dietary peptides binding to lymphocyte receptors ans tissue enzymes are major instigators of autoimmunity in autism. *International Journal of Immunopathology and Pharmacology*, 16(3), 189–199.

Wake, E. (2003). People with profound and multiple disabilities. In Gates, B. (ed.), *Learning Disabilities: Toward Inclusion* (4th edition). London: Churchill Livingstone; 243–280.

White, R., & Bradnam, V. (2007). *Handbook of Drug Administration via Enteral Feeding Tubes*. London: Pharmaceutical Press.

Williams, S. (2005). Nutritional Screening by District Nurses. *JCN Online*, 19(5), 1–10. Available at: http://jcn.co.uk (accessed 5 July 2006).

Wright, C. (2002). Screening for undernutrition in the community. *JCN Online*, 16(4), 1–8. Available at: http://jcn.co.uk (accessed 5 July 2006).

Yang, D., Fontaine, K.R., Wang, C., & Allison, D.B. (2003). Weight loss causes increased mortality. *Obesity Reviews*, 4(1), 9–11.

Chapter 16

CONTINENCE

Jillian Pawlyn and Shirley Budd

Introduction

Although incontinence mainly affects women and older people, it is also recognised that people with long-term physical disabilities, neurological conditions and intellectual disabilities are also likely to have continence support needs and access to services may pose problems (DH, 2000). According to Earnshaw & Bates (2001), an estimated 3 million people suffer from urinary incontinence in the UK many of whom have an intellectual disability.

The development of continence where bladder and bowels are controlled is a complex learnt skill. Toilet training success relies on a development/maturational process. People with intellectual disabilities can benefit from developing habits and routines as well as prompting to use the toilet. Frequent acknowledgement of the desired behaviour will often result in the development of continence skills. It cannot be assumed that family and carers know how to achieve these skills; therefore professionals providing support and advice need the knowledge and skills to be able to complete a continence assessment, understand the issues of the individual and then be able to provide a care plan that will promote continence, manage incontinence appropriately and promote the health and well-being of patients and clients.

Learning objectives

At the end of this chapter the reader will:

- have an understanding of what continence is;
- have an appreciation of the factors that impact on the person with profound intellectual and multiple disabilities;
- develop knowledge of the key aspects of assessment, treatment and management; and
- be able to recognise factors that contribute to incontinence.

Continence products are now readily available on the shelves of supermarkets and on the high street. Information is available through the Internet at the touch of a button. This helps families and carers to manage incontinence but where do they find help to promote continence? Since 1994, the British government, Continence Advisory Services, charitable organisations such as The Continence Foundation, InContact and companies who manufacture pad products or treatments have endeavoured to raise awareness that treatment and support can be accessed (Getliffe & Dolman, 2003). However, Norton et al. (1988, cited in Igbedioh, 2007) identify that it frequently remains a taboo subject where 25% of women wait more than 5 years before they seek help. There is also a lack of awareness that continence may be treated and this includes the vulnerable group of people who have intellectual disabilities. Access to free pad products from the NHS and a lack of resources helps to maintain this status quo.

One of the challenges faced by service providers is identifying their client group. It is incredibly difficult to measure the prevalence of incontinence accurately because the definitions of different degrees of incontinence are in part subjective and people are likely to under-report the problem because of its associated embarrassment.

It is difficult to identify how many people with an intellectual disability have a continence support need as few studies have been conducted identifying the continence support needs of people living independently or with support in the community, and it is particularly difficult to specifically identify how many of these are people with complex needs.

Mencap explored issues relating to access to health services for and by people who have an intellectual disability. In relation to continence services they reported that 7% of the people supported by the carers had used continence services in the last 12 months. Most individuals were more likely to be receiving a service up to the age of 19 (55%), and afterwards this reduced to 45%. The report identified concerns about lack of availability of specialist continence services and the supply of continence products allocated to an individual is often too inflexible. The report identifies that 'some people had not automatically been informed about the existence of the service by their GP and had purchased continence supplies themselves. Others had difficulty getting a service until the community learning disability nurse intervened' (1998: p. 4).

Two years later the Department of Health (2000) identified for adult men and women living in institutional care an estimated one in three in residential homes and almost two in every three in nursing homes will have a continence support need. In institutional care the prevalence of regular faecal incontinence is about 25%.

A study conducted by Cassidy et al. (2002) administered health checks to 69 people with an intellectual disability aged between 3 and 66 years. Results identified that 31% had urinary continence problems and 26% had faecal continence problems primarily constipation and overflow.

Frustratingly Stenson and Danaher reported 'Despite the availability of much research on treatments to promote continence, the problems of under-reporting and under-treatment of urinary incontinence continue' (2005: p. 14). Marketing of provider services and increased potency of commissioners improve awareness within the public domain of service availability for incontinence support and treatment. Ultimately, the goal must be to raise the awareness within the general population to promote the needs of continence services encouraging the commissioning of appropriately qualified professionals, in particular the specialist areas such as intellectual disabilities.

This chapter will provide information and tools to facilitate identification of people who require a continence assessment. The tools will help provide a holistic assessment for people with complex needs, promote continence with healthy bladder and bowel function and provide various options available to manage incontinence. Assessment processes have developed with the publication and dissemination of urinary continence care pathway (Bayliss et al., 2000). The original assessment tool has been adapted and used across the UK aiming to improve knowledge and skills required for assessment (Appendix 16.1).

What is continence?

Continence is described as having the ability to store urine in the bladder or faeces in the bowel and to excrete voluntarily where and when it is socially appropriate (White, 1997, cited in Getliffe & Dolman, 1997, p. 11).

Achievement of continence therefore requires the physical ability and skills to store and excrete voluntarily. This includes being able to understand where and when it is socially appropriate to do so.

Incontinence is defined as '*a condition where involuntary loss of urine is a social or hygienic problem and is objectively demonstrable*' (Abrams et al., 1988, cited in Abrams et al., 1999, p. 200).

Normal bladder

Getliffe & Dolman (1997) identify that a typically developed individual has voluntary control over signals and is therefore able to inhibit messages to empty the bladder and void at a chosen place and time. Most adults void between 4 and 6 hourly intervals during the day usually with no need to void at night; however, the person with complex needs may have impaired neurology, resultant in profound intellectual impairment. They may also experience additional neurological impairments similar to those of the non-disabled population, i.e. multiple sclerosis, cerebral palsy, CVA, dementia, all of which will have an additional impact on the functioning of the bladder.

Normal bowel

Normal bowel function is of bowel opening between three times a week to three times a day, and needing to strain on less than 25% of occasions to achieve emptying (Thompson et al., 1999, cited in Norton & Chelvanayagam (2004, p. 238). Ideally, the bowel should produce soft-formed stools, which are comfortable to pass. Food arriving in the stomach triggers a pressure wave in the colon called the gastro-colic reflex that can lead to the need to empty the bowel. Consequently, eating a meal should encourage peristalsis eventually leading to a bowel movement within 30 minutes following a meal. Food usually takes 1–3 days to be processed.

DH (2000) recognised that people with intellectual disabilities are more likely to encounter problems with incontinence or have difficulties accessing professional support. Ultimately this may impact on care needs. As the person with complex needs develops physically managing personal hygiene, including changing pad products becomes increasingly difficult and this creates lifestyle limitations such as places that a person with complex needs can go to.

The significantly impaired intellect of a person with complex needs means they are unlikely to achieve continence independently. The person may also have neurological or physical inability to achieve continence and impaired ability to communicate, all of which further inhibit the ability to achieve continence.

Stanley stated, '*Given the subtle co-ordination of voluntary actions required to achieve continence, it is both necessary and useful to consider the neurological domains on continence relative to learning disability. People with a learning disability have impaired neurology: this will directly impact on their manifestation of incontinence and their ability to respond to and overcome continence*' (1996: p. 495).

Specific areas of concern identified by Shanley & Starrs (1993) for people who have complex needs include: increased level of immobility leading to weakened abdominal and pelvic floor muscles; reduced gastric motility; diet may lack sufficient roughage and dietary fibre leading to an increased risk of constipation; dehydration when the person receives insufficient fluids; they may be in a recumbent position for prolonged periods of time resulting in reduction in stimulation to defecate and there may be specific neurological damage affecting the nerve supply to the gastrointestinal tract.

Assessment

Why is continence assessment necessary?

Assessment is vital for patients to identify the underlying cause and contributory factors. Once a diagnosis is made, a treatment plan can be developed (Colley, 2003). Consideration must be made of bladder and bowel dysfunction that may affect any typically developed person. This may include stress urinary incontinence caused by a pelvic floor dysfunction, overactive bladder indicated by frequency, urgency and urge incontinence and outflow obstruction or voiding difficulties resulting in urinary retention usually caused by prostate enlargement or neurological problems. In order to support the person with complex needs it is essential that a thorough assessment be carried out (Appendix 16.1). The key aspects of any continence assessment include taking a history, physical examination, urine testing and an understanding of contributory factors (DH, 2000). This will require collaborative working with family and carers.

The nurse faces many challenges when assessing the person with a complex needs. First of all you must establish effective communication. How does the person communicate their symptoms? (Appendix 16.2) For some individuals going to the toilet is a painful and frightening experience, this may be due to presence of a urinary tract infection (UTI), constipation or learnt behaviour. Shanley & Starrs identify that this distress or pain may be communicated to the carers in a number of ways, for example crying (often without tears), vocalisations, facial expressions, undirected aggression (self injurious behaviour (SIB)), movement disorders (unexplained fidgeting, restlessness), a reluctance to move, or eating disorder (loss of appetite) (1993: p. 261). A Person Centred Plan (PCP; Circles Network, 2005) is a valuable tool to support assessment of a person with complex needs. A comprehensive PCP identifies how others interpret the communication of the person with complex needs; it is essential that communication relating to toilet routines is included in the PCP. Tools which can assist the assessment of pain and distress include the PPP (Paediatric Pain Profile) (University College, London/Institute of Child Health and Royal College of Nursing Institute, 2003) and DisDAT (Disability Distress Assessment Tool) (Regnard et al., 2007). Using the appropriate communication tool for the individual enables the reinforcing of an appropriate toilet routine, which will ultimately reinforce the desired behaviour. This process must include a clearly documented plan that is shared with the family/carers. This will provide support and information to reinforce the daily activities and routines required to develop continence skills. Ongoing support is required to encourage collaborative working, as the family/carers will have their own knowledge and expertise that a professional can guide.

Methods of assessment

Urinalysis

Urinalysis is a simple, non-invasive screening test when using the chemically impregnated squares such a Multistix®. The urine sample should be fresh and collected in a clean dry receptacle free from contaminants as urine is an excellent culture medium (Fillingham & Douglas, 2004).

There are likely to be difficulties obtaining a clean specimen, these include posture and mobility affecting one's position whilst seated on the toilet and for some individuals who already wear continence pads there is the difficulty of collecting urine specimen from a pad. To facilitate this process the Uricol™, urine pad collection pack is available (Appendix 16.3). Urinalysis provides an opportunity to screen for conditions such as diabetes, urine infections and to assess the level of hydration. Assessment of urine should include observations such as clarity concentration of urine and the smell of urine. An infection may be noted by cloudy offensive smelling urine, but may also be noted by a change in behaviour, for example increased confusion an expression of pain on voiding and loss of appetite.

Frequency and volume

Continence assessment is conducted through the use of a 3-day bladder diary (Appendix 16.4) with a record of food and drink consumed during the 3 days. For the

**Fluid intake
matrix to determine suggested volume
intake per 24 hours**

REFERENCE:

Abrams P. & Klevmark B. (1996) Frequency Volume Charts – a indispensable part of lower urinary tract assessment. *Scandinavian Journal of Urology and Nephrology Supplement*, 179, 47–53

Patient's weight Stones	kgs	MLS	Fluid OZ'S	Pints	Mugs
6	38	1190	42	2.1	4
7	45	1275	49	2.5	5
8	51	1446	56	2.75	5–6
9	57	1786	63	3.1	6
10	64	1981	70	3.5	7
11	70	2179	77	3.75	7–8
12	76	2377	84	4.2	8
13	83	2575	91	4.5	9
14	89	2773	98	4.9	10

This matrix is to be used as a guideline and broadly it is suggested that patient's fall within a margin of error of +/– 10% – the guideline applies to body frame and gross obesity should not be taken as a guide for increasing fluid. Activity levels should be taken into account.

Figure 16.1 Fluid intake matrix. (Reproduced from the Sheffield Integrated Continence Service with permission of Sheffield PCT).

person with complex needs success of recording relies on the carer, so it is essential to consider the carers' literacy skills. Fluid input and output should be measured (Figure 16.1). For some individuals it is difficult to obtain accurate measurements of volume voided; this may be due to episodes of urinary incontinence, carers may have difficulty obtaining a urine specimen while the person sits on the toilet, or the individual already wears incontinence pads or pants. In this situation it would be advisable to consider measuring the volume of urine passed by weighing the pad, 1 gm = 1 mL. Siltberg et al. (1997) indicate that pad weighing testing may be useful for assessing the severity of urinary incontinence. A pad-weighing test (12–48 hours) will give an indication of average volume voided, which will inform the assessment of volumes voided. Normal bladder capacity is 400–600 mLs and the first sensation to void usually occurs at 150–250 mLs. (Getliffe & Dolman 2003, p. 47)

Frequency can be determined by charting the number of occasions the person passes urine (incidence of incontinence) or using an enuresis alarm. Enuresis alarms are useful for recording when a person begins to pass urine, recording the number of occasions the alarm activates will provide a baseline of frequency (Malem, 2006).

Normal number of voids varies between individuals. Seven times per 24 hours is the average (Getliffe & Dolman 2003, p. 31).

Medication review

It is important to consider the side effects of medication and whether this is impacting on continence comfort or mobility. Before making any changes to the medication dosage it is important to determine a baseline. Their usual diet and fluid intake, their usual behaviour and whether the carer considers that the behaviour is associated with toilet routines; the person's usual toilet behaviour/routine, and the usual presentation of stool and the normal stool form. The Bristol Stool form scale is an essential tool to assist with identification of stool form and texture (Figure 16.2).

There is no single definition of constipation, but it is generally described as infrequent defecation, often with straining and passage of hard, uncomfortable stool (Thompson et al., 1999).

Useful tools to assist with assessing constipation include Fluid Intake Matrix (Figure 16.1) for recording fluid intake and output; Fibre Scoring Sheet (Figure 16.3) for rating the amount of fibre consumed and the Bowel Habit Diary (Figure 16.4) for recording bowel routine and result.

Medication which may effect continence

Having an awareness of side effects and observing for side effects is an important part of continence assessment, treatment and management.

Diuretics, sedatives, tranquillisers, hypnotics, antidepressants, beta-blockers all have the potential to influence continence.

For further reading about medication refer to:

Electronic Medicines Compendium – http://emc.medicines.org.uk/.
British National Formulary – http://www.bnf.org.uk/bnf/.

Further resources to support assessment are identified in Appendix 16.5.

Treatment

Pelvic floor exercises

In order to develop a good technique it is necessary to have an understanding of the sensations your body produces when passing urine or stools. It also requires the individual to be able to visualise bodily functions in order to pinpoint the relevant muscle groups. For this reason pelvic floor exercises are unsuitable for people with profound intellectual and multiple disabilities.

Fluid intake

It is important to measure and record the person's fluid intake, this is especially important if they have difficulty with lip seal or swallowing (see Chapter 14) or

THE BRISTOL STOOL FORM SCALE

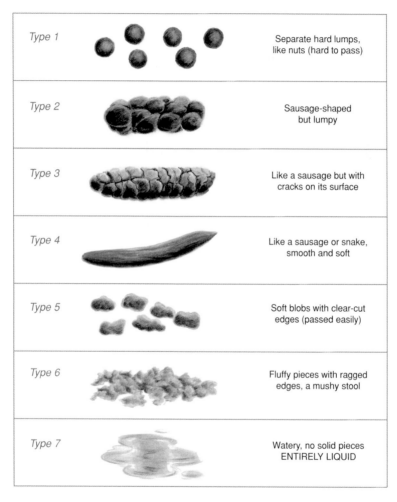

Type 1	Separate hard lumps, like nuts (hard to pass)
Type 2	Sausage-shaped but lumpy
Type 3	Like a sausage but with cracks on its surface
Type 4	Like a sausage or snake, smooth and soft
Type 5	Soft blobs with clear-cut edges (passed easily)
Type 6	Fluffy pieces with ragged edges, a mushy stool
Type 7	Watery, no solid pieces ENTIRELY LIQUID

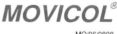

MOVICOL®

MO/06/0808

Figure 16.2 Bristol Stool form scale. (Reproduced by kind permission of Dr K.W. Heaton, Reader in Medicine at the University of Bristol. © 2000 Norgine Pharmaceuticals Ltd.)

Fibre scoring sheet

Rate your diet for fibre

Pick the foods you eat at home and find your score

SCORE	1	2	3	
FOOD				Write your score here
BREAD	White	Brown	Wholemeal/ Granary	
BREAKFAST CEREAL 3 times per week or more	Rarely or never eat or eat sugar coated cereal, e.g. Frosties	Corn Flakes Rice Crispies Cheerios Special K	Bran Flakes Weetabix Shredded Wheat Muesli, Shreddies	
POTATOES PASTA RICE	Rarely or never eat	Eat potatoes, white rice or pasta most days	Eat potatoes in jackets, brown rice or pasta most days	
PULSES BEANS NUTS	Rarely or never eat	Once a week or less	Three times a week or more	
VEGETABLES ALL KINDS OTHER THAN PULSES, POTATOES AND BEANS	Less than once a week	1–3 times per week	Daily	
FRUIT ALL KINDS	Less than once a week	1–3 times per week	Daily	
			YOUR TOTAL SCORE:	

	Score Guide
0-12:	Increase your fibre
13-17:	Good
18:	Excellent

Figure 16.3 Fibre scoring sheet. (Reproduced from the Sheffield Integrated Continence Service with permission of Sheffield PCT.)

Sheffield's Integrated Continence Services NHS

BOWEL HABIT DIARY

NAME..

DATE STARTED..................................

DATE	TIME	The Bristol Stool from scale Hard Type	Normal Type	Soft Type	Watery Type	Stool/faecal leakage? YES/NO	Time spent on toilet	Did you strain a lot?	Did you have pain/discomfort?	Laxative/anti-diarrhoea taken?

Figure 16.4 Bowel habit diary. (Reproduced from the Sheffield Integrated Continence Service with permission of Sheffield PCT.)

posture or mobility difficulties (see Chapter 17) as their actual fluid intake may be reduced through spillage. Conversely over drinking (poly-dipsia) may be a component of an obsessive or challenging behaviour (Emerson, 2001). Modifying a person's fluid intake or diet in order to treat incontinence should only be done after a thorough assessment and under the supervision of an appropriately qualified health care professional, for example District Nurse (D/N), continence Nurse Specialist or dietician. Certain drinks have diuretic properties, for example coffee, tea, alcohol, cola, chocolate. Some foods when consumed in large quantities may have a stimulant effect on the bowel, for example rhubarb, prunes and bran fibre (Appendix 16.6).

Drug therapy

Drugs may be used to treat constipation and overactive bladder symptoms.

Constipation should ideally be addressed by adjusting diet and fluid intake, a thorough assessment will indicate if this is possible.

The main types of medication used to facilitate a comfortable bowel movement include the following:

- Bulk-forming laxatives such as ispaghula husk, which will help to speed the transit time of the stool. Foods such as Weetabix™ and porridge may have a similar effect as they are also predominantly soluble fibre.
- Stimulant laxatives such as Senna, which, encourage peristalsis by stimulating the nerves in the bowel also reduce water reabsorption which will help the stool to remain soft.
- Osmotic laxatives such as Lactulose and Movicol™ soften the stool by drawing fluid into the stool.

Medications used to treat an overactive bladder are called antimuscarinics. They work by inhibiting the action of acetylcholine, which may reduce the frequency of bladder muscle contractions. These drugs include oxybutenin hydrochloride, detrusitol, trospium chloride, propiverine and solifenacin. An explanation should be given to carers/family of the benefits and side effects of these drugs. The aim of the drugs is to reduce frequency by provoking a more relaxed bladder muscle and therefore increase the bladder capacity. They reduce urgency by blocking the chemical acetylcholine and therefore inhibit unprovoked bladder contractions.

Posture

For people with complex needs there must be an assessment of functional ability. This should include postural difficulties focusing on physical positioning, use of positioning equipment and individual for comfort is essential (see Chapter 17).

The aim here is to achieve optimum position for voiding (Figure 16.5). Having a supported and comfortable position whilst on the toilet promotes voiding. Support

Correct position for opening your bowels

Step one

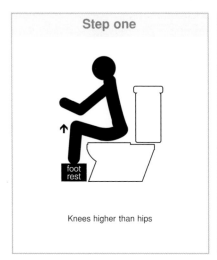

Knees higher than hips

Step two

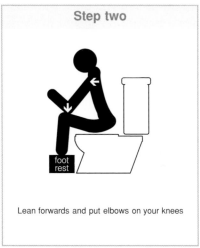

Lean forwards and put elbows on your knees

Step three

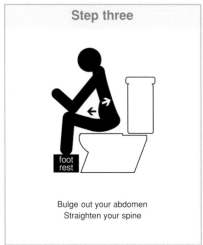

Bulge out your abdomen
Straighten your spine

Correct position

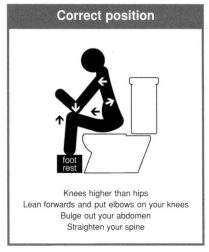

Knees higher than hips
Lean forwards and put elbows on your knees
Bulge out your abdomen
Straighten your spine

Figure 16.5 Correct position for opening your bowels. (Reproduced by kind permission of Ray Addison, Nurse Consultant in Bladder and Bowel Dysfunction and Wendy Ness, Colorectal Nurse Specialist. © 2004 Norgine Ltd.)

for assessment and promotion of continence in these situations may be gained from an occupational therapist or physiotherapist. As well as considering comfortable posture it is also important to consider the comfort of the environment, is the room warm enough, sufficiently ventilated, is it a pleasant environment and does it provide the necessary degree of privacy. Finally is the room large enough for support staff to assist the person safely and with dignity? These are aspects which are important to address both at home and in the community. '*The lack of suitable changing facilities in toilets for people with disabilities is one of the most restrictive practical problems preventing families from going out*' (PAMIS, undated); this inadequacy is being challenged on a national scale by the Changing Places campaign. Changing Places seeks to ensure that 'standard accessible toilets' (disabled toilets) are made fully accessible to all.

Bladder retraining – timed toilet routine

Stanley emphasised that '*little attempt was made to increase toileting skills in people with a severe or profound learning disability until the 1960s*' (1997b: p. 14). During the 1970s behaviour modification of toileting habits became popular with the inception of the behaviourist approach (Azrin & Foxx, 1971). For many toilet-training programmes a 30-day baseline was considered necessary prior to intervention. Interventions were developed following functional analysis; the desired behaviour was reinforced by the use of immediate tangible reinforcements, often edible. There was also often a potentially punitive response to accidents. All interventions needed to be consistently applied by all carers/therapists. There is differing opinion on the success of long-term interventions from behavioural approaches (Stanley, 1997a, cited in Getliffe & Dolman, 1997). Timed toileting appears to have the most successful prolonged effect. However, it is extremely disruptive to the lifestyle of the individual and carer supporting them and success is often sabotaged by non-compliance. Consequently, the benefits of prompted timed toileting should be explained to gain consent and ongoing compliance as the alternative is long–term use of pad products with all the indignity of a person needing to have personal hygiene attended to frequently and the amount of time that this may consume.

Bradley et al. (1995) identify key benefits gaining continence for the individual, their carer and services supporting them. Benefits for the individual include increased opportunity to engage in more prolonged activities, greater comfort, less incidence of skin irritation and less exposure to risks associated with moving and handling. Eligibility for other services and accommodation can increase. All of which contribute to increased self-esteem and greater quality of life (see Chapter 2).

Benefits to the carer include increased opportunity for time to be spent in more pleasurable activities with the client.

Benefits to health services include savings on resources, particularly purchase of continence products. (Please refer to Appendix 16.7 for further guidance on toilet training.)

Management

Achievement of social continence via managed continence is achieved by establishing regular times for going to the toilet, planning the changing of pads, the use of other appliances or very infrequently surgery (Halliday, 1990).

Prompted voiding

Prompted voiding is useful with individuals who either do not recognise the need to void or may be prone to self-neglect. The individual is prompted to visit the toilet but only visits the toilet if they wish. Through repeated experience, some individuals learn the routine of going to the toilet, although they may not recognise the urge or call to stool. Reward/praise should be given to reward successful outcomes. Using readily available printed charts or simple homemade charts may make recording of success easier and more enjoyable. Using disposable pad products does not raise awareness of being wet, as their aim is to lock the urine away in the pad within the super absorbent granules. Using cotton pants under the pad product next to the skin may enhance awareness of being wet. These will need to be changed frequently to maintain the sensation of being wet at each void. Refer to Stanley (1997a) for more detail on behaviour modification to achieve continence.

Timed voiding

This is when assisted toileting occurs within a fixed schedule. The frequency is calculated from a baseline frequency volume chart. This would have been completed during the continence assessment. Timed voiding is especially useful for individuals who have underactive bladders. Utilising gastrocolic reflex can assist bowel action following meal times. Toileting should be explained and encouraged as ignoring the call to stool will often result in constipation.

Aids and appliances

For many people the most suitable method of management is through containment where urine is either soaked up or contained and where faeces are contained.

Pads and pants. These are available in a range of sizes and absorbencies. People with learning difficulties [sic] may have needs well above the average and will need large quantities of pads to provide adequate containment (DH, 2000).

Pads are now available as reusable or disposable items. With the increase in product ranges and selecting the appropriate size, shape and absorbency many individuals no longer experience skin soreness. With many products it is inadvisable to use creams or lotions on sore skin as this impedes the effectiveness of the product and may result in leakage, always consult manufacturer if in doubt. It is advisable that assessments be completed in conjunction with the District Nurse or Continence

Nurse Specialist thereby encouraging collaborative working and a knowledge exchange about the client and their individual situation.

Urine sheaths. For male use only, these are usually self-adhesive, are available in a range of sizes, and include sheaths, which are non-latex and therefore, reducing the likelihood of sensitivity. A skilled practitioner should provide the assessment to ensure success by provision of the correct size product and education support to enable a good application technique by carers/relatives. When sheaths fail there is a loss of confidence that is hard to regain. The local continence service will be able to advice on the best way to facilitate a specialist assessment for sheaths. Specialist bespoke devices can be made but there is now such a large choice of routinely manufactured sheath products that the need for bespoke products has been greatly reduced. A referral for bespoke products is usually made following an initial assessment.

Intermittent self-catheterisation. This is where a special catheter is inserted into the bladder at intervals during the day to empty residual urine from the bladder; this prevents the bladder from becoming over distended, helping to reduce infection and minimise urinary incontinence (Barton, 2000). Intermittent self-catheterisation (ISC) is usually considered for individuals who have overflow incontinence, retention, residual urine, unsuitable for surgery, who are aware of their own body and willing and motivated to understand the technique. Given the nature of profound intellectual and multiple disabilities, it would be necessary that the carer would perform this intervention following assessment and support provided by the local Continence Nurse Specialist/Continence Advisory Service.

Indwelling catheters. This intervention is usually a 'last resort' and only considered for long-term use if the carer is unable to carry out ISC. Catheters and sheaths are connected to a leg bag during the day, which is linked to a bedside drainage bag overnight. Because of the high risk of infection associated with indwelling catheters and the risks of trauma to the urethra if forcibly removed by the confused individual they are infrequently used.

A great deal of support and explanation needs to be given to the carer considering catheterisation or ISC to avoid misunderstanding or 'abuse'.

Rectal plugs. There is variability in success reported, anal plugs can be difficult to tolerate; however, if tolerated they can be helpful in preventing incontinence (Deutekom & Dobben, 2005). However, this is an invasive management method for faecal incontinence requiring an understanding of the procedure thus requiring informed consent. As an invasive procedure it is less suitable for use with a person who has profound intellectual and multiple disabilities. In this situation a less invasive method is more appropriate and a continence pad would be a more suitable choice.

Further resources are identified in Appendix 16.8.

Conclusion

The minimum requirements for a person with profound intellectual and multiple disabilities to achieve managed continence are:

- carer awareness regarding communication and individual's continence needs;
- physical environment – warm, comfortable, pleasant, space to move, equipment available and suitable;
- comprehensive continence assessment taking into consideration cognitive skills, mobility and dexterity. This should be reviewed regularly or when change indicates;
- the ability to store urine in the bladder for at least an hour;
- the ability to sit and void/open bowels on the toilet or pass urine into a urine collection appliance;
- regular review of medication, at least annually (see your local primary care trust (PCT) medicines management policy).
- co-operation from the person with profound intellectual and multiple disabilities with their carers to follow through the plan; and
- collaborative working so that everyone involved follows the agreed plan.

People with profound intellectual and multiple disabilities have the same rights as every one else including the right to dignity. Neglect may occur by lack of a continence assessment and application of a conservative management plan, which will promote dependence on pad products probably for life.

This situation may also be the final straw for family/carers trying to care for a person with profound intellectual and multiple disabilities. Incontinence will cause limitations on lifestyle, stress, a loss of sleep and risks such as moving and handling along with many other challenging issues.

To promote continence an appropriately qualified and skilled person will provide the assessment and a clear plan of action will be documented in the person centred plan. There should be evidence of collaborative working crossing boundaries between all the services that are involved, including social services, health care, housing and education plus provision of ongoing support for the carers.

Appendix 16.1 Learning disability continence care pathway assessment tool.

Surname:	Forename/s:	Date of birth:
Ethnicity:	1st Language:	m/f
Address:		Post code:
		Tel:
GP:	Practice name:	Telephone:
Health supporter/carer name:	Health supporter /carer availability:	Telephone:
Assessor name: Designation:	Date of assessment	Telephone:
Other health care professionals involved	Contact details	Telephone:

TICK APPROPRIATE BOX:		Other (state), e.g. Colorectal	
Urological	Gynaecological	Neurological	Cardiovascular
Learning Disability	Mental Health/EMI	Physical Disability	Neoplasm (tumour)

Main medical diagnosis:

Have you discussed with the patient/carer   Assessment   Y   N
                                                   Treatment   Y   N
                                                   Management   Y   N

When did your bladder problem start?

What help have you had so far with your bladder problem?

How does your bladder problem affect your life?
Does your bladder problem stop you from doing things that you really want to do? (Circle the choice)
(Prompt card could be used here)

a lot   moderately   a little   not at all

NB: Before starting assessment send out fluid charts/food diary/bowel diary (check to see which is most appropriate for the person)
Send out the symptom profile (1 or 2) – to be completed by (1) health supporter/carer or if appropriate fill in with the (2) person

STANDARD STATEMENT	VARIANCE FROM STANDARD STATEMENT AND REASON/COMMENTS	Initial	Date
Person drinks _____ Amount and type of fluid per day – check fluid matrix. (Weight =)			
If person drinks volumes outside parameters of fluid matrix, advise them to drink appropriate amount	*Give copy of fluid matrix*		
Urinalysis performed: -	*Request sample taken to GP/practice nurse for testing/screening* Check UTI history / symptoms		
GLUCOSE			
KETONE			
S. GRAVITY			
BLOOD			
PH			
PROTEIN			
NITRITE			
LEUCOCYTES			
If leucocytes / nitrite, or symptoms of UTI present, take MSU, refer to GP and discontinue this assessment until treated	*If recurrent infections present – may indicate residual urine?*		
To check the bladders working capacity need 2–5 measures of urine. (Complete bladder diary)	*Expected bladder capacity 300–500 ml. If less than this may need to look at bladder retraining to help increase capacity?*		
Person has no bowel problems Frequency Volume Stools passed easily Bristol Stool form no.	*May need to commence on bowel care pathway?*		
Patient takes varied diet and fluids without assistance or risk	*May need to provide information on healthy diet – fibre leaflet/referral to dietician?*		
Person is not taking medication on list provided or consider referral to GP for review	*See list*		

STANDARD STATEMENT	VARIANCE FROM STANDARD STATEMENT AND REASON/COMMENTS	Initial	Date
Person has no mobility, dexterity or sensory problems, i.e. hearing/visual/or may find being touched difficult. Person knows what to do immediately after urination, e.g. shake penis / wipe self/ wash hands			
Person has no signs of cognitive dysfunction/ psychological issues	*Give out leaflet to assist with toilet training routines if information required.*		
Person able to communicate personal needs and wishes clearly			
Person presents with no behaviours which may inhibit or prevent them from using toilet independently			
The person's environment does not prevent them from using the toilet			
If pad products required the products used are successful			
The person is demonstrating signs of bladder awareness.	*Give information on readiness for toilet training*		
Document Symptom Profile guidelines recommended to be followed.			

The person is unable to commence on a Care Pathway because:

NB: For advice on using care pathway please contact The Oxfordshire Continence Advisory Service on telephone number: 01993 209434.

TO BE COMPLETED BY ALL STAFF USING THE PATHWAY

SIGN TO CONFIRM THAT YOU HAVE MET ALL STANDARDS OR RECORDED VARIANCES

FULL NAME	DESIGNATION	INITIALS	SIGN	DATE

SYMPTOM PROFILE

PLEASE READ THROUGH ALL STATEMENTS BEFORE TICKING OR ANSWERING THOSE
MOST RELEVANT, FEEL FREE TO ADD COMMENTS

Bladder

When you are active/laughing/sneezing are your clothes/pants damp?	Yes / No / Sometimes
Are your clothes ever damp or smelling of urine?	Yes / No / Sometimes
How many times are you up in the night? _____	

Do you have to rush to the toilet or need to go quickly?	Yes or No
Would you describe your bladder as shouting for attention?	Yes or No
Do you leak moderate or large amounts or urine before reaching the toilet?	Yes or No
Do you go to the toilet frequently?	Yes or No
Are you up multiple times in the night or very wet?	Yes or No
Have you always had a bladder problem?	Yes or No

Does the flow of urine sound loud and strong?	Yes or No
Do you strain to pass urine?	Yes or No
Does your urine flow stop and start?	Yes or No
Is the flow of urine weak and slow?	Yes or No
Do you stand/sit on the toilet for a longer period of time?	Yes or No
Do you dribble urine on to your cbthes or appear to be dribbling all the time?	Yes or No
Is this frequency or leaking quite new?	Yes or No

Do you demonstrate signs of bladder awareness?	Yes or No
Do you know when you need to have a wee?	Yes or No
Do you remain dry for at least an hour?	Yes or No
Do you pull at your pad or demonstrate discomfort?	Yes or No
If Yes, when and how often does this happen? _____	
Can you indicate when you are wet or soiled?	Yes or No

Bowels

Has constipation been a problem?	Yes or No
If Yes, when and how often does this happen?	_____
Has diarrhoea been an ongoing problem?	Yes or No
If Yes, when and how often does this happen?	_____
Frequency of bowel movement	_____
Size of stool & stool number (see stool chart)	_____
Any stools in the toilet	Yes or No
Any stools passed during the night	Yes or No
Commenced on bowel care pathway	Yes or No
Other comments	_____

_____
_____
_____

Reproduced from the Continence Care Pathways Development Group & Ridgeway Partnership with Permission of Sheffield PCT.

Appendix 16.2 Symptom profile.

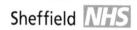

Adult Continence Guidelines: Sheffield's Integrated Continence Service (SICS) 2716837

If **ANY** symptoms are ticked follow guidelines in white box first then follow the guidelines for each coloured box that has 1 or more ticks (more than 1 box may have ticks)

---

1. Perform urinalysis. If positive, take MSU and send to Microbiology for MC&S
2. Observe:
   a. Skin condition: if red use 3M™ Cavilon™ Durable Barrier Cream; if broken use 3M™ Cavilon™ No Sting Barrier Film.
   b. If vaginal or rectal prolapse seen at rest/with cough refer to GP.
   c. Ask patient to tighten pelvic floor muscles: if lift and puckering observed teach/encourage pelvic floor exercises as per leaflet.
3. Mobility problems? Refer to Therapy Services on 2716363 for PT or OT home visit

---

1. Note catheter details in catheter care diary/follow care pathway. Any problems? Refer to Continence Service.
2. Note stoma care needs in plan of care and refer to Stoma team

---

STRESS URINARY INCONTINENCE
Observe genital area, ask patient to tighten pelvic floor muscles:
- If upward and inward puckering seen then give Pelvic Floor Exercise Leaflet and encourage daily pelvic floor exercises; teach patient to tighten pelvic floor muscles quickly before they sneeze, cough, lift etc to prevent leakage.
- If lift not observed: refer mobile patients for Women's Health Physiotherapy to attend clinic, ring Continence Service; if not mobile refer to Link Nurse or Continence Service for home joint nurse visit

Please note: Severe leakage is 4 or more times per day (assessed by Bladder Diary).
Only provide pads for **severe** leakage.

URGENCY/URGE INCONTINENCE
1. Give Urgency/Urge incontinence leaflet, encourage patient to follow advice
2. Assess fluid intake/output via bladder diary for 3 days. Give fluid advice leaflet.
3. Refer to GP for possible anti-cholinergics
Provide pads if required   Consider referral to Link Nurse or Continence Service for joint home visit.

NEUROPATHIC/OUTFLOW OBSTRUCTION
1. Scan bladder to assess for residual. Post-void volume greater than 100 ml: refer to Continence Service
2. Refer to Link Nurse or Continence Service for joint visit. Provide pads if required
3. Pain with voiding? Do MSU: treat infection if present; if no infection present refer to GP.
4. Blood in urine?   Refer to GP immediately

BOWELS
1. Maintain bowel habit diary.
2. If faecal impaction suspected refer to GP for joint management
3. If passive faecal incontinence suspected refer to GP for joint management and give Bowel Care Leaflet + Urgency/Urge Incontinence Leaflet + encourage pelvic floor exercises
4. If constipation suspected or rectum is full/partially full follow Constipation guidelines:
   a. Assess dietary/fluid intake: encourage high fibre diet and water intake (fluid matrix chart)
   b. Encourage gentle exercise – immobility makes constipation worse.
   c. Use laxatives, suppositories and enemas as prescribed
5. If rectal prolapse seen refer to GP
6. If any change in bowel habit or blood/mucus in stool refer to GP
7. Provide pads if required
8. Consider referral to Continence Service for further nursing support

---

Reproduced from the Sheffield Integrated Continence Service with Permission of Sheffield PCT.

Appendix 16.3 Taking a urine specimen – urine collection pad.

Ridgeway Partnership
Oxfordshire Learning Disability **NHS**
NHS Trust

When attempting to collect urine from a person who is unable to provide a midstream clean catch urine specimen or wears a continence pad to maintain their continence then it is advisable that a urine collection pad is used which aims to collect a clean specimen of urine.

The pads that have been found to be suitable for this method are the Uricol urine collection pack (Newcastle pack). This is a sterile pack containing two urine collection pads, 5 mL syringe and a urine specimen container.

1. Wash the person's genital area using soap and water as usual and dry, but do not put any cream or talcum powder on afterwards.

2. Open the pad out and place inside ordinary clean pants or a fresh disposable pad so that it covers the front of the person's genitals. Check every 10 minutes or so to see if the pad is wet.

3. As soon as the pad is wet, remove and replace it. **If the pad is soiled (faeces) you will have to start again.** Remember to wash and dry your hands, put on new gloves before handling the used continence pad.

4. Lay the pad down, wet side up. Take a 5 mL syringe and place the tip of the syringe on to the wet pad and pull up the plunger, extracting urine from the pad. Repeat this across the pad until the syringe is full. Hold the top of the syringe over the open urine bottle and press the plunger down hard to squeeze out the urine.

5. You may have to repeat step 4 until you have sufficient urine to cover the bottom of the urine bottle.

6. Put the cap on the bottle and make sure it is labelled with the name date and time of taking. As the pad results in artificially low white cell counts, ensure that you write on the request form that it is a pad urine sample.

If you have any problems or need further advice regarding taking specimens/investigations contact your district nurse **OR**

The local Continence Advisory Service

Uricol urine collection packs (Newcastle pack), Available from the district nurse.
Ordered from NHS logistics catalogue under the heading of "Urine drainage systems/collectors" at £0.67 per pack Supplier Code FSW106.

Appendix 16.4 Bladder diary.

NHS

Patient's Name ....

Sheffield's Integrated Continence Services

Date of Birth   ....

Date   ....

It is important that you fill in this form to help us understand the problems you are having with your bladder.

In The white box is for the amount you drink. A teacup or small glass is about 150 mL but a mug or larger glass is about 200 mL. Record how much you drank in the white box nearest to the time you had your drink.

Out The grey box is for you to measure the amount of urine you pass. Use a small jug to measure the urine you passed, preferably in milliliters. Write this down in the grey box nearest to the time you went to the toilet. If you are out of the house and not able to measure, just put a cross (X) in the box.

Wets If you are wet, please put Wet or (W) in the blue box at the time you leak Please record even small wets.

Example:

	Day 1			Day 2			Day 3		
Time	In	Out	Wet	In	Out	Wet	In	Out	Wet
7.00		250 mL						250 mL	
8.00	200 mL		W	200 mL			100 mL		
9.00	200 mL				X	Wet			W

Please note down the following on your chart overleaf:

When did you go to bed and get up?

When did you change your pad?

PIL 742 06-05 RHH

Bladder Diary

Name:

Time	Day 1 In	Day 1 Out	Day 1 Wet	Day 2 In	Day 2 Out	Day 2 Wet	Day 3 In	Day 3 Out	Day 3 Wet
7.00 am									
8.00									
9.00									
10.00									
11.00									
12.00 noon									
1.00 pm									
2.00									
3.00									
4.00									
5.00									
6.00									
7.00									
8.00									
9.00									
10.00									
11.00									
12.00 midnight									
1.00 am									
2.00									
3.00									
4.00									
5.00									
6.00									

Appendix 16.5 Resources for assessing continence.

Dobson, P., & Weaver, A. (2006). Nocturnal enuresis: systems for assessment. *Nursing Times*, 102(12), 49–52.

Gilbert, R. (2006). Taking a midstream specimen of urine. *Nursing Times*, 102(18), 22–23.

Wilson, L. (2005) Urinalysis. *Nursing Standard*, 19(35), 51–54.

Tools to assist assessment

Paediatric Pain Profile (PPP) – http://www.ppprofile.org.uk/ – The Paediatric Pain Profile (PPP) is a behaviour rating scale for assessing pain in children with severe physical and learning impairments, it is also suitable for use with adults with profound learning disability.

DisDat – www.disdat.co.uk – Disability Distress Assessment Tool is a tool to help identify distress cues in people who have severely limited communication due to cognitive impairment or physical illness. The tool is used to describe a person's usual cues when they are content, thus enabling identification and recognition of cues when they are distressed.

Person Centred Planning – Resources available from the Circles Network. http://www.circlesnetwork.org.uk/what_is_person_centred_planning.htm.

Appendix 16.6 Food and drinks which can irritate the bladder.

Sheffield Integrated Continence Service

NHS

Food and drinks which can irritate the bladder.

Oranges, Tomatoes, Cola and other fizzy drinks, Alcohol, Tea, Coffee, and Chocolate/hot chocolate drinks.

 Oranges

 Tomatoes

 Cola and other fizzy drinks

 Alcohol

 Tea

 Coffee

 Hot Chocolate

*To summarise, **any** drink containing alcohol, caffeine or is carbonated.*

Drinks which DON'T Irritate the Bladder

NHS

Water, Milk, Diluted fruit juice (Cranberry Juice is recommended), Milkshake, Decaffeinated Tea and Decaffeinated Coffee.

Water

Diluted fruit juice
(Cranberry juice is recommended)

Milk

Milk shake

Decaffeinated tea

Decaffeinated coffee

Reproduced from the Sheffield Integrated Continence Service with Permission of Sheffield PCT.

Appendix 16.7 Routines to assist toilet training.

Sheffield **NHS**

Primary Care Trust

Guidelines to help determine the readiness skills required prior to commencing toilet training.

Children and adults with learning disabilities are often able to achieve toilet training success. Due to their disabilities, such as problems with language, it may not be so easy to see when they are ready to start toilet training. This leaflet may help you begin a toilet training regime suited to the person you are caring for when they are demonstrating signs that they are ready. These are only guidelines.

The person you support may not demonstrate all the signs at once, but any sign being demonstrated provides a good place to start.

People with learning disabilities may still have treatable conditions that anyone may complain of, so a complete continence assessment is recommended.

- This should include urinalysis to provide routine screening and to test for a urine infection. Indications of a urinary tract infection may include a demonstration of pain when passing urine, cloudy or offensive smelling urine.
- An enlarged prostate may cause difficulty with passing urine indicated by frequency, urgency and needing to use the toilet multiple times in the night.
- Severe constipation may cause difficulty emptying the bladder. An assessment by the GP or community nurse will help to resolve this.

Development

- Maturation of the bladder function so that the person can go for at least an hour without passing urine.
- The person is able to delay wetting until they reach the toilet.

Physical development

- The person achieves mobility that enables them to reach the toilet. (Note: Continence of bladder and bowel may still be achieved even with difficulties with cognition or mobility.)
- The person has motor skills that enable them to sit on the toilet/commode. O.T. assessments and specialist equipment are available.

Communication Skills

- The person is able to express when they are uncomfortable or have voided/passed stools into their pad product.
- The person demonstrates an interest/understanding of the toilet/commode.
- The person demonstrates and develops an understanding of the routine.

Cognitive development

- The person demonstrates an awareness of being wet or soiled.
- The person demonstrates an understanding/awareness of when they are about to pass urine/stools.
- The person begins to demonstrate an understanding so that at times they are able to pass urine and faeces into the toilet/commode.
- The person understands and co-operates with basic instructions.
- The person is happy to sit on the toilet/commode for at least 2 minutes.

Basic toilet training routines that may help the person develop continence skills

Essential points

Do not let the toilet training period be a stressful time. Choose a time when you feel able to cope and when your patient/client is settled. Do not worry if it is not this year, it could be next year. By trying you are always making the routine comfortable and eventually they will realise what they are doing.

Spring and summer are a good time, particularly the summer holidays. Also, remember you can recruit other carer environments such as college or day care for support. You can also make toilet training part of your patient/client's care plan.

Decide on the length of time that you want to spend focusing on toilet training.

Do not start if you feel you may have a challenge, for example house move, school change, changes with other patients/clients.

Focus on one routine change at a time, for example sleep routine, meal times as well as toilet training. Do not overload yourself or your patient/client. Life can sometimes be challenging enough.

Use the support system that you have, for example family, carers, school, daytime support services.

Toilet training is all about setting up a comfortable routine for your patient/client.

Decide how many times a day you can follow this routine through.

Consolidate each part of the routine with verbal communication/ picture exchange communication system (PECS). Praise each minor or partial success.

Small rewards may help reinforce the routine. This will depend on your patient's/client's level of understanding, so it may be praise, a small reward such as a sweet or part of a larger reward such as a part of a toy. Think where you can start this routine. Look at your patient/client's current routine. Is there any time you see your patient/client can regularly go to the toilet? You can modify this routine.

Your patient/client should be drinking 6–8 cups of water-based fluid a day. This should be monitored and encouraged. It is difficult for the bladder to perform normally or to prevent constipation if the person is dehydrated. Dehydration may also cause confusion or a lack of concentration. Too much fluid may make it very difficult to achieve continence as the bladder will rapidly and frequently fill.

Regardless of age do anything associated with voiding close to the toilet or in the toilet/bathroom, such as changing the pad.

321

Make the toilet a fun and comfortable room. Put up favourite pictures and take toys and books into the room. Encourage your patient/client to sit on the toilet when possible so that they can be relaxed with the toilet when you do start toilet training.

Store pads in the toilet room or nearby. Not in the bathroom as this is a damp room.

The basic routine

Decide on the toilet routine, keep to it and tell others involved in the care intervention, this will assist continuity of care.

Toilet training can take a long time, it is important that you feel relaxed and remain positive for the duration of the intervention.

Choose a frequency for the toileting routine. Hourly to two hourly is good. Do not do this more frequently than hourly unless you want to do intensive toilet training for a short period of time, i.e. a week.

Break the routine down into small steps. Reinforce the routine at each stage. If school/daycare has pictures to help you, use these. You should use the same pictures as school/daycare anyway. Simple stick man figures showing each action may be enough.

Starting the routine

a. Start the routine with the communication process using a fun story, rhyme or song.
b. Trousers down, possibly remove pad. Then sitting on the toilet for no longer than 5–10 minutes. This may be an activity that you build up the length of time.
c. If they can only sit down for 10 seconds then praise this achievement, the aim is to gradually increase the time they are able to sit by a few seconds each time they return to the toilet; praise each success.
d. Wipe bottom and pubic area. If the pad is clean and dry then it can be reused, replace on the person. If it is wet or soiled then replace with a clean pad. Flush toilet. Then wash and dry hands.

Alternatively you may put cotton pants on under the pad. This allows your patient/client to feel wet after urinating but the pad protects the furniture etc. These pants need to be changed very regularly.

Removing the pad altogether will obviously give you some extra laundry so only do this for a short period as a more intensive toilet training routine or longer term when you feel able to manage the intervention.

Removing the pad will help you to identify urination habits. The patient/client should be able to last 45–60 minutes without being wet. This demonstrates that they do have some bladder control with an adequate bladder capacity.

By building up routines that become habits your patient/client can learn to be clean and dry. This may happen quickly or may take months. It will take as long as your patient/client needs.

Give your patient/client lots of praise and praise the desired behaviour, for example sitting on the toilet, or passing urine when stood by or sat on the toilet.

Adjusting a routine

If they already know when they are passing urine or faeces but their routine is to do this into the nappy then you can change their routine. Albert's example is very good.

If you do not have a similar opportunity then the following are tips that you can use to adjust routines.

You can also ask for shaped pads that are held in place by stretch pants or a belted disposable pad product. This helps to provide quick access.

At an age as early as possible get them regularly sitting on the toilet. Boys can use a jug more easily so this can be a good tool. There is also a discreet fold-up male urinal available on prescription. Telephone Manfred Sauer[1] for information: 0191 2910166. Encourage your patient/client to flush the toilet once and wash their hands. You can overlay your hands over theirs for this.

You can add something interesting into the toilet to help their concentration. This may be something to aim at, such as cornflakes or coloured popcorn, or coloured ping pong balls that should not flush away. Finally, stay calm and give your patient/client a comfortable and relaxed atmosphere to help them feel confident.

Albert's[2] story as told by his mother

We started by trying to find a time when Albert regularly had a wee. The only time I knew he did this was in the bath. This was maybe something to do with getting into the water. So we only put a small amount of water in to start with allowed Albert to wee and then emptied it. Then he had his bath. Then I started catching his wee in a jug. He would be kneeling first and then standing. It took time for him to get used to this. Once he was happy with this every time he appeared to need a wee I would catch it in the jug. We gradually moved nearer to the toilet until I was holding the jug over the toilet. Each time he performed in the jug I would empty it into the toilet. I always gave lots of praise when he performed. I took him every hour or so just in case.

Once he got used to going into the jug over the toilet I got him used to doing it into the jug over any toilet. Remember to take your time until each stage becomes a comfortable routine. I took the jug out with us in a bag when we went out. We even took it on the plane when we went to America. He coped OK with this as the jug stayed the same all the time. Eventually, I would pull the jug away and he would pass urine into the toilet. He then got to the point when he went to the toilet on his own. First thing in the morning came first and when he arrived home from school as he used to hold it in all day.

Now he goes regularly where ever we go unless he is a bit worried or unsettled. In this situation he waits until he gets home.

The next stage is to take the pad away for the more solid version. This we will have to do very gradually by firstly getting him to stay in the bathroom/toilet while he performs. Then we sat him on the toilet with a pad on to perform and then gradually undoing the pad whilst sitting on the toilet. Eventually taking the pad away completely. The stools should be tipped into the toilet to let him see where the motion is disposed of so that he knows where it should go. Get him to flush the toilet as well.

Albert knew he was ready to do this as he did not like wearing a pad to school and when wearing pants would hold it in till he came home. It took at least 6 months to get him happily dry.

---

[1] http://www.manfredsauer.co.uk/home.asp
[2] Pseudonym used to protect the identity of the person.

Reproduced from the Shiffield Integrated Continence Service with Permission of Sheffield PCT.

Appendix 16.8 Resources for managing continence.

Bradley, A., & Lambe, L. (2006). *Helping People with Learning Disabilities Manage Continence: A Workbook for Support Workers and Carers*. Kidderminster: The British Institute of Learning Disabilities (BILD).

Bradley, A., & Lambe, L. (2006). *Supporting Continence Management: A Reader for Managers*. Kidderminster: The British Institute of Learning Disabilities (BILD).

Deutekom, M., & Dobben, A. (2005). Plugs for containing faecal incontinence. *Cochrane Database of Systematic Reviews* (3). Available at: http://www.mrw.interscience.wiley.com/cochrane/clsysrev/articles/CD005086/frame.html (accessed 25/07/07).

Norton, C., & Kamm, M.A. (1999). *Bowel Control: Information and Practical Advice*. Beaconsfield: Beaconsfield Publishers.

Stanley, R. (1996). Treatment of continence in people with learning disabilities: 1. *British Journal of Nursing*, 5(6), 364–368.

To request copies of the Continence Assessment Tool and other materials produced by Sheffield Integrated Continence Service please write to:

Shirley Budd
Continence Advisory Service,
7 Edmund Road,
Sheffield
S2 4AE
0114 2716837
shirley.budd@nhs.net

Further reading

ACA (2000). *Notes on Good Practice*. Available at: http://www.notesongoodpractice.co.uk/ACA_Notes_on_Good_Practice_Full.pdf (accessed 6 August 2007).

Böhmer, C.J.M., Taminiau, J., Klinkenberg-Knol, E., & Meuwissen, S. (2001). The prevalence of constipation in institutionalized people with intellectual disability. *Journal of Intellectual Disability Research*, 3(45), 212–218.

Bradley, M., Ferris, W., & Barr, O. (1995). Continence promotion in adults with learning disabilities. *Nursing Times*, 91(39), 38–39.

Brazzelli, M., & Griffiths, P. (2006). Behavioural and cognitive interventions with or without other treatments for the management of faecal incontinence in children. *Cochrane Database of Systematic Reviews* (2). Available at: http://www.mrw.interscience.wiley.com/cochrane/clsysrev/articles/CD002240/frame.html (accessed 25 July 2007).

Chiarelli, P., & Markwell, S. (1992). *Let's Get Things Moving – Overcoming Constipation*. Rushcutters Bay, NSW: Gore and Osment.

Clark, J. (2006). Intimate care: theory, research, practice. *Learning Disability Practice*, 9(10), 12–17.

Dobson, P., & Weaver, A. (2006). Nocturnal enuresis: systems for assessment. *Nursing Times*, 102(12), 49–51.

Grieve, T. (1998). Continence promotion among children with severe disabilities. *Nursing Times*, 94(41), 58–59.

Newman, D.K. (2005). *Continence Promotion: Prevention, Education and Organisation.* Available at: http://www.icsoffice.org/documents/ici_pdfs_3/v1.pdf/chap1.pdf (accessed 1 July 2008).

NICE (2006). *Urinary incontinence: the management of urinary incontinence in women.* Available at: http://guidance.nice.org.uk/CG40/?cg91526 (accessed 26 March 2007).

NICE (2007). *Faecal incontinence: the management of faecal incontinence in adults.* Available at: http://guidance.nice.org.uk/CG49 (accessed 21 September 2007).

NICE (2007). *Injectable bulking agents for faecal incontinence.* Available at: http://guidance.nice.org.uk/IPG210 (accessed 21 September 2007).

NICE (2007). *Urinary tract infection in children: diagnosis, treatment and long-term management.* Available at: http://guidance.nice.org.uk/CG54 (accessed 21 September 2007).

NICE (under development). *Irritable bowel syndrome in adults: diagnosis and management of irritable bowel syndrome in primary care.* Available at: http://guidance.nice.org.uk/page.aspx?o=4291060 (accessed 25 July 2007).

NICE (under development). *Prostate cancer: diagnosis and treatment.* Available at: http://guidance.nice.org.uk/page.aspx?o=guidelines.inprogress.prostatecancer&c=91526 (accessed 25 July 2007).

Powell, M., & Rigby, D. (2000). Management of bowel dysfunction: evacuation difficulties. *Nursing Standard*, 14(47), 47–51.

Useful websites

Association for Continence Advice (ACA) – http://www.aca.uk.com/.
The ACA is a membership organisation for health and social care professionals concerned with the progression of care for continence.
Bowel Control – http://www.bowelcontrol.org.uk/index.html.
An NHS supported website which aims to give you information about possible causes and treatments of faecal incontinence, and some ideas on practical self-help measures.
Changing Places – http://www.changing-places.org/.
National campaign for *fully accessible* toilets.
ERIC – http://www.eric.org.uk/.
Education and Resources for Improving Childhood Continence (ERIC) website provides information to Kids, Parents & Professionals childhood continence.
InContact – http://www.incontact.org/.
InContact is a national organisation that provides information and support to people with bladder and bowel problems, their carers and health professionals that support them.
NHS Direct – http://www.nhsdirect.nhs.uk/.
Website operated by NHS Direct supplying health information.
For further information on Urinary incontinence visit NHS Direct
Health Encyclopaedia > A-Z > Urinary incontinence
Health Encyclopaedia > A-Z > Faecal incontinence

References

Abrams, P., Blaivas, J.G., Stanton, S.L., & Anderson, J.T. (1988). The standardisation of terminology of lower urinary tract function. *Scandinavian Journal of Urology & Nephrology*

Supplement, 114, 5–19. Cited in Abrams, P., Khoury, S., & Wein, A. (eds). (1999). *Incontinence 1st International Consultation on Incontinence June 28-July 1, 1998 Monaco.* Plymouth: Health Publication; 200.

Azrin, N., & Foxx, R. (1971). A rapid method of toilet training the institutionally retarded. *Journal of Applied Behaviour Analysis*, 4, 89–99.

Barton, R. (2000). Intermittent self-catheterisation. *Nursing Standard*, 15(9), 47–52.

Bayliss, V., Cherry, M., Locke, R., & Salter, L. (2000). Pathways for continence care: development of the pathways. *British Journal of Nursing*, 9(17), 1165–1172.

Bradley, M., Ferris, W., & Barr, O. (1995). Continence promotion in adults with learning disabilities. *Nursing Times*, 91(39), 38–9.

Cassidy, G., Martin, D.M., Martin, G.H.B., & Roy, A. (2002). Health checks for people with learning disabilities – community learning disability teams working with general practitioners and primary health care teams. *Journal of Learning Disabilities*, 6(2), 123–136.

Circles Network (2005). *What is person centred planning?* Available at: http://www.circlesnetwork.org.uk/what_is_person_centred_planning.htm (accessed 6 August 2007).

Colley, W. (2003). The assessment of continence problems in adults. *Nursing Times*, 99(29), 50–51.

Department of Health (2000). *Good Practice in Continence Services*. London: Department of Health.

Deutekom, M., & Dobben, A. (2005). Plugs for containing faecal incontinence. *Cochrane Database of Systematic Reviews* (3). Available at: http://www.mrw.interscience.wiley.com/cochrane/clsysrev/articles/CD005086/frame.html (accessed 25 July 2007).

Earnshaw, K., & Bates, A. (2001). Continuing professional development: continence. *Learning Disability Practice*, 4(2), 33–39.

Emerson, E. (2001). *Challenging Behaviour: Analysis and Intervention in People with Severe Intellectual Disabilities*. Cambridge: Cambridge University Press.

Fillingham, S., & Douglas, J. (eds). (2004). *Urological Nursing* (3rd edition). London: Baillière Tindall.

Getliffe, K., & Dolman, M. (eds). (1997). *Promoting Continence: A Clinical and Research Resource*. London: Bailliere Tindall.

Getliffe, K., & Dolman, M. (eds). (2003). *Promoting Continence: A Clinical and Research Resource* (2nd edition). Edinburgh: Baillière Tindall.

Halliday, P. (1990). The management of continence. In Hogg, J., Sebba, J., & Lambe, L. (eds), *Profound Mental Retardation and Multiple Impairment: Volume 3 – Medical and Physical Care and Management*. London: Chapman & Hall.

Malem Medical (2006). *Enuresis alarms (bedwetting alarms), bladder stimulator, vibrating watch and sit up alarms*. Available at: http://www.malemmedical.co.uk/ (accessed 6 August 2007).

Mencap (1998). *The NHS – Health for All? People with Learning Disabilities and Health Care*. London: Mencap.

Norton, C., & Chelvanayagam, S. (eds). (2004). *Bowel Continence Nursing*. Beaconsfield: Beaconsfield Publishers.

Norton, P.A., Macdonald, L.D., Sedgwick, P.M., & Stanton, S.L. (1988). Distress and delay associated with urinary incontinence, frequency and urgency in women. *British Medical Journal*, 297, 1187–1189. Cited in Igbedioh, C. (2007). Changing practice through a national incontinence audit. *Continence U.K.*, 1(2), 49–55.

PAMIS (undated) *Campaigns: Changing Places – Accessible Loos for All*. Available at: http://www.dundee.ac.uk/pamis/campaigns.htm (accessed 28 September 2007).

Regnard, C., Reynolds, J., Watson, B., Matthews, D., Gibson, L., & Clarke, C. (2007). Understanding distress in people with severe communication difficulties: developing and assessing the Disability Distress Assessment Tool (DisDAT). *Journal of Intellectual Disability Research*, 51(4), 277–292.

Shanley, E., & Starrs, T. (eds). (1993). *Learning Disabilities: A Handbook of Care*. Edinburgh: Churchill Livingstone.

Siltberg, H., Victor, A., & Larsson, G. (1997). Pad weighing tests: the best way to quantify urine loss in patients with incontinence. *Acta obstetricia et gynecologica Scandinavica*, (Suppl), 166, 28–32.

Stanley, R. (1996). Treatment of continence in people with learning disabilities: 2. *British Journal of Nursing*, 5(8), 492–498.

Stanley, R. (1997a). *Modifying the behaviours of incontinence: achieving functional change in toileting*. In Getliffe, K., & Dolman, M. (eds), *Promoting Continence: A Clinical and Research Resource*. London: Baillière Tindall; 342–374.

Stanley, R. (1997b). Treatment of continence in people with learning disabilities: 3. *British Journal of Nursing*, 6(1), 12, 14, 16, 18–19, 22.

Stenson, A., & Danaher, T. (2005). Continence issues for people with learning disabilities. *Learning Disability Practice*, 8(9), 10–14.

Thompson, W.G., Longstretch, G.F., Drossman, D.A., Heaton, K.W., Irvine, E.J., & Müller-Lissner, S.A. (1999). Functional bowel disorders and functional abdominal pain. *Gut*, 45(Suppl II), II43–II47.

University College, London/Institute of Child Health and Royal College of Nursing Institute (2003). *Paediatric Pain Profile*. London: University College, London/Institute of Child Health and Royal College of Nursing Institute.

White, H. (1997). Incontinence in perspective. In Getliffe, K., & Dolman, M. (eds), *Promoting Continence: A Clinical and Research Resource*. London: Baillière Tindall; 1–22.

Chapter 17

MOBILITY, POSTURE AND COMFORT

Sarah Hill and Liz Goldsmith

Introduction

Protection of body shape is a fundamental need for any individual with movement difficulties. Many people with complex and continuing healthcare needs have difficulty moving and controlling their own body and so are at risk of developing changes in body shape. This chapter will introduce a number of key concepts; however, it should be understood that there are complex risks associated with therapeutic positioning, particularly at night. Training and advice should be sought before its introduction.

Learning objectives

- To understand the principles of protection of body shape.
- To be able to identify individuals at risk of developing changes in body shape.
- To be aware of equipment that may be needed to support individuals.
- To be aware of the social factors relating to the introduction of therapeutic positioning.
- To be aware of thermal regulation issues and their implications.
- To understand the role of measurement of body symmetry as an objective outcome measure of intervention.

The principles of postural care

Protection of body shape using postural care requires a 24-hour approach, which without the use of night-time support as well as adequate support during the day will not be effective. Much has been written in relation to seating and for the purposes of this chapter, we will focus on developments in therapeutic positioning in the lying position. If supported positions at night are used in conjunction with adequate seating and comprehensive equipment provision, people are given the best chance of avoiding body shape distortion and participating in the world around them.

> Out of 8760 hours of the year, a person may spend approximately:-
> 1140 hours in school or attending services during the day;
> 7620 hours with their family and personal assistants;
> 3640 hours in bed if they go to bed at 10 pm and get up at 8 am.

Children are in bed three to four times longer than they are in school, yet previously resources were allocated to those activities which take place during the day when commissioners can 'see what they are getting'. Current trends within Health and Social Care Policy towards self-directed support emphasise self management and personalisation of services.

> *Improving care for people with a long term condition is one of the biggest challenges facing health and social care organisations and demands wholesale change in the way they think, train and deliver/design services. The role of self care is crucial in people maintaining good health and taking care of their condition.* (Department of Health, 2006: *preface*).

In the past, distorted body shape has been synonymous with people who have complex and continuing healthcare needs. In order to make progress we must challenge this concept and raise our expectations. We must expect to grow straight children and help adults to be as straight and comfortable as possible.

Evidence of body shape distortion in previous generations shows that the principles of postural care are not intuitive. Families and personal assistants (PAs) need accessible training, support and equipment to self-manage effective postural care safely and humanely. Failing to protect body shape leads to a loss of mobility which increases the need for specialised equipment, support and surgery. Most importantly it leads to pain, discomfort and secondary health complications for the individual. In terms of safer practice, failing to protect body shape exposes individuals to obvious risks which could be guarded against (Bolitho v City & Hackney Health Authority, 1997).

The emphasis on night-time positioning stems from an understanding of the difficulties faced by individuals with limited movement at night. Kotagal et al. (1994) found that children who cannot control their movements have limited changes in position through the night and become trapped in one position. The position adopted is often one in which the person originally felt comfortable, safe and secure; however, this position may distort joints, limbs and ultimately the internal organs.

The following x-rays demonstrate the impact that distortion of body shape has on an individual's health and their ability to participate in life (Figure 17.1).

Fred was born in the late 1950s and from the age of 18 months lived in an institution with over 1200 other people. Individuals that knew him tell us that at this age he was able to move if he was lying on his back, but that he would go around in circles. This suggests some asymmetry in his movement and muscle tone (Figure 17.2).

This x-ray shows that Fred's body shape has changed slightly, it appears that his chest is wider on his right hand side and his spine has started to curve; this is called a scoliosis. Measurement of body symmetry would have identified early, preventable rotational distortion at this stage (Figure 17.3).

This disturbing image shows how Fred's body shape has deteriorated further. Growth spurts experienced during puberty compound any existing body shape distortion. Fred's chest has continued to change shape to the extent that his pelvis now impacts on his ribs and the contents of Fred's abdomen are invading the space usually reserved for the heart and lungs. This led to Fred having difficulty in breathing and swallowing, referred to as dysphagia, it is important to recognise that a safe swallow is only the first stage of a successful digestive process. He had joint dislocations, pressure sores, open wounds, septicaemia, painful trapped wind and faecal impaction (Figure 17.4).

This x-ray was taken shortly before Fred died a slow death from multiple, severe, painful complications. Sadly, although the institution in which Fred stayed has been consigned to the history books these images and experiences are still commonplace.

Over the past 10 years it has been found that distortion can be prevented in children and that for adults, restoration to relative symmetry can be achieved. This is due to an improved understanding of biomechanical forces, the availability of new equipment, use of supported symmetrical postures at night time and importantly training, trusting and supporting families and PAs to self-manage this care (Goldsmith & Hill, 2001).

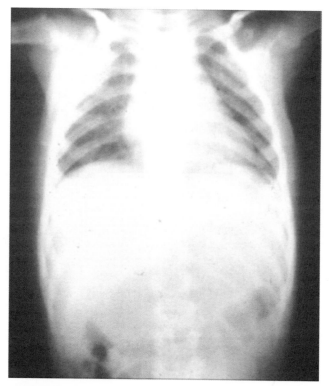

Figure 17.1 Fred aged 3. (Reproduced by kind permission of Anna Goldsmith on behalf of PCSP (UK) Ltd.)

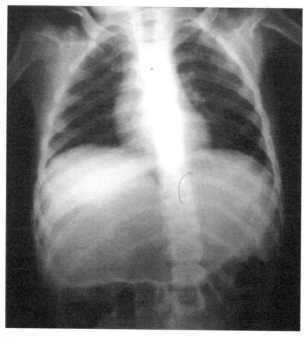

Figure 17.2 Fred aged 10. (Reproduced by kind permission of Anna Goldsmith on behalf of PCSP (UK) Ltd.)

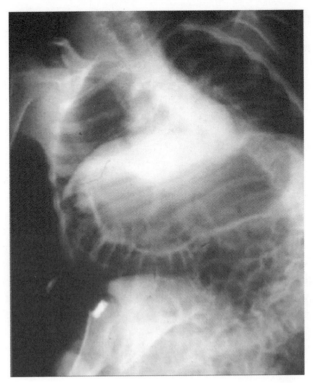

Figure 17.3 Fred aged 17. (Reproduced by kind permission of Anna Goldsmith on behalf of PCSP (UK) Ltd.)

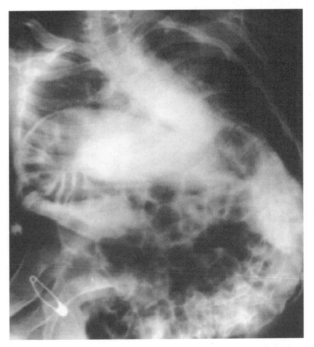

Figure 17.4 Fred aged 23. (Reproduced by kind permission of Anna Goldsmith on behalf of PCSP (UK) Ltd.)

A person-centred care pathway

The following person-centred care pathway *I Got Life: In Control of my Body* (Hill & Goldsmith, 2006) provides a framework for the introduction of self-management.

In 1976, a seminal article was published which identified the lying position as a cause of what was then termed 'deformity' (Fulford & Brown, 1976), such terminology has negative connotations for many and so should be avoided. The article called for therapeutic intervention and yet in 2007, despite the findings of the Audit Commission report (2002) many families do not receive either structured training and support or a reliable source of equipment. Language is vitally important in this field as partnership working between professionals, family carers and PAs is central. Complex and confusing scientific terminology should be made accessible and care should be taken to ensure that everyone understands the terms being used.

Success relies on families' own daily effort and may entail behavioural change within intimate and emotive aspects of their private lives. This Care Pathway offers a structure in which families and PAs are supported to take control, making the concepts of compliance and non-compliance invalid. No one else is qualified to make decisions about when and how to use therapeutic positioning, particularly at night time.

Family led variance reporting

Variance reporting involves keeping a record of any reasons why the strategy was not able to follow its expected course. This process should be led by the person, family and PAs wherever possible and should take place after each stage of the pathway.

It is expected that the person supporting individuals and their families to self manage postural care is qualified to do so. There are a number of undergraduate qualifications available to all. These relate to postural care, person-centred care pathway development and the measurement of body symmetry (Hill & Goldsmith, 2004) (Figure 17.5).

Step 1: identification of need

The Mansfield checklist of need for postural care (Goldsmith, 2000)

The Mansfield checklist of need for postural care was designed to be used by both professionals and family carers. Any person who finds it difficult to vary and control their position during the day or at night may be in need of postural care (Figure 17.6).

The next step is for all those involved to decide together whether use of the Postural Care Pathway would be helpful to the individual.

The Care Pathway process map is divided into five steps:-

Step 1

(a) Identification of need

(b) Identification of stakeholders and building relationships

(c) Baseline measures of body symmetry

(d) Making a plan

Step 2

Establishing trusting relationships through accredited and

quality-assured value training.

The social model

Step 3

Empowerment of families and personal

assistants through accredited and quality-

assured training

Step 4

Establishing Individualised funding where possible and equipment

acquisition

Step 5

Ongoing support, measurement and keeping in touch

Variance reporting

Throughout this process variance reporting will be led by the person, family and personal

assistants.

Figure 17.5 Structure of the pathway.

Tick ☑ the box which best describes their situation:-

Is the person limited to a restricted number of positions?   Yes ☐ No ☐

Does the head seem to turn mainly to one side?   Yes ☐ No ☐

Does the body seem to fall sideways?   Yes ☐ No ☐

Does the body seem to fall forwards or backwards?   Yes ☐ No ☐

Do the knees seem to fall mainly to one side?   Yes ☐ No ☐

Do the knees seem to fall inwards or outwards?   Yes ☐ No ☐

Is the body shape already asymmetric?   Yes ☐ No ☐

Ticks in any of the "yes" boxes indicate that this individual may need physical support to protect and restore their body shape, muscle tone and quality of life.

Figure 17.6 The Mansfield checklist of need for postural care (Goldsmith, 2000).

Identification of stakeholders and building relationships

If it is agreed that being on the postural care pathway would be helpful, make a list of all the people who will need to help, either directly or indirectly.

Consider all the individuals, including professionals, who can help or who need to be informed that the individual is on the Postural Care Pathway.

Efforts need to be made to build trusting, helpful relationships with everyone concerned. Making a plan as well as recording progress and variance can be very helpful (Table 17.1).

Baseline measures of body symmetry

What is it? Who needs it?. Taking measurements of body symmetry when protecting and restoring body shape is like weighing yourself when you are on a diet. It tells you where you are starting from, the progress you are making and what you need to do to succeed.

There are three procedures, called the Goldsmith Indices of Body Symmetry (Goldsmith et al., 1992) which have been tested for reliability and validity.

Some or all of the measures can be gently taken, or a bit at a time. Wherever possible the individual concerned should be supported to decide whether they wish to have the measurements taken, if this is not possible those who care for them and

Table 17.1 Identification of stakeholders and building relationships.

Name/role	Help needed Describe how this person needs to help to make postural care successful	Action Describe what action could be taken to develop a trusting, helpful relationship with this person

know them best would decide. An advocate for the individual always takes part in the procedures in order that the individual is protected.

Measurement can be used both as the basis for objective evidence of service provision and to direct care planning.

Making a plan

As a result of measuring body symmetry, plans can be made as to how the body can be protected and restored by providing postural care. A report about what the measurements mean and what to do on a daily basis is completed. Illustrations and photographs are useful to help everyone understand what is needed.

Step 2: establishing trusting relationships and working in partnership (Hill & Goldsmith, 2004)

People who need postural care may well have other complex needs and require constant physical support to help them. Many family members, PAs and clinicians will therefore be permitted to lay hands on the individual for a variety of reasons. This licence to handle another person's body needs to be carefully thought about and strictly regulated. *It doesn't happen to disabled children,* identified that disabled children were 3.8 times more likely to be physically abused than non-disabled children. '*We still come across situations where child care professionals do not believe anyone would abuse a disabled child; where the child's pain and distress is not recognised; where abusive practices are seen to be necessary because of the child's impairment.*' (National Working Group on Child Protection and Disability, 2003, p. 43). Donal MacIntyre's investigative work demonstrates that these concerns are as valid in the care of both adults and older people (MacIntyre, undated).

Success in protecting body shape depends on inspiring the person and those caring for them. They need to understand that body shape distortion is not inevitable and protecting the body can make a difference. Families decide how they can apply theoretical approaches to the realities of their situation and family life. Families need to be assured that professionals recognise that they are paid to *help* the family, appreciate the family's expertise, respect their decisions and can be trusted to work in partnership.

Training issues that are considered when supporting professionals to act in harmony with families and PAs, in the person's best interest may include:

1. The ways the individual can tell us if they are in pain and how they can indicate their consent. An adapted version of the Paediatric Pain Profile can be used to analyse and record the impact of intervention. (University College, London/ Institute of Child Health and Royal College of Nursing Institute, 2003);
2. The vulnerability of the individual;
3. The vulnerability of the family group;
4. Whether an individual can cope with what is being done to them and whether the intervention is justified;

5. Risk and benefit analysis of strategies for the individual with consideration of the possibility that activities are proposed to meet the emotional needs or ambitions of others.

Step 3: empowerment of families and personal assistants through accredited and quality assured postural care training
(Hill & Goldsmith, 2004).

Training and investment in those closest to the individual is essential if we are to create an environment in which true partnership working can take place. There is a great deal of anecdotal evidence that at present families face difficulties obtaining funding and support for training.

There are particular risks associated with the introduction of night-time positioning which are partly due to the complex nature of disability and health status of those involved. Providing accurate therapeutic positioning at night is a complex form of physical therapy, particularly because the family needs to introduce behavioural change into intimate and emotive aspects of their life. Success usually comes about as a result of gentle, sensitive introduction and by respecting the *Gateway to Sleep*, the usual habits that help the person to feel comfortable and safe to go to sleep. Most mistakes are made by expecting too much change, too soon with too little training and support. The decision to introduce night-time positioning is ultimately that of the individual, their family and PAs, no one else is qualified to make the decisions involved.

The following checklist is designed to support safety planning (Figure 17.7):

Is the person happy? (If they are not happy it may affect their ability to sleep which will be damaging to them.)
Do they have epilepsy? (Think about the type of seizures, when they are likely to happen and if the person's safety will be affected by their position.)
Can they breathe safely? (Think about the position of head and neck and the long-term effect of the combined force on the chest, consider the possibilities and consequences of aspiration, reflux,etc.)
Are continence issues resolved? Are they comfortable with regard to temperature? (Think about difficulties with controlling temperature and using different materials, consider the temperature chart.)
Are there any new pressure areas resulting from a change in body position? (Think about where the weight of th body used to be taken habitually and where it is taken in the new position. Is there any pressure as a result of spasm or bony prominences?)
Are there any problems with circulation? (Think about the position of the limbs and how the circulation can get through. Think about the effect of gravity on the limbs.)
Are there any other issues which need to be thought about in order to make sure any change of support and posture will be introduced safely and humanely?

Figure 17.7 Checklist to support safety planning.

Temperature regulation is a common issue for individuals with neurological impairment. Everyone needs adjustment of conditions to achieve a comfortable temperature at night. We adjust room temperature by switching heating or air conditioning on or off and by opening and closing windows whilst electric blankets and hot water bottles may be used for warmth. We alter our clothing and the number and type of coverings we use and if we are able to move, we kick off bedclothes or pull them back on during the night. This is called 'heat seeking and heat avoidance behaviour'. The individual unable to move efficiently sometimes needs help to make these adjustments. For those with complex neurological conditions, reflex control of thermoregulation may be disturbed and numerous other factors may interfere with achieving thermal comfort.

Many new materials can be used to help manage thermal comfort but, particularly if the person is unable to communicate effectively, care must be taken when introducing changes to make sure that the individual is at a temperature that is comfortable for them. It is important to recognise that:-

- Some individuals will show the signs of having a high temperature, i.e. warm skin, flushing and sweating when in fact their core temperature is low. Their skin response may be inappropriate and misleading due to neurological or cardiovascular problems. Use an aural thermometer to find core body temperature and remember that the helpful response may well be counter-intuitive.
- Inadequate nutritional status will influence the individual's ability to generate heat and disseminate it appropriately.
- Hormone levels have an effect on temperature generation and control.
- A lowering of body temperature will often occur naturally in the early hours of the morning.
- For some people increased body heat may induce febrile convulsions.
- Epileptic arousals may be increased if the individual's temperature is unstable.
- Muscle relaxants will inhibit the individual's ability to generate heat whilst making them appear relaxed and comfortable. Similarly anti-cholinergic drugs, used to prevent excess salivation for example, will also inhibit sweating.

Getting it right for an individual can be complicated, particularly when those providing care are short of sleep. Sleep disturbance and deprivation has been identified by families as a major factor in caring for their relative with complex needs. *No Ordinary Life* (Mencap, 2001) acknowledged that families were disturbed 3 times per night on average and that service providers were dismissive of the lack of sleep families experience.

Sleep deprivation is a recognised method of torture all over the world and most have experienced the disintegration of ability and morale which results from periods of lack of sleep. Perhaps the most commonly recognised situation is that of parents with a new born baby. However, for those caring in an ongoing situation there is often no end in sight. Additional contributory factors complicate the introduction of therapeutic night-time positioning:-

- Many families have been through periods of extreme stress with regards to life-threatening complications for the individual they care for and as a result they are particularly sensitive to any ominous signs and symptoms. The intensity of their relationship with a person who is completely dependent on them adds another layer of potency to the anxiety felt and the emotional overlay.
- Research shows that the physical factors which contribute to sleep disturbance are multiple and have been identified in both The Mansfield Project (Goldsmith, 2000) and work carried out to monitor sleep abnormalities in people with cerebral palsy (Kotagal et al.,1994).
- Individuals unable to change position effectively can become trapped in destructive postures at night in which the joints are stressed and painful with the result that body structures are damaged. This may lead to those providing care needing to change the position of the individual regularly.
- Individuals with neurological impairment may struggle to control their body temperature. For many families the option of sleeping with the individual and carrying out heat seeking and heat avoidance behaviour for them may make the difference between being constantly disturbed or being able to catch some sleep. Understanding of the issues involved, careful monitoring of core temperature, a comprehensive collection of different, good quality covers, support surfaces and night wear are basic requirements for families to manage thermal comfort.
- For some individuals sleep apnoea, in which breathing is interrupted, may be an ongoing problem. This may be of a central origin in which the messages to keep breathing are unreliable or it may be obstructive in which the airway becomes closed (see Chapter 12). Both of these occurrences are frightening and potentially life threatening and therefore careful monitoring is necessary. Apnoea alarms are commercially available as well as CCTV and are used by some families. Again, the option of sleeping with or nearby the individual is favoured by many.
- Nocturnal seizures will sometimes take a form which is dangerous for the individual with regards to physical security and length and type of seizure. Many families require specialist support and monitoring of medication to ensure the individual is as safe as possible.
- Some individuals will experience disturbance of circadian rhythms, particularly those with visual problems. The pattern of sleeping during the night and being awake during the day will be disturbed. Some may cat nap throughout the 24-hour period. Behavioural work to promote a consistent sleeping period may be beneficial to all the family.
- Reflux will influence the position in which the person is most comfortable and safe. For many a degree of tilt for the whole bed will be necessary to help prevent or reduce reflux (see Chapter 12 & 14). A symmetrical position with as little hip flexion as possible should be achieved so that the tilt does not induce distortion of body shape. If an individual vomits frequently the position in which they are supported should be carefully considered along with their ability to clear their airway. Although a side-lying posture may cause asymmetrical rotational

distortions in the long term it may be necessary to use the position in order to keep the individual safe in the short term. A careful and sensitive assessment of risk and benefit will need to be carried out by all involved.

Sleep is a complex, delicate and sophisticated function. For some people with neurological problems the damage may mean that they are unable to sleep consistently. Behaviours may be affected by any of the complications listed above or other factors. For families coping with complex sleep issues it is important that professionals have a thorough understanding of both the contributory factors as well as potential solutions. The utmost respect must be shown at all times for the family's survival strategies.

Step 4: equipment acquisition and funding

Families and PAs need training and support to use equipment effectively. They need to understand what equipment is needed and why they need it. They will also know what best suits their own personal situation and this knowledge must be taken into account, *'Given enough information and the chance to talk things over with peers, ordinary people are more than capable of understanding complex issues and making meaningful choices about them.'* (Surowiekcki, 2004, p. 260).

The following list of equipment is not exhaustive but may be used as a starting point when thinking about possible equipment need.

1 Wheelchair
2 Alternative seating
3 Standing frame
4 Walking aid
5 Support for the lying posture during the day
6 Support for the lying posture during the night
7 Moving and handling equipment
8 Equipment to assist personal care
9 Orthotics

It is important that families, PAs and professionals collaborate to develop a reasoned statement of equipment needs, costs and sources of funding with a record of dates acquired. At present equipment funding sources vary both between regions and between Children's and Adult services and development of an efficient and equitable system is essential (Table 17.2).

'Independence through user led services … is about defining our own needs … being responsible for our own lives.' (Mason, 2005, p. 66). With adequate training

Table 17.2 Table for recording equipment funding sources.

Equipment	Why it is needed	Cost/funding source	Date acquired

and support families know the equipment that best suits their needs. A self-directed approach requires services to establish efficient funding routes, including direct funding to enable families to source vital equipment when it is needed.

Step 5: Ongoing support, measurement and keeping in touch

Measurement of body symmetry should continue to be used at appropriate intervals depending on progress. This Care Pathway operates an open door policy with regards to ongoing contact, as the need for postural care is ongoing it is not appropriate for individuals to be discharged from sources of support although levels of contact naturally reduce as appropriate equipment is acquired and empowerment to self manage is established (Hill & Goldsmith, 2006).

Conclusion: the care pathway in action

An example of one young man's experience of postural care: James's story

This story is about James. He is 19 years old and lives at home with his parents and brother. He is a football fan and avidly follows the highs and lows of his favourite team, Coventry City. James was born at 24 weeks and has complex, ongoing medical needs; he is profoundly deaf and understands British Sign Language. James's movement difficulties mean that he needs the Care Pathway process described earlier (Figure 17.8).

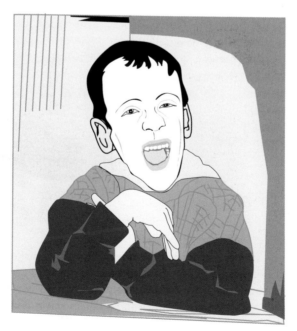

Figure 17.8 'Ready for Action, aged 5!'.

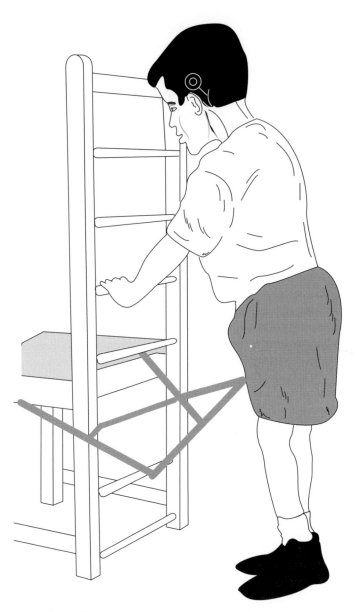

Figure 17.9 'Standing up'.

When James was young he could bear weight on his legs and hold himself up. This had tremendous benefits for both James and his family (Figure 17.9).

James finds it hard to control his movements and so in order to feel in control he used to sleep on his tummy. He felt safe and secure in this position. At this stage simple advice and support would have enabled James to be supported comfortably, securely and symmetrically on his back, with his hips and knees straight and his

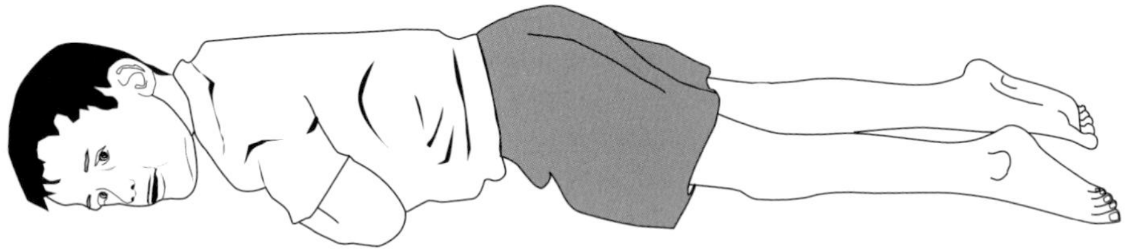

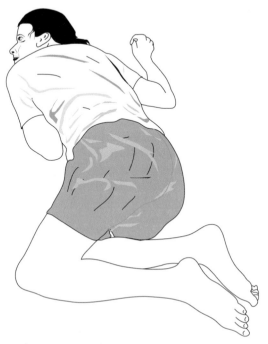

Figure 17.10 'Lying on my tummy'.

arms in front of him thereby protecting his body shape and ability to function (Figure 17.10).

James used to tuck his arm underneath his chest and twist his knees to the side. This is a very common position for people to become trapped in when asleep and results in rotational distortion of the whole body and loss of arm function.

As James grew he continued to sleep in this position and it became more and more difficult for him to get out of it (Figure 17.11).

James's legs were bent at his hips and his knees when he was asleep and he gradually found it more difficult to straighten them in the day (Figure 17.12).

The inability to straighten his legs meant that James could only lie in certain positions and so a vicious circle was created. It became more difficult for James sit comfortably, to bear weight in standing and to use his arms (Figure 17.13).

Figure 17.11 'Trapped on my tummy', aged 19.

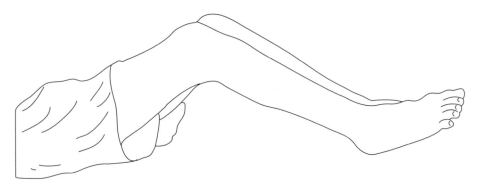

Figure 17.12   'Bent knees'.

James did not sleep well at night because he could not get comfortable so this affected his whole family as he would have to wake his dad, mum or brother to help him. James's physical condition was deteriorating, his legs were starting to give way when he was being transferred and his parents were dreading the introduction of hoists and other equipment in their home. The impact on James's life would have been devastating. At present James's friends can take him out, even if there is only one of them, as he is able to help when he is transferring. Everyone was worrying about how they would cope should his condition deteriorate further.

By chance, at 19 years old James and his family became aware of self-directed postural care through *I Got Life: In Control of my Body* (Hill & Goldsmith, 2006) (Figure 17.14).

James now sleeps on his back so that over the years, as he relaxes in sleep, his knees will gradually straighten and his arms will become used to being in front of him so that he can use them better. The benefits for him and his family have been enormous; James is getting a good night's sleep, so his family are getting a good night's sleep. Although James needs a lot of equipment at present he will use less as his body recovers.

James has been provided with a walker recently which supports him so his legs are getting stronger (Figure 17.15).

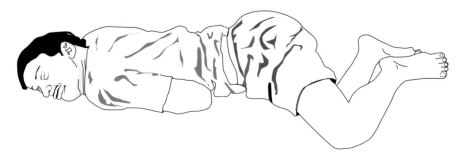

Figure 17.13   'Not good for my legs, pelvis, arms, neck, chest'.

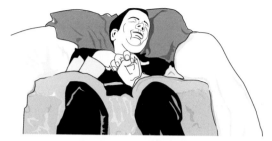

Figure 17.14 'Relax'.

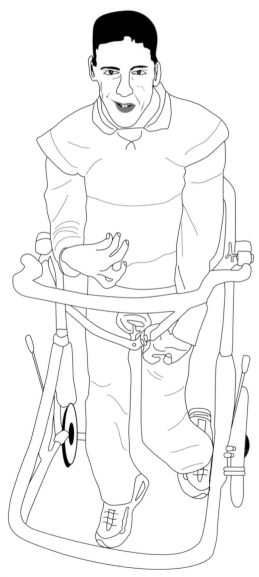

Figure 17.15 'Back on my feet'.

He is more flexible in the mornings and has less pain in his knees throughout the day. James and his family are in the early stages but the future looks bright.

James is involved in training healthcare professionals, families and self advocates to understand the benefits of therapeutic positioning at night and the need for it to be routine that families learn how to take control of postural care in the very early stages before damage is done and solutions are simple in both behavioural and equipment terms. He and his family are hopeful that by sharing their story others will benefit from this gentle, respectful and effective therapy.

With thanks to our great friends James, Debbie, Liam and Joe – a family in a million!

References

Audit Commission (2002). *Fully Equipped: Assisting Independence*. Wetherby: Audit Commission.

Bolitho v City & Hackney Health Authority (1997). Judgements – House of Lords. Available at: http://www.publications.parliament.uk/pa/ld199798/ldjudgmt/jd971113/boli01.htm (accessed 19 September 2007).

Department of Health (DH) (2006). *Supporting People with Long Term Conditions to Self Care: A Guide to Developing Local Strategies and Good Practice*. London: DH.

Fulford, G.E., & Brown, J. K. (1976). Position as a cause of deformity in children with cerebral palsy. *Developmental Medicine and Child Neurology*, 18, 305–314.

Goldsmith, J., & Hill, D. (2001). 'Biomechanics of distortion of the immobile chest' and 'biomechanics of regaining equilibrium of the immobile chest'. *Proceedings Manual, Canadian Seating and Mobility Conference*, 89–92, 102–105.

Goldsmith, L., Golding, R.M., Garstang, R.A., & Macrae, A.W. (1992). A technique to measure windswept deformity. *Physiotherapy*, 78(4), 235–242.

Goldsmith, S. (2000). The Mansfield project. *The Journal of the Chartered Society of Physiotherapy*, 86(10), 528–534.

Hill, S., & Goldsmith, L. (2004). *The postural care skills programme*. Available at: http://www.posturalcareskills.com (accessed 19 September 2007).

Hill, S., & Goldsmith, L. (2006). *I got life – a person led postural care pathway*. Available at: http://www.library.nhs.uk/pathways/ViewResource.aspx?resID=123913&tabID=288 (accessed 11 January 2007).

Kotagal, S., Gibbons, V.P., & Stith, J.A. (1994). Sleep abnormalities in patients with severe cerebral palsy. *Developmental Medicine and Child Neurology*, 36, 304–311.

MacIntyre, D. (Undated). *Official Website of Donal MacIntyre: Care Home Page*. Available at: http://macintyre.com/content/view/24/78/ (accessed 19 September 2007).

Mason, M. (2005). *Incurably Human*. Nottingham: Inclusive Solutions UK Limited.

Mencap (2001). *No Ordinary Life*. London: Mencap.

National Working Group on Child Protection and Disability (2003). *It Doesn't Happen to Disabled Children: Child Protection and Disabled Children.* London: NSPCC.

Surowiekcki, J. (2004). *The Wisdom of Crowds.* London: Doubleday.

University College, London/Institute of Child Health and Royal College of Nursing Institute (2003). *Paediatric Pain Profile.* London: University College, London/Institute of Child Health and Royal College of Nursing Institute.

Chapter 18

PROFOUND INTELLECTUAL AND MULTIPLE DISABILITIES: MEETING COMPLEX NEEDS THROUGH COMPLEX MEANS

Steven Carnaby and Jillian Pawlyn

Introduction

This concluding chapter attempts to draw together some of the ideas raised by contributors to this book by considering the 'philosophy' towards people with profound intellectual and multiple disabilities (PIMD). Thinking about *how* people are perceived enables us to consider the rationale behind the dominant approaches to their support, both historical and current. We suggest that the apparent 'invisibility' of people with PIMD within and without support services may have its roots in industrial and post-industrial societal attitudes, but that services and professionals are also prone to ignoring the particular needs of this population. In adopting a stance of honest acknowledgement and appreciation of the highly complex nature of individual lifestyles, we suggest that support can indeed become 'person-centred' for *all* people with intellectual disabilities.

People with PIMD: invisible citizens?

One of the issues that led to the development of this book concerns visibility – or rather, *in*visibility. It remains our personal view that people with PIMD are largely invisible on many levels, be that in the literature describing best practice in supporting people with intellectual disabilities, within services themselves or in terms of citizenship and taking a rightful place in society.

Invisibility might be seen as a concrete symbol of discrimination. The idea that a group of people is so unimportant that their very existence is more or less unknown is a powerful one. This phenomenon has been observed by others (e.g. Samuel & Pritchard, 2001; Mencap, 2007) and is certainly borne out by our own clinical experience over the years. However, wider society perhaps takes its cues on how to understand, think about and respond to people with PIMD from those purporting to be responsible for their care and support or otherwise representing them in some way. The messages conveyed by services and professionals working within them are therefore crucial if there is to be any attempt at addressing discrimination.

One way of thinking about the tendency for people with PIMD to be invisible within services and the literature describing and evaluating them concerns the principles upon which service supports are built; the development of community-based service models aiming to promote social inclusion necessarily involves the implementation of normalisation and ordinary living principles, which by definition focus on independence, skill acquisition and age appropriateness (see Szivos, 1992; Carnaby, 1998). For many people with intellectual disabilities, the increasing emphasis on social integration and citizenship has led to a wider range of opportunities and access to an enhanced quality of life that aims to be directly comparable to that assumed and enjoyed by the general population. The 'ordinariness' of everyday life is emphasised, aiming to avoid stigmatisation of those with disabilities – in practice by avoiding where possible any references to 'special' or 'different' treatment.

Historically, prejudice and assumption has been felt to colour the opportunities made available for people with intellectual disabilities, thereby impeding their right to an equitable life. O'Brien & Tyne (1981) used 'vicious' and 'virtuous' circles, respectively, to illustrate the impact of this social prejudice and how it can be addressed by making a shift in perception (see Figures 18.1 and 18.2).

However, the population of people with intellectual disabilities, like so many subgroups identified within wider society, comprise an incredibly diverse range of individuals who differ in terms of ethnicity, culture, family and socioeconomic context and above all perhaps, in terms of their cognitive abilities. While evidence suggests that people with intellectual disabilities are more vulnerable to inequalities in areas of health, employment, education and housing, it is still the case that if and where adequate support is available those at the 'cognitively more able' end of the intellectual disability spectrum may well have partners, be parents, be employed or at college and have wide and varied social networks – all of which together would make it difficult to distinguish their lifestyles and experiences from those of the general population. Ordinary living principles continue to inform the ways in which society is challenged to be genuinely inclusive.

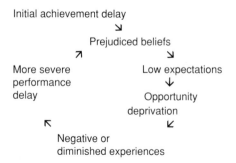

Figure 18.1 The 'vicious circle' (O'Brien & Tyne, 1981).

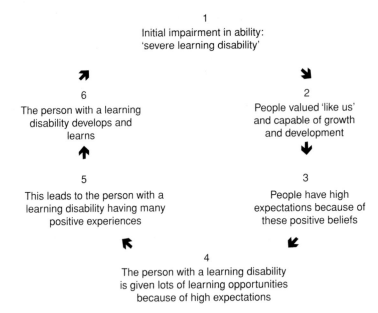

Figure 18.2 The 'virtuous circle' (O'Brien & Tyne, 1981).

There are those, however, who doubt that 'ordinary living' is available to all in its current form or that society is genuinely inclusive, requiring the government to set social inclusion as the key objective (Department of Health, 2001; 2007). People with the most limited levels of cognitive ability also have a right to citizenship and a place in society, but it is unlikely that applying normalisation and ordinary living principles in its usual form to the lives of people with PIMD without particular care and sensitivity will enable this to happen. While the blanket goal of increased independence may be highly appropriate for many, a failure to acknowledge the likelihood of a need for planned dependence for people with PIMD[1] can be detrimental at best, and fatal if ignored – as many of the chapters in this book testify.

One criticism of the models described above in Figures 18.1 and 18.2 might be that the emphasis is placed on the societal perspective. It is within the gift of 'society' to perceive people with disabilities from either a perspective informed by biased prejudice or from one based on positive expectation. Bartlett & Bunning (1997) have returned the focus to the individual, providing a helpful development of these ideas. Whilst acknowledging the role of prejudice and assumption, they suggest that the shift in perception can accelerate beyond the point of helpfulness, leading to an overestimation of an individual's abilities. Such a misjudgement can

---

[1] See how the concept of 'planned dependence' translates into exciting opportunities that encourage the development of self-esteem in schools, for example Mallett, A. & Taylor, J. (2001). A review of the curriculum for pupils with profound and multiple learning disabilities. *Tizard Learning Disability Review*, 6(2), 22–29.

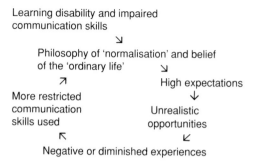

Figure 18.3 The 'overestimation career' (Bartlett & Bunning, 1997).

equally lead to the provision of inappropriate opportunities and the development of learned helplessness (for individuals and their supporters alike) as the expectation of development and progress is not fulfilled (see Figure 18.3).

Arguably, here lies the present day difficulty with supporting people with PIMD effectively: attaining an accurate profile of what the individual needs across all levels of functioning and experience in order to properly meet those highly complex needs.

As with many attempts at effecting change, the move against institutionalisation for people with intellectual disabilities – an extreme conceptualisation of people as lacking and, at its most pernicious, less than human – warranted thinking and related action that gave a strong message in order for change to occur. Such was the degree of entrenchment with regard to anybody deemed unable to live in industrial society. Transferring people's lives to community settings symbolised the need to 'rehumanise' people with intellectual disabilities as citizens and above all, as individuals. But social inclusion and integration for *all* requires consideration of the impact on subjective experience, and here is where services have struggled to evaluate this for people with the most limited levels of cognitive functioning and the most complex of additional disabilities and related health issues. Now, it is time to fully acknowledge what is reality for people living their own lives, accepting and valuing that difference.

Person-centred planning has the potential to enable supporters to do this, as person-centeredness by definition needs to begin with the person and what they need (see Chapter 6). However, failing to fully comprehend the person's experience and what they need is arguably more likely unless there is a commitment to an honest acceptance of the individual's developmental functioning and emotional understanding. This is what we would define as being person-centred, and does not in any way negate the need for identifying individual strengths and positive achievements. On the contrary, it is likely that by mapping the complexities regarding impact of sensory and physical disabilities and the nature of related health issues, it will be easier to then frame achievement and attainment within more appropriate scales of progress that are meaningful for that person, within his or her individualised context.

Meeting complex needs

We propose then an extension to the models presented above by introducing focus on 'getting to know the person' through transdisciplinary assessment as outlined in Chapter 7 (see Figure 18.4). The emphasis here is on an assessment cycle – assessment as intervention – that enables a continuous and rigorous gathering of information and monitoring of support that ensures a holistic approach and decreases the likelihood of symptomatic change in behaviour going unnoticed.

It is proposed then that we accept that an individual with PIMD is likely to have a wide range of complex needs requiring assessment and intervention through complex means. 'Complexity' in this context relates to interconnected or interwoven ideas; the organisation of this book has attempted to convey the principle that 'complex' is not just about 'difficulty' but more about relating concepts and phenomena to each other in ways that provide meaning.

In order for this to be achieved and translated into person-centred action, there may need to be certain adjustments to the ways in which support services are delivered to people with intellectual disabilities, something of a journey towards a more systemic way of working. For example, professionals will need to work alongside families and informal carers in a truly collaborative – rather than tokenistic – relationship, which is likely to require good facilitation in order to address any disagreements and differences in opinion. Steering groups that enable joint discussion and sharing of ideas and experiences can help to foster this collaboration. Clinical staff will need to reconsider their criteria for referral towards a more proactive, preventative model rather than only be involved once issues have been brought to their attention. When measuring outcomes, more flexibility will be needed to design individualised tools and ways of measurement that attempt to capture the

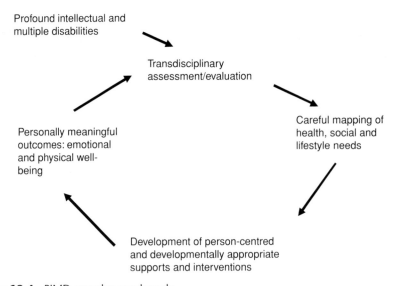

Figure 18.4 PIMD complex needs cycle.

unique nature of what is likely to be in place. Setting up and maintaining databases can help to monitor people with PIMD in a named area and track interventions and assessments, flagging up pathways for continuing care. Commissioners may need to review decision-making processes regarding priority of need and the competences required by tendering providers. Training officers will need to develop programmes that are able to cover the wide range of issues and concerns raised by working proactively with people across professional boundaries using a developmental approach.

We hope that this book helps in some way to convince practitioners, clinicians, commissioners and families that the complex needs of people with PIMD can be ignored no longer, and that by using complex means so much more can be done to increase the likelihood that in the twenty-first century they are enjoying an acceptable quality of life.

References

Bartlett, C., & Bunning, K. (1997). The importance of communication partnerships: a study to investigate the communicative exchanges between staff and adults with learning disabilities. *British Journal of Learning Disabilities*, 25, 148–152.

Carnaby, S. (1998). Reflections on social integration for people with intellectual disability: Does interdependence have a role? *Journal of Intellectual Disability Research*, 12(3), 219–228.

Department of Health (2001). *Valuing People*. London: HMSO.

Department of Health (2007). *Valuing People: The Next Steps*. London: HMSO.

Mencap (2007). *Death by Indifference*. London: Mencap.

O'Brien, J., & Tyne, A. (1981). *The Principle of Normalisation: A Foundation for Effective Services*. London: The Campaign for People with Mental Handicaps.

Samuel, J., & Pritchard, M. (2001). The ignored minority: meeting the needs of people with profound learning disability. *Tizard Learning Disability Review*, 6(2), 34–44.

Szivos, S. (1992). The limits to integration? In H. Brown & H. Smith. (eds), *Normalisation: A Reader for the Nineties*. London: Routledge.

INDEX